Essays on International Health:
Collected Papers

By

Ralph Andreano

Professor of Economics (Emeritus)
University of Wisconsin
Madison, WI

1stBooks - rev. 7/5/01

TABLE OF CONTENTS

INTRODUCTION

This book collects twelve papers of mine written over a period of the past 20 years. Some of these have been published and slightly updated for this volume. A few of the unpublished papers have been altered a bit more in order to put them into the context of the issues of today. My earliest work in the economics of health dates from 1973, but the collection gathered in this volume is representative of my work as a whole.

The first three papers in this collection ("Reflections....","New Paradigm....", and "Challenges of HFA....") are related to my active career as a health economist who worked mostly in poor countries, often for the World Health Organization. I was not in the purest sense a research scholar. I wrote dozens of papers for the World Health Organization and for health ministries in the developing world. Only a few of these saw publication and most were in the form of Memos to Administrators, other analysts, Ministers of Health, and other governmental agencies. My main concern has always been that of being a problem solver for health care finance and system issues in developing countries. As such one must interact with the leading international health agencies such as WHO, as well as government officials. I often strayed beyond these limitations, but the key way to affect governmental policies in health was always through some affected institution or agency. A lot of my work, therefore, did not result in publication in the leading journals of the day. These three papers all are about themes in international health policy that emanated from the World Health Organizations' policy of what was known as "Health For All By the Year 2000." The Health For All movement, as it came to be called, was based on an historic meeting in 1978 of all the countries of the world, organized by WHO, and held in the then city of Alma Ata in the Soviet Union. A declaration known as the Alma Ata Declaration outlined a focus on how health care should be structured and what were the keys and important elements to improved health. It singled out what was then and is now called Primary Health Care as the key means to attain the best health in poor countries. Health care systems in the developing world were highly tilted toward acute, or hospital-based care. What the Alma Ata Declaration called for was a shifting of emphasis and resources toward Primary Health Care (PHC), which it defined in some particular ways, as the way for health levels to be elevated in the poorest countries of the World. Nearly every country signed the Alma Ata Declaration and its principles of PHC were adopted widely in the developing world. It was, and still is a momentous document. It defined health research and health policy until the most very recent times. The current policy direction of WHO, still pays lip service to the goals and aims of Alma Ata, but its focus is on other things. These first three papers reflect my thinking and to a certain extent, my assessment of the policy aspects of Health for All and the key tool of Primary Health Care. Primary Health Care should be the principal focus of health services in a country. Primary health care included things such as safe water, nutrition, disease prevention methods, and other aspects of care that aimed to prevent ill health among populations and to fight poor health with the best combination of treatment interventions. Primary Health Care was thought to be a more simplified but still relevant means to deliver better health to poor people. And there was a belief that this would be cheaper than Acute, hospital-based, care services. Acute Care is highly intensive care and uses methods that are both expensive and frequently invasive. The signers of the Alma Alta Declaration believed that Primary Health Care was not only cheaper, but also better. In any case, these three papers are my commentary on much of what was occurring in this policy environment and was based heavily on my own experiences in assisting developing countries and writing policy papers for WHO. Throughout all the papers in this volume, however, the issues of Health For All by the Year 2000 as a governing principle of international health policy is a constant theme. In one way or another nearly all the papers touch on one or more dimensions of Health for All as well as Primary Health Care. It is just that these three papers put forth my own take and theory about these matters and how I approached using, thinking about, and criticizing these concepts.

The next series of papers, four in all, relate to the topic: the economics of tropical diseases. I first became interested in applying the tools of economics to health care issues by a research project that dealt with the economic impacts of tropical diseases. Some colleagues and myself were the first to study whether or not the presence of parasitic diseases affected how hard people worked (compared to those without the disease), how it affected the performance of school children, and on the birth rate. The locale of this research was the Caribbean island country of St. Lucia. The book which resulted from this project (Disease and Development, University of Wisconsin Press, 1973 with my then colleague Burton A. Weisbrod as the key author of this study. Others were Robert Baldwin, Allen Kelly, an anthropologist, Leonard Glick and myself.

I give this brief background so that the reader may be able to put into context these four papers. At the time, and even today, the extent to which disease influences human behavior as well as economic behavior is a fundamental issue. While these papers are from the past, they do cover the issues that yet today are current. The current resurgence of Malaria and the worldwide pandemic of HIV-AIDS contain the same theoretical and measurement issues that are explored in these papers. Therefore, the papers are of some interest to current concerns.

The first paper ("Economic Issues...") is a survey of the topics and the theoretical basis for analyzing economic impacts of disease. The second paper on Schistosomiasis in China was written as President Nixon had earlier opened up American interests to China. At the time the paper was being written, the view held in the West, though never really confirmed, was that China had eradicated this parasitic disease. The eradication of Schistosomiasis was celebrated in a poem of Mao Tse Tsung called: "Farewell to the God of Plague." I include this paper for its historical interest since at the time access to Chinese research resources was non-existent and there was considerable skepticism in the West that China had, indeed, eradicated Schistosomiasis. As subsequent events transpired, this disbelief about eradication was confirmed. My paper is just a small contribution to this debate and it was done without access to the original sources that were unavailable at the time to a Western economist.

The next paper, an analysis of the WHO Program in Malaria Eradication, was written for WHO and is an examination of the background and thinking of such a momentous policy choice as to believe that the eradication of Malaria was possible. This paper was written well after the time that the WHO Policy of Global Eradication of Malaria had been changed to a policy of containment. But in the context of international health policy, what WHO does and thinks, has enormous impact on what countries do. So the background for this paper was to ask whether or not when WHO decided on the policy of Global Eradication of Malaria, they had approached this policy through use of the right planning and analysis, especially the kind of issues economists would think were important to the formulation of such a major policy initiative.

Finally, the last paper done jointly with my long-time colleague Thomas Helminiak is as complete a survey of the economics literature on the impacts of parasitic diseases on the major variables of economic life and activity as existed at the time, and perhaps even today. It was delivered at an International Meeting in Manila. This paper is included since these issues still seem relevant for the reigning parasitic and autoimmune diseases of the present.

The remaining five papers can be thought of in two groups. The first three papers ("The Phenomena of...","Notes on Health Sector Reform,", "Health Economics...Global....") are all unpublished papers but were delivered at very high level meetings of one kind or another or were written for a particular audience. These papers have a flavor of the health policy issues that have dominated international health policy debates in the 1990's. Nearly all scholars, and practitioners in the field such as my self, came to realize that Health For All and Primary Health Care had problems. Public, or so-called "free" health care systems were failing all over the developing world and many of us believed that reform of the health sector was the key policy activity of the decade. The World Bank solidified this outlook in its World Development Report for 1993 that was exclusively on world health systems and health care. These three papers were, in a sense, my commentary of what was happening and represent my thinking of the time. I believe my thinking was in the mainstream, so in a sense, these papers are a comment on the events as they were happening in the developing countries. I also did many missions to developing countries during the 1990's and these papers reflect a lot of what I said to Ministers of Health during this period.

The paper on "The Phenomena of Health Care Reform" was given at a meeting in Mexico at the time just before the presidential elections of that time. Other papers on other social and economic topics were given at this meeting. The meeting served, in a limited way at least, as a session on background of key issues likely to face the next president of Mexico. In this paper I survey all areas of the world and report on what has and/or is happening with reform of the health sector. The paper is a broad sweep of changes in both the industrialized and developing worlds.

The paper, Notes on Health Sector Reform has three parts to it. First is the main paper, and then another called "More Notes on" and yet one more called "Notes on Economics of Governance". All three papers are meant to be read successively and therefore are grouped as one paper in this collection. These papers were written for a particular purpose but reflect the debate of the times, still going on, about how and in what ways developing countries could successfully reform their health systems in order to better serve the health needs of their populations. This paper is a summation of my thinking and a survey of others as well. As the reader may notice, there is a direct linkage between the first three papers of this volume, especially the paper on a New Paradigm for Health, and these papers on health reform. The barriers to the production of good health in poor countries are immense and new ways of thinking about reform of the finance and delivery systems are of very great importance. This paper, or these papers, constitute my thinking on the topic and I believe it is very much relevant to the debate that is still going on in international health policy circles.

The last two of the remaining 5 papers ("Are we Spending...." And "The Role of the Private sector...") also deserve some special comment. The first of these papers was given to a conference in the Gulf states (Saudi Arabia, United Arab Emirates, Oman, Qatar, Yemen, Kuwait), all of which have spending profiles for health care very similar to industrialized countries. This meeting was, in a sense, to let the Ministers of Health of these states understand the forces behind rising health expenditures worldwide as well as in their own countries. What has become obvious to me after a quarter century of work in this field is that the problems in health care systems between the industrialized and non-industrialized worlds are very comparable. The industrialized countries are richer, of course, but their systems are no less inefficient and costly than those found in poor countries. At this meeting of Ministers of Health of the Gulf States, my paper surveys the topic for them so as to place their own experiences in the context of what is happening around the world. Over the course of my career I have done quite a few missions to the Gulf states for the World Health Organization and typically the problems they have and still face is how to get control of a vast "free" system that is primarily based on acute care, hospital centered, medicine. When oil revenues are rising, the costs of this system seem bearable. But when oil revenues fall, the costs seem "excessive." This paper was presented at a time of falling oil revenues.

The last paper, on the "Role of the Private Sector", again done with my long-time colleague Thomas Helminiak was given at a conference organized by the Asian Development Bank on the private markets in health care in the Asian region. This paper reflects my long-standing point of view about the role of private health markets in the financing and delivery of health services in the developing world. I was giving such advice to countries in the 1970's but no one really was interested in that point of view at that time as Health for All dominated all policy thinking. But in the 1990's when my advice was quite similar, the audience was much greater for what I had to say. There have been a number of papers since ours was done documenting the role of private health markets in poor countries, but this paper still seems quite current and relevant to the current discussion of the topic.

All things considered, the papers collected in this volume are representative of my work over the past quarter century on the economics of health. I have almost as large a number as collected in this volume that could still be published or re-published. Perhaps I might put out a companion volume to this one later. But for the present, the hope is that this collection will shed some light on the historical dimensions of international health policy as well as cast a point of view on the debates of today.

Ralph Andreano
Madison, Wisconsin
Date Feb. 15, 2001

Acknowledgements

I have had the benefit of lots of help throughout my career but I want to single out several individuals in particular. One is my long-time associate and colleague, Dr. Thomas Helminiak. He is the co-author of two of the papers in this volume. But his collaboration with my work extends well beyond these two articles. He was once a student of mine and is a valued and lasting friend. My long-standing friend, associate, and some-time colleague, Dr. Dev Ray, now retired from the World Health Organization has been my window into the world of health care in the developing countries. Many of the papers in this collection resulted from discussions with Dr. Ray and often were written for him in connection with some activity he had undertaken in his capacity as a high official of the World Health Organization. I thank both these splendid people for all they have done for me. I want also to thank Dawn Duren for her considerable assistance in the preparation of this volume.

SELECTION 1

REFLECTIONS ON THE ECONOMIST AND HEALTH ECONOMICS IN AN INTERNATIONAL SETTING[1]

INTRODUCTION

As a practicing economist in health it is very difficult to separate the interactive roles played by research and practical field experience. As an academic economist the first test one must meet is that of research productivity; experience with how research findings and basic theorems of western economics actually work should inform the research scientist and produce 'better' research. After some 25 years of engaging in this process I am still not sure I know how it works, or how it should work. When asked for a contribution to this special issue of *Social Science and Medicine*, I have had the opportunity to rethink the past quarter century of active work as an academic economist in international health. I have asked myself: what have I done that has made life better? These are humbling questions and somehow the potential answers I could muster seem, today, trivial.

For the past decade or so, however, there has been an organizing principle that has conditioned my research as well as my active life in the field. That principle has been the Health For All (HFA) By the Year 2000 declaration at Alma Ata in 1978. (All of these are often given the shorthand designation of: HFA/2000/PHC, meaning, Health For All by the year 2000 through Primary Health Care.) It has been a difficult principle to reconcile with one's training as an economist. The usual paradigms western trained economists are equipped with have enormous difficulty finding both relevance and applicability to the Alma Ata Declaration. A decade plus later and a call by a new Director-General (DG) of World Health Organization (WHO) for a 'new paradigm' for health has forced a closer reconciliation of my economist precepts with the principles of Alma Ata.[2] What follows is a crude adjustment of these values. I am not sure if other Western economists have had the same difficulties as I over the past decade, but it has been frustrating and sometimes very disappointing to reconcile the two—the economist and the 'true believer'—in research, in policy analysis, and especially in work in the field with countries.

---

[1]This article was originally published in *Social Science and Medicine*, Vol. 36, No. 2, pp. 137-141, 1993.
[2]Speech of the Director-General, WHO, Executive Board, January 1991, and World Health Assembly, May 1991.

THE PRINCIPLES OF ALMA ATA THROUGH AN ECONOMIST'S MIRROR

As I viewed the principles of Alma Ata what was emphasized was market failure; consequently markets, as expressed in individual freedoms, were minimally noted compared to the enhanced role of governments to correct failures. Economists in talking about market failure include only issues related to the ability of markets to get goods produced at market prices that reflect appropriate social prices; equity issues are considered a separate problem. Alma Ata principles, however, have an implicit damning of markets and give particular emphasis to the failure of markets to produce equity. In my economist's mirror, my paradigm is just the opposite: it emphasizes *government failures* in equity, in productive efficiency, in nearly every sense and entails *market successes.* Everything is somehow oversimplified and generalizations are a dime a dozen. But I have come to realize that the ten plus years since Alma Ata seemed to fit the explanatory power in the economist's tool kit rather than the underlying principles, which promoted the Health For All movement.

In many senses, the pursuit of HFA and the strategy and tactics subsequently urged upon the world health community has accomplished much to be proud about. But, realistically, the world today is not much closer to HFA than it was a decade ago. Why? HFA posed five basic values: (1) social justice; (2) universal access to care; (3) community involvement; (4) resource availability; and (5) health as a central part of economic development. The realities are: (1) individual rights and preferences received muted expression in these values, running counter to the lessons of human experience, as well as to principles of rational behavior; (2) resource availability differed materially and significantly from what was anticipated; (3) access to care is uneven and skewed (and probably always will be); (4) expansion of private health care markets gave expression to the unequal distribution of income as well as the failures in quality and access of direct government-provided services, and (5) the role of government proved more complex, less predictable and less well able to manage macro-economic conditions that were required to operationalize HFA. The reasons the basic principles of Alma Ata and HFA were not achieved are multiple and complex; and no single source alone can explain such an intricate and elusive goal. But, the original paradigm of Alma Ata was that—with fundamental values of social justice and equity exposed and with a legitimate expression of equity (HFA) and methods for attainment of Primary Health Care (PHC)—the world would embrace these values, methods and goals; and the resources necessary for success would be available or become available.

But, on the whole and aside from notable and important exceptions, this did not happen. The infrastructure for PHC proved as fragile and weak as the rest of the health system infrastructure. World economic conditions changed drastically in the decade following Alma Ata; and this change was to the substantial disadvantage of the developing countries. The resources available for HFA did not expand but stabilized or declined. Health inequalities grew wider, as did the world income distribution. Management capacities within countries and in the international network of health, including WHO, proved as weak and fragile as a country's health infrastructure. The ease of shifting health care systems, from acute care-based to primary and preventive care-based, naively implied in the original paradigm, proved difficult (if not impossible) and was largely intractable to well-meaning government policies that tried to effect this transition.

Similarly, the willingness of individuals and communities to have their own preferences for health care (and other things as well) expressed by others (e.g. planners, other government officials, etc.) proved to be not acceptable. And individual preferences, as expressed in the health arena, created strong impetus for private health care delivery and finance systems to be expanded outside the official channels of government health institutions. The original paradigm of HFA did not allow for. nor appreciate, the power of individual preferences and private markets. The central role for health in economic development anticipated in the original paradigm of HFA was shown to be naive; the reality has proved otherwise.

A LOOK AT ALMA ATA IN THE ECONOMISTS MIRROR

Other observers may well disagree with my characterizations (simplification?) of the principles of Alma Ata and my naturally cursory review of what has happened since. The principles that have governed my work as an economist may be no better than any one else's but I do believe they have some explanatory power of what has gone wrong and where international health work may now be headed. The economist's paradigm—an overworked and almost useless term but I use it nonetheless because of its current usage in international health—rests on individual and collective rights. It emphasizes the primacy of markets and the limits of governmental actions and roles. I hesitate to call this a paradigm but it is certainly a set of values and beliefs that are orthogonal to the principles of Alma Ata. But let me pose it as if it can be stated as a paradigm with three intended anchors: (1) individual rights and responsibilities; (2) social (or societal) actions and consequences; and (3) the functions and limits of collective actions and governmental roles and policies. These principles are interrelated and each affects negatively and positively upon the other. Individual rights and responsibilities can produce private benefits (to the individual) but social costs, i.e. costs borne by the rest of society. An example: individuals in pursuit of the highest level of health (within their resources) for themselves and their families, can create health service demands at odds with community or societal benefits.

Demand for physician services, high technology and drugs may advance individual health, but these could be at variance with what might be the best use of scarce medical resources by society: Social consequences (costs) are then produced as a result of individual actions. Similarly, private companies, as well as individuals, may generate pollution of the air and water of their surrounding communities. These social costs are not self-correcting and will require some collective action, either by government to protect the rights of others, or by individual actions that mitigate the pervasiveness of the social consequences. The role of government, therefore, is to design policies that while protecting individual rights. restrict them enough to mitigate their social costs. That is one set of relationships.

Another set of relationships involves the social costs and infringements on individual rights resulting from ill-designed collective actions of government and exogenous social factors. Government actions and policies frequently impinge on individual rights and produce unintended social consequences. Poor macro-economic management of the economy is one example. Restrictions on individual actions and rights through prohibitive laws governing personal behavior are another. In another example, illuminated in recent events, the major air, water and environmental pollution produced by the centrally planned economies are extensive. Major social costs were produced by government policies and individual rights were compromised. Now that such economies are no longer centrally planned, the social costs of the earlier actions are still there. Who will pay to mitigate these costs? Similarly, exogenous social factors, such as the economic effects of rapid population growth, can constrain individual rights and require reorientation of individual behavior, as well as governmental policies and actions.

The three interrelated elements—individual rights and responsibilities, social costs and consequences and the role of government (with its functions, limits and impacts) can form a 'paradigm' useful for redefining international health work. A paradigm is an organized model, both explaining past and current behavior and capable of defining future behavior. A paradigm as a model, is an abstraction, and is only useful if it has power to define and explain individual behaviors and social actions. Whether or not the 3 principles noted above constitute a 'real' paradigm is, in my view, not important. They do, however, provide a different way of viewing what has happened since Alma Ata and perhaps offer some insights into future directions.

THE NEW PRINCIPLES AND THE OLD

Let me return to the somewhat simplified principles articulated earlier as representation of Alma Ata and Health For All. How do they look in the new mirror?

Social justice

The term social justice has universal acceptance, but its attainment is elusive and unmeasurable. Similarly, in health care it is a value to which all societies aspire but few achieve. Who decides when social justice has been attained? Governments? People? Statistics? In the new 'paradigm', social justice is the joint pursuit of individual aspirations, with the role of government to protect the individual from abuses and social costs (sometimes the consequences of the individual's own actions). In pursuit of economic development, irreplaceable resources can become exhausted. This process has generated wages, incomes and profits, but future generations may suffer ecological and environmental damage, which circumscribe their rights, threaten their quality of life and inhibit their income growth. Social justice in the present, by the measure of the new 'paradigm', requires a balancing of individual rights and unintended social consequences from the exercise of those rights. A key role for government is to functionally promote and maintain this balance—and, when imbalance occurs, to use its power to correct the abuses. For social justice in the new 'paradigm' individual rights must be respected; but it is the duty of government to mitigate, through public policy, social costs to levels that populations accept as being 'socially just'. Another important component of social justice is the empowerment of individuals and their actions rather than expanded collective actions. Individuals through the exercise of democratic values and institutions can contain the excesses and mismanagement of governments.

Universal access to care

In the new principle individuals and governments bear the joint responsibility of ensuring access to care. Individuals who can afford to pay for care should pay and government or the voluntary and willing actions of individuals should protect those who cannot. It is not necessary for government to be the sole producer or provider of services, to all groups. But, it is responsible for ensuring access to care either through insurance, financial subsidy or other means. Access to care will always be uneven and skewed, because of different individual preferences, circumstances and incomes. But, the floor should be solid and the average quality high enough for a society to say: "We are satisfied that all have a minimum level of access to care; none in our society are going without needed care." The role of government is to produce care that would otherwise not be produced (those things with positive externalities, such as immunizations, vector control, health education) and to create policies that reinforce individual actions and, as needed, correct the negative consequences of individual actions. Vulnerable and high-risk groups, who have not achieved the average level of care considered basic, are the joint responsibility of individuals and governments. But, the role of government must be more broadly considered: it need not be the producer of care to accept its share of responsibility for ensuring the provision of that care.

Community involvement

Community involvement was, perhaps, one of the most innovative and yet most naive of all the HFA values. Communities, however, though they have a life of their own, are largely composed of different and unique individuals and, in some sense, each with a different incentive system conditioning their behavior. In the new 'paradigm', individual involvement is the core (if this collectively interacts with community values so much the better). But, individuals should be—and want to be—free to act in their own way and with their own means. The energy, the resource raising potential and other dynamic aspects that stem from community involvement start at the most basic level first: the individual. The role of government is to ensure through its policies that resources, actions and accomplishments are leveraged in the communities, but within the context of protection and adherence to individual rights and freedoms.

Resources availability

Alma Ata principles assumed resources would be there and could be transformed into health care systems based on primary health care. Not only did this not happen but the original principles did not have internal to it mechanisms for it to happen. The new principles say resources for health must be generated internally with certain exceptions. For the most part, success in health in each country will depend on its ability to generate resources internally. Individuals also have important responsibilities. Individuals could be able to have access to the level of care and the technology of care they can afford. Health may be a right, but it is a right that people—who can afford to do so—should (and really they want to) pay for from their own resources.

The role of government

Government's role is to balance social costs and private benefits and to be the ultimate protector of equity—for those who are vulnerable, unable to pay, or are in high-risk situations. Concurrently, the generation of resources for health internally is a key function of governments: it must examine its ownership of health services against competing alternatives and better opportunities for use of government generated resources. When governments must operate health services, they must be required to do so efficiently. Governments must fashion what balance between public and private sector roles they wish to maintain; but there is a key role to be played by private initiative, actions and markets. These distinctions were not a prominent part of the original values of Health For All.

Health as a central part of development

As with the resource availability factor, this element of the original HFA failed. It failed for three reasons: (1) It did not have operational significance; (2) It was not self-evident to macro planners; and (3) The health sector itself—PHC and the total system—underperformed relative to expectations. The infrastructures for PHC and the health system proved fragile and insufficient to perform at a level comparable with other inputs crucial to the process of economic development (e.g. transport, education, banking, exports). Health infrastructures will inevitably be strengthened if private initiatives and public policies defining a new role for governments in health care catch on and become standard fare. Health has to earn its role as a central input to the development process—not through assertion of its importance, but from a demonstration of its effectiveness and performance.[3]

THE POWER OF THE PRINCIPLE

The key aspect that emerges from this economist's mirror of principles is that it places health in a wider social, political and economic framework. If economic development is enhanced, as it is through the exercise of individual initiatives and supportive collective actions and policies of government, why shouldn't the same relationships be valid for health? The answer, of course, is that they are. Some generalizations seem relevant.

---

[3]The new 'paradigm' for health being proposed here also has ramifications for other aspects of social policy (e.g. education and social welfare) and, also, for macro economic management policies. Governments cannot force economic development or generate substantial economic growth through centralized management from above. The power of individual behavior and preferences on consumer behavior, the incentive structure facing producers and entrepreneurs and the building blocks of human resources (education, health and other social means) have proved more powerful engines of development than forced savings policies by centralized governments.

1. Improved health comes from the interaction of individual actions and choices supported, but not dominated by collective actions or governmental policies.
2. Building sustainable health systems depends on the willingness and preferences of individuals not dominated by collective actions or governmental policies.
3. Governments need not be the sole providers of care, unless individuals express this as their clear preference; no one is better situated than government to raise resources (through taxation) and to protect society from social consequences of individuals and collective actions.
4. Individual preferences for health care matter; private markets for health care exist because of this.
5. No one, except government, has the power to constrain individual behavior and to control consequences.

Some countries will not have sufficient resources to build sustainable health systems unless and until their economies develop. Their economies will not develop unless they place the burden for its development squarely on the shoulders of the people. Sustainable health systems become essential inputs to the larger development process. Similarly, there is now a rationale and a stricture for intensified cooperation with countries that fit the category of most vulnerable and least developed, both economically and from a health perspective. Such countries cannot generate sufficient resources for health from internal efficiencies or individual actions to provide that basic floor of access consistent with HFA as a goal; outside assistance is called for. Where social costs and consequences transcend national boundaries international aid is relevant. Certain diseases, such as AIDS, malaria and others, fit this category. The building of health systems to contain these diseases cannot be from internal resources alone: These social costs have no national boundary. To make health systems sustainable, in such cases, requires more resources than can be internally generated. But the additional resources need not only come from governmental or public sources: private sources are just as supportable.

Examining the reflections in the mirror at yet another level of application to health is to look at some of the major aspects of modern health care systems. Take as an example science and technology: countries again are on different points of a spectrum from complete to nil. How science and technology will be used in support of—or to build—sustainable systems of care depend on individual as well as collective actions and decisions. Countries will define where they want to be and then will find the path which optimizes their resources, maintains the integrity of individual values and does not produce social spill-over effects that constrain the development of a supportable system of care.

Because individual preferences, rights and values are central, this also means that private markets are also essential. For health systems the existence and value of private markets has major implications. It means that individuals who can afford to pay for care should do so, whether the health system is public or private. Therefore, user charges in public systems are appropriate (subject to usual caveats and conditions), but private health care markets will also exist, because of differences in preferences, incomes and tastes of individuals. Government's role is to ensure that private systems meet quality standards; and government should not be diverted from its role in correcting market failures and protecting equity. Again, countries will be on different points of the spectrum. There is no single mix between public and private, between what services government produces, or what role government may play in the financing of services, or how the standards of protection of equity in access and finance will be applied. These are for countries to decide: each must, through an interaction of individual values and governmental norms, decide what is the optimal path.

At the level of individual countries, there is not a lessened role for government, but rather a more pointed, more opportunistic, a more efficient role. (By government, we include all levels, from the center down to a village council.) Governments have the power to tax, to regulate, to prescribe rules and norms, to circumscribe individual behavior and, above all, to protect. Protection goes beyond security, in the defense sense, to that of individual rights and the amelioration of unintended social costs. Protection also implies correction of inequities and the general advancement of social welfare of individuals and the country.

In the developing world, governments and Ministries of Health (MOHs) have believed the direct provision of health services to be the duty of government. The rationale for this is equity and the belief that provision of health care is a fundamental right—and, therefore, a fundamental obligation of governments. Provision of services across the board, as data now show, is not equitable, nor is it perceived by people as something that government must do. First, in public systems great inequities exist in access and cost, because of supply imbalances and travel and waiting time. The same quality of services is not there for each and every individual. Second, people continuously bypass public health services; and those who do so, buy care in private markets. Private markets can be those operated for profit (pharmacies, clinics, hospitals, etc.) and not for profit. People have traditionally bypassed public services when private options were available. World-wide data document the extent and pervasiveness of private health care systems in the developing world existing side by side with public ones.

What is suggested in the economist's mirror is that governments need not be the providers and producers of care across the board, available for everyone. This does not work unless it is the fully expressed choice of the people. In most developing countries, 50% or more of a MOH total budget goes to acute care, especially hospitals. Rather, the government's role to protect equity and access to services is most efficiently served if it allows people who can pay to do so and at whatever level they can afford. But, government must protect those who cannot pay; and, it has a variety of means within its vast arsenal of powers to accomplish this. It can produce and own services exclusively for bypassed groups; it can subsidize services produced by others through financial means and according to income; it can promote national insurance and decide the public-private delivery mix it wants to have. All of these options exist and in each country, the country should decide which path is best to optimize its limited resources.

FINAL REFLECTIONS

I do not know if the view of the past or the vision of the future presented here is any better or any more than what was presented at Alma Ata. I have been trying to reconcile my personal belief and hope for the ideals of Alma Ata with the realities of a western trained economist. There are many different 'truths' and about as many different paths to it. The path described here is one economist's attempt—I speak only for myself—to try to understand what has happened and what could happen.

Acknowledgements

Some of the ideas expressed have been scrutinized and challenged during the past 15 years by Dr Dev Ray, WHO Geneva. 1 thank him for educating me. My long time colleague, Thomas Helminiak and I have a longer and conceptually tighter and less personal, paper called 'The New Paradigm for Health' in which some of the ideas expressed here are elaborated further. Many thanks to him as well. All errors and responsibilities are mine.

SELECTION 2

A NEW PARADIGM IN HEALTH[4]

Paradigms are the favorite toys of economists: we use them even when they don't seem useful. So, yet another try at one may be dismissed easily. But I hope not. Health care systems worldwide are under close examination. Finance, insurance, and coverage issues dominate reform debates in many countries. The U.S.A., where reform impulses are closer to the surface than perhaps elsewhere, shows the poverty of creative thinking about health care systems. The major issues in the U.S.A. debate are how to fix a system that is wasteful and inefficient, inequitable by most standards, and consumes annually nearly 1/8th of the country's national wealth. The U.S. system is thought to be a private one, but that is true only on the delivery side: on the expenditure side almost half originates in the public sector. In other parts of the industrialized world, those systems that on both the expenditure and delivery side are mostly public, there are reform efforts to make them behave more like private systems with recommendations for various types of internal market competition. These systems are also thought to be inefficient and wasteful of resources and inequitable as well. Some believe not enough of national resources are devoted to health; others too much. In the developing world, with few exceptions, the picture is much the same. Private systems (for profit and not for profit) have grown enormously; public systems have stagnated and seem wasteful as well as inequitable. Governments in poor countries spend most of their resources on acute care and almost nothing on primary care; the same is true in the industrialized countries. The more one looks at health care systems around the world the more their problems and shortcomings converge. There is a difference in scale (both scope and size) between the poor and rich countries. But the problems look similar and the same potential solutions keep reappearing. In a modest attempt to help advance thinking about reform and organization of health care delivery and finance systems, I propose a 'new paradigm.' This paradigm is really not 'new' nor is it a 'solution' for countries to adopt: rather it is a framework for countries to organize their thinking and to sort out what values are important and must be maintained. To be sure an opposing paradigm, prescribing a minimal role for government and/or unfettered operation of the free market, is what usually has tempered debates on health care reform: health care is a basic right, therefore let government do it. Or, health care markets are mostly like all other markets, let competition prevail. An intermediate paradigm based on

---

[4]This article was originally published as an Editorial in *Social Science and Medicine*, Vol. 36, No. 4, pp. iii-v, 1993.

expressions of equitable and just societies with dominant roles for collective action did also leave room for both private markets. Our modest effort here to define a 'new paradigm' draws upon all of these conceptual foundations.

A NEW PARADIGM

As all seem to know, a paradigm is an organized model capable of explaining past and/or current behavior and offering a roadmap for future behavior. A paradigm as a model is an abstraction and it is only useful if it has the power to define and explain. The paradigm for health proposed here is based on three interrelated spheres of behavior and actions: (1) individual rights and responsibilities; (2) social (or societal) actions and consequences; and (3) the functions and limits of collective actions and governmental roles and policies. These principles are interrelated and each affects negatively and positively upon the other. One can think of the paradigm as three interconnected spheres such as a Venn diagram.

Individual rights and responsibilities, if fully exercised, can produce private benefits (to the individual) but social costs, i.e. costs borne by the rest of society. These social costs are not self-correcting and require some collective action, either by government to protect the rights of others, or by individual actions that prompt governmental and/or private responses. The role of government, therefore, is to design policies that while protecting individual rights restrict them enough to minimize the social costs of some individual behaviors. That is one set of relationships in the paradigm. Another set involves the social costs and infringements on individual rights resulting from ill-designed collective actions of government and/or exogenous social factors. Government actions and policies frequently impinge on individual rights and produce unintended social consequences. Poor macroeconomic management of the economy is one example. Restrictions on individual actions and rights through prohibitive laws governing personal behaviour are another. Another example is the extensive and major air, water and environmental pollution produced by the centrally planned economies. Major social costs were produced by government policies and individual rights (and health) were compromised. Now that such economies are no longer centrally planned, the social costs of the earlier actions are still there. Who will pay to mitigate these costs? In the original framework, individuals, or even organized groups of individuals, had no means of expressing their distaste for the social costs of pollution. And the centrally planned economies did not include these costs to the rest of the economy or to individuals (persons and firms). Similarly, exogenous social factors, such as the economic effects of rapid population growth, can constrain individual rights and require reorientation of individual behavior. Rapid population growth can also shape or restrict governmental policies and actions. The three interrelated elements—individual rights and responsibilities, social costs and consequences and the role of government (with its functions, limits and impacts) form a paradigm useful for redefining how policies and interventions in health might be framed.

THE ROLE OF INDIVIDUALS

At yet another level, recent world events seem insightful. Individuals are pressing for recognition of their rights everywhere—as consumers, as voters, as producers, etc. People want to be able to exert their own choices and not be told by government that they have no choices. The drive around the world for democratic values, protection of human rights and the rights of individuals to be free to choose what they do, how they do it and when they do it has never been stronger. The new paradigm says that individual rights and freedoms do matter. Individual choices are important, not only for the value that people place on having such choice, but for the economic efficiency and societal gain that can result.

Because individual preferences, rights and values are central to the paradigm, this also means that private markets are also essential. For health systems the existence and value of private markets has some major implications. It means that individuals who can afford to pay for care should do so, whether the health system is public or private. The paradigm suggests that user charges in public systems are appropriate (subject to usual caveats and conditions), and that private health care markets will also exist, because of differences in preferences, incomes and tastes of individuals. Government's role, however, is to insure that private systems meet quality standards; and government should not be diverted from its role in correcting market failures and protecting equity. The paradigm predicts no single mix between public and private, between what precise services are produced by government, or what exact role government may play in the financing of services, or how the standards of protection of equity in access and finance will be applied: These are for countries to decide: each must, through an interaction of individual values and governmental norms, decide what is the optimal path.

Individual rights, actions, and responsibilities are not without limits, under the paradigm. The paradigm says the people and their governments set these limits by custom, religion, traditions and history. Individual rights either in the market place or in personal values are not unlimited. The basic restriction is that the exercise of individual rights must not produce net social costs, or diminish the rights of others. Government is the means to balance and adjudicate these limits.

THE ROLE OF GOVERNMENTS

People and government make their own institutions, rules and futures. The new paradigm puts health in the most central role it has ever had in economic development. Health of a population is the basic building block for human resources. Human resources, plus physical resources, plus wise government policies are what produces economic development. This is the essence and the core of the new paradigm: health is a central input to economic development. But, the paradigm says that health is an individual and a collective responsibility. To generate resources for health is an individual and a state responsibility: the people and their government are responsible for each other; their futures and their welfares are inextricably interwoven. One cannot improve without the other. What the paradigm says is that governments must use their limited resources for health wisely and put their power and their resources on the right things: mitigation of social costs, protection of equity and insurance of individual choices, freedoms and responsibilities.

The problem that governments have is being able to interpret—in some real world pragmatic fashion, with some explicit guidelines—where the optimal tradeoff point lies, between individual choice and competitive markets on the one side and, on the other, social/collective choice and government decision-making. The decision rule seems simple, but in practice is difficult. Government's role is to balance social costs and private benefits and to be the ultimate protector of equity—for those who are vulnerable, unable to pay, or are in high-risk situations. Concurrently, the generation of resources for health is a key function of governments: it must examine its ownership of health services against competing alternatives and better opportunities for use of government generated resources. When governments must operate health services, they must be required to do so efficiently. Governments must fashion what balance between the public and private sector they wish to maintain; but in the new paradigm there is a key role to be played by private initiative, actions and markets and governments.

The key aspect of governmental roles that the paradigm addresses is where, or to what, and in what manner government's power will be applied. The paradigm implies not a lessened role for government, but a rationale for a more efficiently opportunistic one. The paradigm does not lessen government's power to tax, to regulate, to control and to redress imbalances. What the paradigm does forecast is a way to use governmental powers to advance health where its impact can be greatest and where its efficiency can be at a peak in optimizing the use of its limited resources. The paradigm says that governments cannot do everything for everybody and for all things. Like individuals in the paradigm, government must be free to make choices. And the choices are where to bring government powers to bear to do the most good with the least misuse of resources.

The new paradigm suggests that governments need to be the providers and producers of care across the board, available for everyone. This does not work unless it is the fully expressed choice of the people. In most developing countries, 50% or more of a MOH total budget goes to acute care, especially hospitals. The new paradigm questions the grounds for this role for government, Government need not be the sole provider, or provider of last resort to all, in order for it to protect health as a right or to protect and promote social justice and equity.

The government's role to protect equity and access to services is most efficiently served if it allows people who can pay to do so and at whatever level they can afford. But, government must protect those who cannot pay; and it has a variety of means within its vast arsenal of powers to accomplish this. It can produce and own services exclusively for bypassed groups; it can subsidize services produced by others through financial means and according to income; it can promote national insurance and decide the public-private delivery mix it wants to have. All of these options exist and the new paradigm is saying that in each country, the country should decide which path is best to optimize its limited resources.

THE PARADIGM AND THE FUTURE

Several predictions can be suggested by the paradigm. Governments must reexamine policies that restrict individual actions, which do not have any negative social consequences (costs). Similarly, individuals must be free to exercise their rights, but always within the boundaries prescribed by society. Also, in translating the paradigm directly to health, it is clear, since responsibility is placed squarely on the population and society, in the poor countries and perhaps even in the rich ones, that resources for health must be generated internally. There are certain cases, consistent with the predictions of the paradigm where this may not be so. Three cases come to mind:

1. Countries of greatest need, where internal capacities are weak or non-existent.
2. Where social consequences of health impacts may transcend national boundaries (AIDS, epidemics).
3. Natural, or man-made emergencies and disasters, (famine, typhoons, nuclear).

Ralph Andreano

THE POWER OF THE PARADIGM

The key aspects of the basic paradigm, as it relates to health, are that it places health in a wider social, political and economic framework. If economic development is enhanced, as it is through the exercise of individual initiatives and supportive collective actions and policies of government, why shouldn't the same relationships be valid for health? The answer, of course, is that they are. Here are some predictions for health that. derive from the basic paradigm:

1. Improved health comes from the interaction of individual actions and choices supported, but not dominated by collective actions and/or governmental policies.
2. Building sustainable health systems depends on the willingness and preferences of individuals not dominated but supported, by collective actions and/or governmental policies.
3. Governments need not be the sole providers of care, unless individuals express this as their clear preference; no one is better situated than government to raise resources (through taxation) and to protect society from the negative social behavior of individuals.
4. Individual preferences for health care matter; private markets for health care exist because of this.
5. No one, except government, has the power to constrain individual behaviour and to control its costs.

CONCLUDING NOTE

I am sure I have stated the obvious and have overstated the power of what I call a new paradigm for health. My intention, nonetheless, is noble. Public policy on health care reform is on the top of the agenda in dozens of countries, rich and poor. What can guide these policies and the proposed interventions? Politics, cultural values, power-groups? Perhaps all of these. But what I am suggesting, perhaps not modestly enough, is that policy changes must be informed by what they assume about individual choices and collective behavior. Governments, if left alone, are seldom wise enough to do the right thing. But then again, neither are individuals! The fact that health care is a 'basic human right' does not mean that government has to be the producer; its overriding obligation is to see that public and private markets insure the attainment of this 'right'. If rich countries, such as the U.S.A., spend too much of the resources and do so inequitably, and at great expenditure levels, this is not an invitation for governments to take over the sector. Private markets are important. Governmental actions and interventions are important. Individual behavior is important. What the new paradigm suggests is that public policy be informed and framed by these interactions.

Ralph Andreano

SELECTION 3

THE CHALLENGES TO HFA AND PHC: AN ECONOMIST'S PERSPECTIVE[5]

PROLOGUE

The retrospectives on the first ten years after Alma Ata are in. A new Director General assumes the leadership of WHO. All who have spoken about the past ten years of HFA find more good things than bad to sum up the achievements of the decade. What leadership role WHO assumes for the next ten years of HFA remains to be seen. My objective in this paper is much more modest than trying to evaluate the past ten years or predict the next decade. What I have to say is, I think, important to any objective appraisal and/or to whatever future there may be for HFA/2000 and PHC. There are some inherent sources of tension in the HFA concepts and like all great rhetorical ideas, purity of motives and clarity of objectives are in the eye of the beholder. As an economist neither my motives nor my objectives in analyzing the challenges to HFA are any purer than anyone else's. In discussions on HFA and in analysis of PHC, economists have received severe criticism from many quarters. Some of this is justified but a lot is just simply rubbish.[6] Economists have no greater hold on the truth than others; but the issues and questions economists, by definition, must deal with, and the analytic methods used, rub many the wrong way. I do not intentionally want to rub anyone the wrong way; my objectives are the same as most—I want a greater effort towards health care in the developing world and a greater result than has thus far been achieved. HFA and PHC are useful organizing principles, but how a country works out its own destiny in health care involves more than these two concepts can contain.

---

[5]Paper prepared and presented at a World Health Organization meeting in Geneva 1-3 August, 1988.

[6]A survey of the general vs. selective concepts of PHC and one in which the economist's analytical framework comes in for severe criticism is offered by Andrew Green and Carol Barker, "Priority Setting and Economic Appraisal: Whose Priorities—the Community or the Economist?" Social Science and Medicine (1988), Vol. 26, No. 9, pp. 919-929. This article covers many of the criticisms leveled at economists but it is, in my judgment, quite unconvincing.

CONTRADICTIONS AND TENSIONS IN HFA AND PHC

The original intent of the Alma Ata declaration and the subsequent elaboration into programmatic principles, in my mind, have created certain contradictions and tensions that make widespread application of the concepts at best insufficient, at worst, trivial. Let me illustrate what I mean. HFA has a strong bias toward equity and perhaps properly so. Yet, in the real world of health care governments cannot usually achieve greater equity in the access, distribution, and costs of services without sacrificing something else. That something else is what economist's would call efficiency.[7] A country's health care system cannot simultaneously be maximally equitable and maximally efficient: a government typically must choose how much equity is to be achieved and how much efficiency should be traded-off to achieve it. (These points are elaborated further in attachment I.) HFA is a concept biased toward equity. But if governments cannot internally generate the resources for redistribution by improved efficiency, how can they tilt their policies toward equity? There is a basic tension here, not easily resolved. To make health care policies to enforce such choices is very difficult to do.[8]

Another fact of HFA and perhaps even PHC is that it is biased toward community level responsibility for health and not toward individuals and families. The current debate on "selective" PHC vs. "comprehensive" PHC is, I think, reflective of the community bias inherent in the original HFA and PHC conceptualizations. The problem for policy is that communities can take an equity approach but be frustrated in generating sufficient resources to maintain the chosen equity level. This could happen because finance and production of community generated resources is basically inefficient. I am not qualified to judge whether or not a community focus on health care is better or worse than other alternatives. What I do know, however, is that people tend to act in his or her own self-interest and community-based schemes usually have a substantial "free-rider" problem (i.e. people who receive benefits of the action but bear none of the costs).

---

[7]There are different types and measures of equity and efficiency, most of which have been examined in R. Andreano and T. Helminiak (1987), "The Role of the Private Sector in Health Care in the Developing Countries," paper prepared for Asian Development Bank. In the present paper I am using the terms in a much more generic way than to illustrate specific policies. (Authors note: This paper is collected in this volume as the last selection.)

[8]A refreshing and searching discussion of the equity/efficiency trade-off in an advanced economy may be found in, Lawrence Malcolm, "Progress Towards Achieving Health for All New Zealanders by the Year 2000," Social Science and Medicine (1987), Vol. 25, No. 5, pp. 473-479.

Also, in my view, there is a decidedly rural bias to HFA and PHC, which masks the equity trade-offs involved. If rural health is of greater priority, all things equal, resources have to be shifted from elsewhere. A rural bias, therefore, greatly complicates the efficiency and equity trade-offs governments necessarily have to confront.

Finally, another source of tension that I see is that PHC proposes the adoption of a new health technology. It is saying to governments that the road to better health (including more equitable access and distribution of health resources) is through a technology—PHC—which is different than populations customarily observe—i.e. the clinical or medically centered acute care model. Again PHC has strong equity overtones because in most developing countries (and developed ones as well) the preponderant distribution of resources is in the medically centered acute care model. So why would people and/or governments want to adopt such a new technology? Health care in this respect is not different from other economic goods. The new technology would be adopted if its price were lower than the existing technology. It could also be adopted if prices are indifferent between the new and the old, but the new technology offers greater quality, equity, or something else the old does not. In general, in my experience, new technology such as PHC is not easily adopted because there is insufficient evidence it is cheaper—all things equal—or of higher quality for a given standardized measure (i.e. life expectancy).[9]

Last, but not least, the HFA and PHC concepts strongly recognize the potential health impacts of intersectoral resources: i.e. water, agriculture, food policy, etc. Again the policy directions of this proper and correct recognition of the importance of intersectoral coordination to governments are at best ambiguous. Health ministries that pursue intersectoral coordination are asking other parts of government policy to trade-off efficiency for equity in its behalf, a result I find generally implausible.

What is the point of dwelling on what, from my point of view, are contradictions or at best tensions in policy inherent in the conceptualization of HFA and PHC? Others, of course, may not see these as tensions in quite the same light as I do.[10] And to dwell on the concepts this way is not to impugn the

---

[9]There is an interesting survey on the cost effectiveness of Community Health Workers as part of the PHC strategy. On the whole the survey found that while CHW average costs were lower than a clinic setting in rural environments, effectiveness was also low. The survey concluded that the cost effectiveness of PHC over comparable medical model alternatives was yet to be proved. See Peter Berman, et al., "Community-Based Health Workers: Head Start or False Start Towards Health For All?" Social Science and Medicine (1987), Vol. 25, No. 5, pp. 443-459.

[10]The contradictions of HFA and PHC concepts I focus on are quite different from these noted by Carl Taylor and Richard Jolly, "The Straw Men of Primary Health Care," (*Social Science and Medicine* (1988), Vol. 26, No. 9, pp. 971-977). They call their

motives or potential usefulness they may have. To me, however, the way to look at HFA and PHC is to ask what kinds of policy signals do these concepts send to governments? How do these concepts get translated into concrete policies? The retrospectives on Alma Ata point to some great successes.[11] But the truth is that health care in the developing world is still nearly as backward and financially precarious as it was ten years ago. What we have to ask of the future is can HFA and PHC still be useful concepts for governments in trying to lift health levels in their countries? By pointing to some of the contradictions and tensions what I am suggesting is that, in some sense, the concepts have sent conflicting signals to governments. Lip service can be paid to HFA and PHC but the reality of a country setting is a far cry from formulating policies toward fulfillment of these high ideals.[12]

WORLD ECONOMIC CONDITIONS AND HEALTH FOR ALL (HFA)

Almost from the date of Alma Ata to the present, world economic conditions have cast a pallor on the potential for working out the contradictions of HFA and for pursuing concrete policies in the developing countries based on these concepts. The rise in oil prices, the accumulation of foreign debt, severe trade and payments imbalances, domestic inflation and other economic problems put resources for health care in a precarious position in most countries.[13] The world economic community since the late 1970's has been trying to adjust their economies to the gigantic dislocations created by changes in world economic conditions. While there is some dispute among scholars about the degree of damage done to health care levels in the developing countries as they tried to cope with debt, trade, and domestic inflation problems, the most damage that was

---

contradictions "misleading points of polarization:" selective *vs.* comprehensive, vertical *vs.* horizontal, top-down *vs.* bottom-up approaches, planned *vs.* participatory approaches, and "technological, magic bullet approaches" *vs.* "building organizational structures" (see especially, pp. 972-973.)

[11] See address by Dr. H. Mahler before World Health Assembly, May 4, 1988 and the summary of the "Ten Years after Alma Ata," WHO Features No. 119, March 1988.

[12] Carl Taylor and Richard Jolly, "The Straw Men of Primary Health Care," suggest that the final and most fundamental question is how can it be ensured that "true equity" will be achieved in reaching those in greatest need? So far as I can tell, the authors don't define what this term is supposed to mean.

[13] See R. Andreano, "Recession: A Salutary Warning," in World Health Forum, Vol.8, 1987, pp. 34-37.

done was that future resources for health were constrained in very severe ways.[14] The basic issue in health care in the developing countries today, whether conceptualized around HFA or PHC, is how can resources be generated to maintain existing levels of health and health care services and where can more resources be accumulated to care for growing populations and deal with wider disparities (equity) and failing and/or rundown public service systems? The challenges of HFA and PHC for the next ten years are inherent in how these concepts can help countries muster the resources. This is why I have dwelled on the policy inconsistencies of the concepts. Today the issue is what set of economic policies for health care the concepts help formulate which can succeed in generating resources required for the future.[15]

A variety of policy advice is being offered to developing countries on what to do to facilitate a transition to these new conditions. The World Bank in a recent report has pinpointed three major problems facing countries and has proposed four policy reforms to deal with these problems. The problems are: allocation: insufficient spending on cost effective health activities, internal inefficiency of public programs, and inequity in the distribution of benefits from health services. The four policy reforms are:

1. Charge users of government health facilities.
2. Provide insurance or other risk coverage.
3. Use non-government resources effectively.
4. Decentralize government health services.[16]

In another paper these issues are further explored within the context of HFA and PHC.[17] I do not have sufficient space in this paper to recount all the details of either study. Instead, let me focus on the two main challenges that seem to impinge mostly on the viability of HFA and PHC. These are:

---

[14]There is a recent IMF study by Peter Heller and Associates that argues on the basis of seven sample countries (Chile, Dominican Republic, Ghana, Kenya, Philippines, Sri Lanka, and Thailand) that poor people, including their levels of health, have been hurt by IMF policies to help such countries adjust their economies to the dislocations created by world economic conditions. See (*WSJ*, Wednesday June 1, 1988). Also see, David E. Bell and Michael R. Reich (eds.), *Health, Nutrition and Economic Crises* (Dover, Mass), 1988.

[15]See David de Ferranti, "Strategies for Paying for Health Services in Developing Countries," World Health Statistics Quarterly, Vol. 17, No. 4, 1984, pp. 428-442.

[16]See World Bank, *Financing Health Services in Developing Countries* (Washington, DC, 1987).

[17]See Selection in this volume: "The Challenges of Health For All".

1. How can governments muster, for the year 2000, the resources necessary for health care maintenance and growth in their countries?
2. How can the concepts of HFA and PHC help them do these things?

RESOURCES FOR HEALTH BY THE YEAR 2000

It is fairly obvious to most observers that the resources for health in most developing countries in the coming decade will be in short supply. External resources for health will not be forthcoming in significant amounts. So if countries are to maintain existing health levels and do so for increasing populations, the resources necessary for maintenance will have to be generated internally. Incremental improvements in health levels beyond pure maintenance will add further strains upon resource availability. So the existing and future pressures on developing world health ministries in pursuit of HFA and in the reorientation of care to PHC will be unbearable and politically explosive. Actual and existing health levels may deteriorate. This is the context that leads to the broad policy prescriptions for reform of health systems proposed by international lending agencies and other economists as well. We do not do justice to the health ministries in the developing world by proposing policies that they have little chance of maintaining. What I want to propose may be just as difficult but, I think, has a better chance for success.

The issue is: Where will resources for Health for All come from in the decade ahead? Developing countries, generally cannot hope to generate such resources from high rates of economic growth. Only a few will be able to do so; the rest of the developing world will be struggling in the decade ahead with economic adjustment policies rather than growth policies. From my perspective the policy agenda needed to successfully address the issue of resource availability is simple, but quite complex politically. The agenda involves three major policy choices:

1. How should governments in the developing world spend their limited resources?
2. What can governments do to generate more resources for how they decide to spend for health?
3. How should governments manage effectively the available resources for whatever policies and objectives they decide to spend?

A brief discussion of each of these questions. *First*, how should governments spend their resources? The issue here is that not everything can be done. You cannot hope to achieve "true equity" (whatever it is!) and be efficient at the same time. You cannot provide equal amounts of hospital services as you do PHC services in rural areas. In economics parlance, the question as I've posed it is this: What is "appropriate" in health care for governments to do and what is "appropriate" to be left to private markets to solve? In health care in the developing world governments, again with few exceptions, have for a variety of reasons (historical, cultural, and/or political) elected to provide most, if not all, health services. And they have usually done so from general tax revenues. In a world where resources are now limited further and demands on the resources approach infinity, is it appropriate for governments to continue providing services that private markets could provide better (i.e. more efficiently)? Government services in the developing countries, provided "free", and for reasons based on equity, are neither actually free (consider travel and/or waiting times, for example) nor equitable (i.e. hospital care, urban-based is favored over PHC, rural-based). Governments could limit themselves to what we economists call "public goods" and let private markets allocate resources through changes in prices and incomes. The theory of public goods applied to health care suggests that governments should provide basic sanitation services, mass campaigns (such as immunizations, nutrition, etc.), individual immunizations (because of the high externalities), health education, and perhaps basic and applied health research. In these instances of public or quasi-public goods, governments could not count on private markets to supply the socially desirable amounts of consumption, i.e. private markets would "fail".

In the developing countries, however, governments provide or attempt to provide public as well as private goods in health care. Public sector activity seems based less on reasons of market failure than on concerns for equity. If equity is not being satisfactorily achieved, however, is it not time for governments to decide to husband their resources so as to pinpoint equity-i.e. by providing public goods to those most in "need" and/or unable to purchase from private markets? Resources "saved" (withdrawn) by governments competing (and doing so poorly) with the private sector, should be reapplied to more specific targets such as public goods, equity, and underprovided goods from the private market. This would be a way to generate huge amounts of resources in the developing countries. The resources could be used to achieve a different level of equity. The private sector (profit and non-profit) can produce these services much more efficiently than can the public sector.[18] So the answer to my first question is this: Governments should get out of the business of providing health care services that duplicate those better provided through private markets and apply the resources "saved" by pinpointing their application to well-defined equity objectives, pure public goods, and controls and regulation (cost and

---

[18]These points are developed with more completeness in Andreano and Helminiak. "The Role of the Private Sector: Paper delivered to an Asian Development Bank Meeting (`1987) (This paper is also reprinted in the present collection).

quality) over the private sector. In an ideal world these things might be done easily; however, in the real world governments cannot close down traditionally provided health services without incredible political risks.[19]

The *second* question may be more grounded in the real world. If governments can't (or are unwilling) to dismantle their systems, how can they still generate more resources? The answer here is also simple: Charge those who can pay something for the services and, most importantly, manage the services more efficiently, i.e. manage them as if they were in the private market. Imposing user charges or cost recovery is controversial politically, but it can and, in my view, should be done. The reality is this: Real resources available for health may decline and if so, existing health levels will as well. Can governments continue to maintain the facade of full services, strain their budgets to meet operating and recurrent costs, and adversely select the population between private and public facilities? Private sector health care is growing in the developing countries and there is precious little governments can (or should) do to prevent this. The sensible policy is to make public facilities, if they are going to be maintained, as competitive from a price and quality standpoint—as the private sector.[20]

My *third* question addresses the status quo: If governments can't or won't change the distribution of production, and can't or won't use incentives for cost recovery, how can they manage their systems better to squeeze out additional resources? There is much that can be suggested on this question but space limitations limit me to discuss just one aspect: How can managerial performance be improved in the public system? The answer is: Improve the reward/incentive structure for managers at all levels. We must look at a health care system in terms of what is motivating its managers: the potential for generating new resources through improved managerial efficiency is enormous. Personnel rules, reward structures for performance, and the panoply of disincentives public employees face all have to be changed if managerial performance is to be improved.[21] The point is this: If governments can't or won't change the financial or the production basis of their health care system, they can gain extraordinary amounts of resources by just managing "what they got" better.

This brief excursion into these three main questions is meant to summarize a lot of the creative thinking now underway in the international health research

---

[19]An excellent analysis of the public vs. private issues in health care is in A. J. Culyer and Bengt Jonsson (eds.), Public and Private Health Services (1986), Basil Blackwell, Oxford).

[20]The discussion on user charges in World Bank (1987), pp. 25-32 is very instructive on the analytical as well as policy issues.

[21]This complex interaction of rewards and incentive is called the "real" system in Andreano and Helminiak (1987), Appendix III, pp. 65-69.

community. It is indicative of current thinking but by no means exhausts the possibilities for new and creative developments in health policy.

THE RELEVANCE OF HFA AND PHC FOR THE FUTURE

I began this paper with a discussion of some of the contradictions and tensions inherent in the basic concepts of HFA and PHC. This was not meant to demean these concepts but to provide a sense of reality about them in terms of the policy signals they send to governments in the developing world. The concepts have served well to focus world attention on the inequitable distribution of health benefits (in poor as well as rich countries) and on a newer technology (PHC) that might successfully compete with the existing medical model on both an access (equity), cost and quality basis. There is no reason to suppose that as concepts they cannot continue to serve as an organizing set of values and ideals to inspire countries. My problem with the concepts is at the operational and policy level. HFA and PHC have to be reshaped as concepts if they are to guide the translation of ideals and values into operational policies. PHC, for example, whether selective or comprehensive has to be able to compete effectively for resources with the existing system. PHC, which just uses the clinical model, does not embody the new technology as developed in the typical concept of PHC. Similarly the strong equity bias of HFA has to be modified: "true equity" (which many supporters of HFA frequently cite as a goal) is non-existent. What equity is meant? Financial? Access? Distributional? Income? HFA must be translated to governments in terms that make the confrontation between equity and efficiency in the financing and delivery of health services meaningful. The future in the developing countries is unlimited wants but limited means; governments must be realistic about resource allocation policies in health care. Everything that "needs" to be done cannot be done. Trade-offs and choices must be made. Equity concerns still should be of paramount importance. But there are many different levels of equity that are socially tolerable or desirable and there is no single policy agenda to achieve equity. Governments must make choices and pinpoint available resources, used efficiently, to those populations not able to be served by private markets. Competitive behavior in public health care systems—using rewards, incentives, and disincentives is not to be avoided just because such advice flows from the pens of economists.[22]

---

[22] Many of these ideas and expressions of concern emerged at the Technical Discussions at the World Health Assembly in 1987. See, "Report of the Technical Discussion on Economic Support for National Health for all Strategies," 40th World Health Assembly, 12 May 1987, Geneva.

The problems are real and the instruments of intervention are limited. Countries should not run from the ideas of new financing methods for health care. Nor should they fear using taxes, subsidies, and user charges as ways to redistribute health benefits and move their production and delivery system towards economic efficiency. Despite what the critics of the economists' way of thinking suggest, consumer demands and preferences do count and do influence the way real resources get allocated. If consumers prefer drugs to preventive changes in life styles, prefer seeing doctors to seeing community health workers, prefer hospitals and clinics to rural health centers, than these preferences will influence any resource allocation choice a government makes. Planning models in health care usually fail because these characteristics are either ignored or underestimated by planners. The future of health care in the developing countries is this: strive for mixed systems—private and public—efficiently financed and managed with governments concentrating on the equity redistributions required when private market solutions fail. Governments should concentrate their resources on achieving acceptable equity solutions and on the production and delivery of public goods in health—those where net externalities are highest in that society. Governments should get out of the business of prescribing which health technologies, i.e. PHC as an example, should be adopted unless the pushing of the technology is in support of an equity objective or a private market failure. In the next retrospective on HFA and PHC held in the year 2000 I hope we will be able to say that health care systems in the developing world are meeting most of the demands of their populations and doing so in ways that are efficient and involve the proper role of governments in health care markets. If HFA and PHC can be translated into policies that will govern resource allocation rules responsive to a country's real resource position, then we will, and should, praise these concepts effusively in the year 2000.

I have written, to this point in the paper, nothing explicitly about nurses in the PHC context. But I think the implications for nursing in the point of view taken in this paper are substantial. If governments are to make health systems more efficient, manpower training and development policies will also have to be changed. Such changes will require that the substitution properties in treatment modalities between nurses and physicians should be encouraged. Perhaps training methods and curricula for training of nurses will have to change as well. The primary health care team needs to maximize the human capital nursing brings to the delivery side; governments need to drop employment restrictions that inhibit efficient allocation of nursing services. I am no expert on nursing, but because the resources for the future have to be generated from internal efficiencies and better management, nurses could and should play a pivotal role.

Acknowledgement—I want to thank my long time research associate Dr. Thomas Helminiak for his careful and helpful comments on this paper. All errors and omissions are, of course, mine.

ATTACHMENT I

EQUITY IN HEALTH: THE CONCEPT OF TRADE-OFFS

The concept of "trade-offs"—the necessity of giving up something in order to obtain (more of) something else is fundamental to economics. For national economies, this concept is often illustrated by a "production possibility frontier." Figure 1 depicts a simplified version of a production possibility (PP) frontier for an economy.

With the available two dimensions of the surface of the figure, just two separate goods (or separate bundles of goods) can be shown. The figure indicates that if all of the economy's resources are devoted to the good(s) measured on the vertical axis, amount A of that good could be produced (and 0 amount of the horizontal axis good). Intermediate positions on the curve AB describe the rate at which either of the two goods must be sacrificed (trade-off) to obtain a given increment in the other. Thus, e.g., if the economy's resources were distributed to produce amount A1 of the one good and B1 of the other (point X on the PP frontier), it could increase the production of the second from B1 to B2 if it is willing to reduce the production of the former from A1 to A2 (at point Y on the PP frontier).

But this assumes that the economy's resources are already operating with maximum achievable efficiency. If, as in Figure 2, instead of operating on the maximum efficiency PP frontier (i.e. on curve AB) the economy is at point Z (on a less efficient PP curve), it could, by improving the production efficiency of the system, achieve more of both goods. This is not easy to do, however.

Within the health sector, it is believed that there is a trade-off between the total amount of health services that can be produced (termed "efficiency") and the degree of equity in the distribution of these services. That is, as we choose to increase the equity of health services distribution, we necessarily must sacrifice some total output of health services—as in moving from X to Y in Figure 1. So, if the health sector is unable (or unwilling) to improve the overall efficiency of the system, it must decide how much additional equity it is willing to produce—at the expense of some, corresponding amount of total health services.

Figure 1: Production Possibility Curves: Maximum System Efficiency

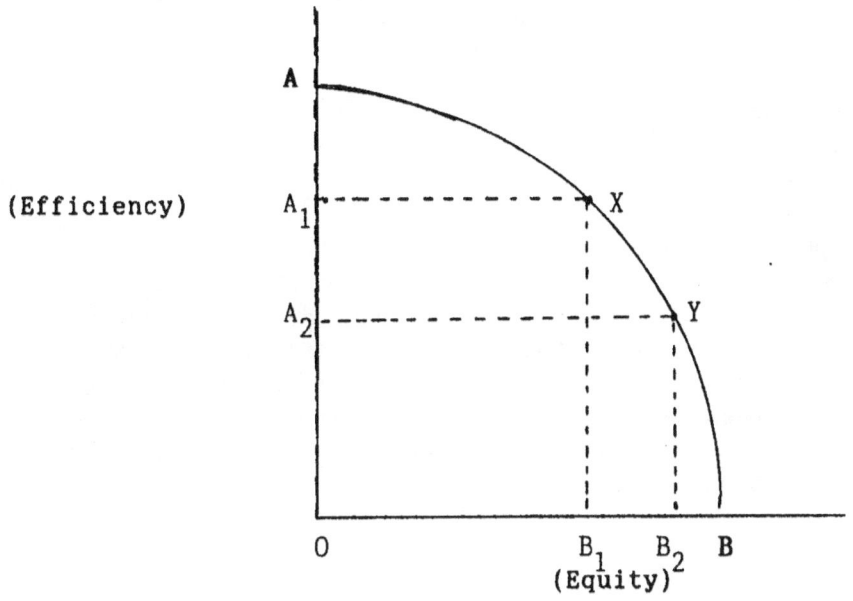

Figure 2: Production Possibility Curves: Less than Maximum System Efficiency

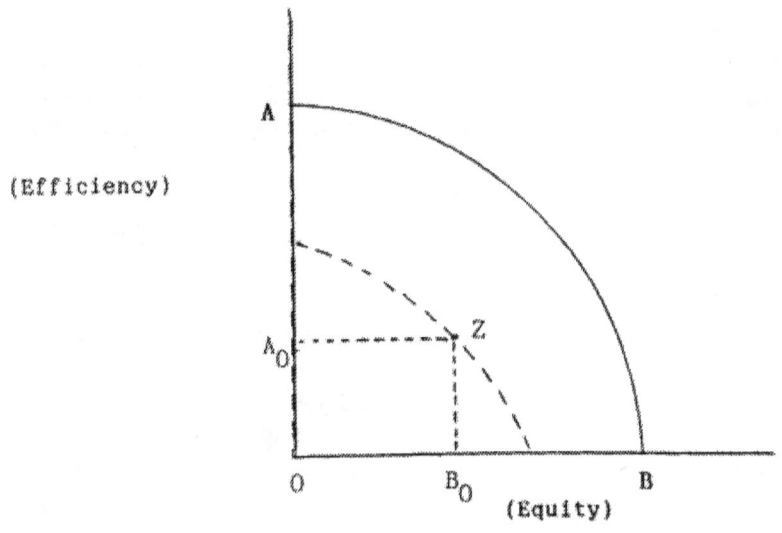

Ralph Andreano

ANNEX II

A FURTHER NOTE ON THE CHOICE OF TECHNOLOGY ISSUE IN PRIMARY HEALTH CARE (PHC)

In the main paper for this meeting I noted a contradiction (or tension) in the concept of PHC regarding the choice of technology. Because of space limitations in the main paper, I could not develop fully the importance of this point. Again, I repeat that by discussing such aspects of PHC, I do not mean to suggest the concept be abandoned or that we reinvent the "hidden" meaning of the original framers of the concept. My principal aim here, as in the main paper, is to use the tools of economic analysis to assist the policy choices countries face as they implement their PHC programs and objectives. There were in the main paper two issues involving the choice of technology: (1) under what conditions can PHC supplant existing medical service delivery technology and (2) what combination of PHC technology is most socially efficient and adoptable? 2 This brief note explores both these issues.

SOME PROBLEMS IN THE TRANSFER OF PHC TECHNOLOGY

Transfer of technology from one country to another is an old and historically important aspect of economic development. In the case of PHC most countries had already one or more pieces of this technology in place. Repackaging into HFA through PHC concepts elevated the technology of PHC into an activist mode, with a better defined social goal of health for-all! But to transfer this technology, as any other, from country to country creates a number of extremely difficult economic problems.

(1) <u>The Relative use of the factors of production—land, labor, and capital— varies enormously across countries</u>.

The full, i.e. comprehensive, PHC package requires that the factors of production be combined efficiently if the technology is to be successfully (i.e. socially optimally) applied. But because the known capital requirement for parts of PHC are high and the labor skill content of other parts of PHC somewhat unknown, successfully transferring the comprehensive package of PHC requires both large quantities of capital and labor. It also requires capital and labor from sectors other than health. Developing countries are usually rich in labor but capital short. That is why many agencies such as UNICEF have opted for what

30

has come to be called "selective" PHC: adopt only those parts of PHC for which, in a given country, available skills and labor supply are adequate and for which outside infusions of capital (e.g. immunizations) can be efficiently applied. The real facts are that the productivity of the resources used in PHC will vary enormously from country to country because the quality and availability of the factors of production vary widely. That is why there is some economic logic attached to breaking the PHC concept into parts of the technology that the factor endowment of a country can support. In some sense, my argument is a supporting point for the Basic Needs approach.[23]

(2) Shelf of Technology in PHC.

If we view PHC, as constituting many different health technologies-which is what "selective" PHC does—then the policy guidance offered to countries is to take something from that shelf that fits local conditions and frame out of it an indigenous PHC technology. The problem here is that PHC is both a technology concept and an equity objective; but as I've pointed out in the main paper these objectives often have to be traded-off.

If, however, we view PHC as offering a Shelf of Technology the task for a country is to identify which technologies it wants to take down from the shelf and apply in its country. I see several other problems, other than those already noted.

(a) The country must have the capacity to select. This means the country must know itself, its factor endowments, and what can or cannot work.

(b) The country must select the parts or all of PHC that suits the prevailing market conditions for the prices and supplies of the factors of production needed for PHC, or parts thereof. In most developing countries the actual market prices of, say, labor, are distorted and do not measure relative scarcities or surpluses. Distorted market signals prevail because of institutional reasons and rigidities. Recurrent cost issues can also be mis-specified because of these market rigidities and distortions.[24]

---

[23] An instructive article, surveying PHC experiences in Nepal, echo's most of the comments noted above. See, Linda Stone, "Primary Health Care for Whom? Village Perspectives from Nepal," *Social Science and Medicine* (1986) Vol. 22, No. 3, pp. 293-302. This article also highlights the community rather than individual focus of PHC, a point prominently made in (2).

[24] See in particular, Mead Over, "The Effect of Scale on Cost Projections for a Primary Health Care Program in a Developing Country," *Social Science and Medicine* (1986), Vol. 22, No. 3, pp. 351-360.

(3) <u>Indigenous Technology of PHC</u>.

Finally, for countries to pick and choose from PHC as a concept or as a collection of technologies will ultimately require an indigenous PHC. Let me mention three notions countries must consider as they transfer PHC into man indigenous set of technologies.

(a) Searching and learning. Countries must be willing to try different combinations and to learn from mistakes in the search for the PHC package best suited to their social objectives and factor endowments.
(b) Continuous Process. In adopting PHC, countries should do so gradually and not shift dramatically the direction of current resources allocated to health care. Abrupt changes are likely to be disruptive and to cause further distortions in markets.
(c) Underutilized knowledge. Countries pursuing PHC should follow their best instincts; there is usually underutilized knowledge about health techniques both in the communities and among individuals. The process of searching and learning, of grafting small but significant changes gradually, and taping the collective wisdom of the people, are all-important ways to building an indigenous PHC.[25]

CONCLUSION

All I've tried to highlight in this brief note are some further ways policy and decision makers in the developing countries already have, or could use to approach PHC. The fundamental point of my main paper is that additional resources for HFA and PHC will have to be generated within a country. To do so their use of resources must be efficient and their use of technology must be innovative, suitable to local conditions, and based on a realistic assessment of the supplies and prices of factor endowments.

---

[25]All three points above are revealed in, Clive S. Gray, "State Sponsored PHC in Africa: The Recurrent Cost of Performing Miracles," *Social Science and Medicine* (1986), Vol. 22, No. 3, pp. 361-368.

SELECTION 4

ECONOMIC ISSUES IN DISEASE CONTROL AND ERADICATION[26]

My paper falls under the *theoretical* rather than the *practical* side of things. Yet, the practical impact of the somewhat abstract approach taken toward the subject is highly significant for at least two reasons:

(1) Governments and donor agencies have undertaken to commit vast amounts of resources to control or eliminate disease. Aside from the humanitarian point of view, the economist asks: have these resources been applied in the most appropriate way so as to maximize the gains to society? And by gains, one means: have the resources applied to control and/or eradication of disease had desirable net effects on improving those attributes important to health and/or economic growth and development?

In this sense, then, an abstract rather than directly pragmatic approach may have some relevance for it can help us determine what is important and how resources can best be applied.

(2) Control of disease is such a complex phenomena, with such innumerable interdependent effects, that some abstraction of such processes has value in helping policy makers to focus on the appropriate parameters of change. It is also necessary to abstract so as to assist in defining the important relationship one wants to measure.

The kind of disease control/eradication I refer to is usually called vertical (i.e. single disease) rather than horizontal (i.e. multiple diseases), though in practice my approach has applicability to both.

We speak of traditional economics and perhaps such economic thinking may be equivalent to what is sometimes referred to as the 'bad' part of traditional medicine, namely the witch doctors. Economists may be the witch doctors of modern health policy in the developing world. Lord knows we have done a lot of damage'—but for better or worse, in disease control as in life, resources are

---

[26]This paper was originally published in *Social Science and Medicine*, Vol. 17, No. 24, pp. 2027-2032, 1983.

limited and the demands infinite as choices must be made. And the theory of choice making is the 'medicine' of economics.

In 1973 my colleagues and I reported the results of our research on the economic impact of schisto on the island of St Lucia. Whatever the merits (and faults) of our study it was the first systematic attempt by economists to theorize and then to test empirically the theory on how specifically the presence or absence of disease affects certain powerful components of economic development. We focused on three effects:

(1) worker productivity
(2) demographic effects—i.e. fertility and birth rates
(3) the performance of school attenders.

My point is that to examine the economic impacts of disease control/eradication, one must first start from some basic theoretical level. In the St Lucia study that theoretical level was related to human capital theory.

That is, growth and development are spurred by improvements in skills and energy (i.e. productivity) just as physical capital contributes to an economy's growth.

The human capital theory suggests, among other things, that growth in human capital can raise the total output of goods and services in an economy. It is also the traditional economic approach to appraising the impact of programs for disease control and/or eradication.

(1) is labor productivity at the margin improved?
(2) is total output over time likely to be increased?
(3) is the stock of human capital increased on balance in ways, which enhance and make possible efficient uses of available physical capital?
(4) is the distribution of income altered and in ways that promote higher savings levels?

The traditional economist's armamentarium to answer these questions is not large—mainly the enumeration of the benefits as compared to costs. We give the policy makers some probabalistic statement that yes if you do such and such, such and such may occur. This analysis can be powerful, however, in informing choices and in influencing the allocation of resources. Indeed, the choices often are between degrees of control, or degrees of eradication rather than either/or.

The formidable task then becomes one of measurement of benefits and of costs. And here the methodological and measurement issues are so complex and so vast that it is impossible to believe that only economists should make such calculations. Yet internal resource allocation in countries requires it, donor agencies demand it.

The following are a few of the methodological measurement problems:

- what is a benefit? how far does one trace the linkage between social and economic factors and control or disease eradication? on workers alone? on the entire household? on non-work activities? That is, what is to be included and what excluded as benefits. The choices can be crucial in determining whether or not a wise allocation of resources will be made or a project undertaken.
- What discount rate should be used to value the benefits? If a program takes 10 years before it achieves any measurable effects; how do we judge whether or not it is worth it today, compared to other uses of the same resources? Here the issue of the social discount rate is crucial.

We shall return to two other classes of measurement difficulties:

(1) The price to be used in calculating the expected benefits of a disease control program? the prices that prevail today or those that would prevail *after* a control or eradication program had altered the distribution of income, the patterns of asset holdings and consumption, etc.?
(2) The so-called 'spillover effects' or 'linkages'; i.e. disease control programs aimed at one target group affect in unintended ways other groups—such spillover effects must be counted but they are difficult to quantify—often such things are not measured.

We should also note how the approach of the target group (or groups) at risk to disease control greatly complicates measurement problems and often makes ambiguous the evaluation of the economic impact of such programs on the improvement in human capital. To the extent that one can evaluate, economic judgment dictates that control programs concentrate on those that produce both health benefits and net gains in output; the latter may take longer to achieve, but these are, nonetheless, the objectives an economist hopes can be achieved by control eradication schemes.

I now posit a simple model as might prevail in rural agriculture, focusing the demand curve for two kinds of labor: peasant families and hired workers on farms owned by peasant families.

The model subsumes an improvement in the health of both classes of workers. Impacting this effect on the supply curve and the demand curve for labor, the model shows that a likely impact of the improvement in health is that total farm output can be increased but total employment may be decreased. Its use as an abstraction is to give direct meaning of how health interventions must be viewed and measured because they can produce positive health benefits, positive output effects, but negative employment effects.

35

It is of great significance that health interventions have negative as well as positive economic effects, a point which is central to any discussion of the economic effects of disease control /eradication.

I shall briefly discuss some of the difficulties in linking health and development before considering some specific calculation problems in assessing the benefits/ costs of control and/or eradication schemes and some general conditions for an increase of output from health intervention.

Empirical research is still in its infancy regarding the precise form and magnitude of linkages between health and development. One has the unusual case with health of consumption and investment, both private and public, being embodied together. Economic research has not been particularly successful in disaggregating these elements or in independently quantifying their economic impacts. But that does not mean such impacts do not exist: it means that our methodology has not advanced sufficiently to have measurement techniques and conceptual models capable of dealing with the simultaneous nature of such relationships. In theory such relationships exist but are so complex that attempts to derive quantitative estimates of a few of them without knowing how to deal with all the others generally results in inconclusive findings.

As was written in 1973 in connection with our study on the economic impact of parasitic disease in St Lucia,

"...When a disease is endemic to an area...its elimination or control can bring about non-marginal changes that will ramify throughout the society and its economy—and the consequences of structural change are very difficult to deal with empirically, given the current state of knowledge. General equilibrium theory in the social sciences exists at a level of abstraction which as yet has relatively little operational value"[1].

The major diseases of Africa, especially the highly important parasitic diseases (malaria, schistosomiasis, onchocerciasis, filariasis, trypanosomiasis, leishmaniasis and others, such as hookworm and ascaris) put millions of people at risk. If one looks at the size of the populations at risk from diseases and the circumstances under which infection occurs, one knows it is not irrational to try to develop health strategies to control the spread of further infection as well as the circumstances and conditions under which the populations at risk are forced to live. As economists, what we are less certain about is the precise form and magnitude control or eradication of such diseases would have on the capacity of people to develop their economy and enhance their material lives. Theoretical evidence exists for thinking so, but empirical evidence is harder to generate. Our thinking has been too narrowly structured. The benefits and costs of single diseases have held our attention when, in fact, it is the dynamic interaction of disease with daily life that ultimately determine the development impact of disease control eradication as one of the components of improving health. The benefit/cost ratios of control programs for any of the major parasitic diseases, for example, will be underestimated simply because all the indirect benefits cannot be captured quantitatively and because it takes time for such benefits to mature. The direct benefits from mortality and morbidity reduction may well be large for diseases such as schisto, oncho and malaria. But even though great, the potential impact on the productivity of labor, the improved security and stability of family life, and qualitative improvements in the human capital stock must all be balanced against potential demographic changes.

The real developmental importance of control or eradication of the parasitic diseases comes from the synergistic effects in a dynamic sense on how life is perceived now, on attitudes toward family and home and on the behavioral attributes of daily life. Under conditions where the environment of the past has now been altered dramatically, will peasant families be able to save more? Will their children be more productive school learners? Will the farmers be more capable, physically and mentally, of accepting new ways of farming? Will families be more receptive to ideas and techniques to control fertility? Will the ability to save what used to be expended in caring for, or avoiding, disease be used to improve life? All these processes largely depend on the stability and security of family life. And the removal of health as a daily, constant barrier around which life must take place will surely have impacts that transcend their sudden removal or reduction. If poor health and disease had previously disrupted daily life, their removal as constraints on other activities must surely be counted as beneficial results.

Development economists, especially those advising donor and granting agencies, have nonetheless asked for more and specific rationales for making investment choices in disease control and/or eradication. Inability to produce hard numbers has had much to do with the paucity of resources such programs have been able to command. Yet, it is not likely that hard numbers will ever be able to capture the real nature of the dynamic relationship health variables have with developmental ones. The literature on this subject is now quite large and one does not wish repeat it here. But there are two calculation problems worth mentioning which reinforce present difficulties in obtaining precision in measuring impacts. We in the industrialized countries are bound up in our quantification work with attaching prices to everything, including disease, health and life itself. But prices that exist in poor countries reflect the initial distribution of income and wealth that exists; if income and wealth were more evenly distributed, demands—and hence prices—would be different. To control or eradicate diseases is to affect the distribution of income. Yet the decision to undertake control or eradication is usually based on calculations made with the prices and markets that prevail now; calculation of benefits will reflect this, but the real benefits would be different, and presumably higher, if the prices that prevailed under a more equal distribution of income were used to make the calculation. This is why conventional calculation methods fail to build a case for larger resource allocations for disease control and health services in the Third World.

Secondly, our conventional calculations have difficulty in knowing how to value what are commonly called 'leakages' or 'spillover effects'. That is, disease control aimed at one population group at risk also confers benefits to others not currently at risk but who could become so given the freedom of migration and the movement both of people and disease vectors. Such spillover benefits (and costs) should also be counted in assessing whether or not economic impacts warrant investment in a disease control or eradication program. But it is difficult to do so and consequently one other neglects to count them, as any appropriate analysis should.

To keep our perspective clear, then, whatever the precise manner in which disease control and health generally interact with components of the development process, one presumes that when all effects reach equilibrium there should be a new capacity for the society to increase output. To do so alone would not ensure a better life unless structural changes, such as the equitable distribution of output gains, ensure that the new development possibilities do not occur at the expense of social equity. In theory, we could produce greater output. Such effects might be looked at in two ways: on people who now enjoy better health being able to do things differently; and on people as embodied factors of production—what economists call human capital. A grouping of direct effects that increase output would include:

(a) An increase in output due to reduced absentee ism from work and school;
(b) An increase in output due to improved mental and physical ability of both children and adults;
(c) An increase in output due to an extension of working lives.

Indirect effects would include:

(a) Reduction in resources previously devoted to care for sick people;
(b) Freeing of resources previously tied up by people trying to avoid disease and illness;
(c) An output increase due to a rise in the birth rate, which had resulted from better health conditions.

The measurement of such direct and indirect output has not proved easy, though in theory one presumes they can and do occur as a consequence of disease control and improved health. There can also be costs, or negative benefits as well, which could offset output gains.

Against this background, it will be useful to present some more abstract configurations of the economic impacts that derive from disease control or eradication. In the developing world context rural development and rural agriculture are the locus of development and growth. This is the development setting in which to interject disease control/eradication. Production and consumption increases in rural areas are dependent on the fate of agriculture.

To illustrate the difficulty is assessing economic impacts of disease and how one measures them, following some earlier work done by development economists (principally Tinbergen and Bhagwati), let me posit three production-ownership models for rural agriculture:

(a) Farmer-owned (families, extended families, etc.; perhaps no labor purchased outside);
(b) Tenant farms/sharecropping—non-farmer owned (also outside labor purchased for seasonal/crop uses);
(c) Collectivism; state owned; no outside labor purchases; no market transactions.

Of the three models, theory suggests that, all things being equal, one gets greater total output from options (a) and (c) (scheme 1).

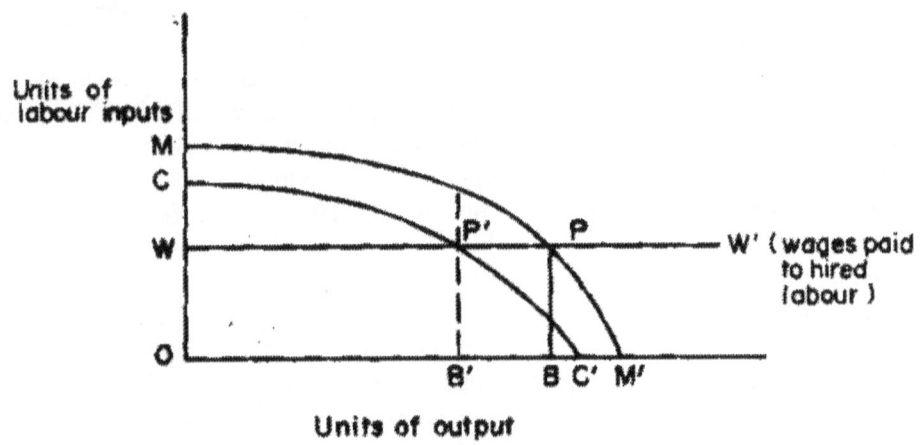

If farm laborers were hired at wage rate (W), a peasant farmer would stop use at Point (P) because at that point the amount of output contributed by a worker is just equal to what it costs to employ him. If option (a) represents an extended or peasant family farm, it would want to continue to work to acquire all the output possible (i.e. the area B'BP'). Thus, if farms are operated only with wage laborers, total output is less. If only peasant farmers operate, total output is greater. If the two are mixed, the peasant farmer would always choose not to purchase hired labor, except in special circumstances.

If one now inserts the presence of disease into rural agriculture—that is if we cojoin a health argument to the graphic description—the result could be as follows. If MM' is the marginal productivity schedule (or demand curve for labor) for 'healthy' peasant farm families, for 'sick' families the schedule is lower, i.e. CC'. Thus, a health intervention, which improves the marginal productivity of each peasant family farm worker, results in a larger total output (BPM'). The impact of a health intervention on the supply curve of hired workers (WW') is less clear in the absence of asset redistribution and given the realities of land ownership in rural areas. If WW' is the supply curve of sick workers, then an improvement in their health would raise the price of hired labor (the supply curve of healthy workers, following our earlier analysis, is presumed to be above WW'). But as their marginal productivity would be greater, the peasant farm operator might consider substituting hired workers for family workers over a greater range of output possibilities. But much would depend on market prices for the output. The realities are such in rural agricultural areas that total employment of healthy hired workers by the peasant farm family would be reduced. The anomalous situation is thus produced where a health intervention produces a positive output effect (i.e. on the peasant family) and a negative employment effect (on the hired workers). Thus, health interventions unaccompanied by other asset redistribution policies or other employment generating opportunities will not on balance be sufficient alone to raise average income levels of all. The difficulty of measuring this in advance so as to judge whether or not the health intervention (disease control) was worth it is difficult to contemplate. Yet such discussions are and must be made.

Under complete collectivization (option c), total output depends only on the average product of labor, not the marginal product. Thus, no individual worker is, in theory, indispensable, so one can always get the same total output. There are, of course, problems with option (c), but it seems to have worked especially well where population density is high, viz. China. Increases in average health levels unaccompanied by asset redistribution in such cases would largely be pointless.

The existence of large proportions of rural populations in 'landless' situations and no sustained employment possibilities makes the 'trickle-down' possibilities of an output/production expansion strategy for improvement in living standards in rural areas quite difficult if not unlikely. Health interventions will produce positive economic impacts and undetermined negative ones as well on the quality and productivity of labor. The analysis that flows out of the simple theorizing performed above, however, suggests that health interventions upon the common work force in rural agriculture must be accompanied by additional employment generating policies, as well as a redistribution of assets. Thus, weighing the benefits against the costs of disease control and/or eradication is insufficient unless the additional (what one thinks of as developmental) impacts on output and employment are also measured.

In Africa and in the Third World generally, disease control/eradication follows the 'target group' or 'group at risk' principle. For economists attempting to evaluate the benefit/cost relationship of various possible health interventions, the target group approach presents formidable measurement issues. Those groups of the population living or working within a defined geographical area which are particularly exposed to a certain degree of risk of contracting or severely suffering from a specific disease or health hazard will thus constitute the 'target group' for any program aimed at reducing that risk.

In certain cases, for example diseases produced by mosquito vectors or by pollution of the water supply, the whole population of a defined geographical area may be the target group for a program of control or prevention. In other cases, such as protein-calorie malnutrition, there will be physiological groups at greatest risk, such as young children and pregnant women. Within these groups, risk may be concentrated in certain social, educational or economic subgroups and be virtually absent in others, e.g. families of cash croppers are often worse off nutritionally than those of farmers on a mixed subsistence, non-cash economy; children whose mothers are educated, and so can work for wages, are often worse off nutritionally than those whose mothers remain at home. In some cases, high risk of certain diseases is associated with rural occupations and in others with certain local ecological conditions.

The 'target group' concept, therefore, is one of identified, higher than average, health risk. Preventive and promotive health programs generally aim at reducing the most important of the various risks operating upon a community's members. For epidemiological and operational reasons, it is not feasible in communicable disease control to withhold protection from any group at health risk within a geographically discrete community merely because it has certain economic, social or other characteristics. Ethical considerations also should bar any such discrimination based upon non-health criteria. Unfortunately, in practice, political, social and economic factors still override the ethical obligations for equity in health to which all health workers and Ministries of Health should be committed. The reality is that resources are limited and choices have to be made if health interventions are to be both efficient *and* equitable.

Conceptually, we have to disaggregate health interventions (read disease control) into two classes of components: (a) those which reduce disease incidence and health risk only; and (b) those that reduce disease and health risk *and* produce positive output and employment effects. As has already been suggested, disaggregation of health into its consumption and investment components is empirically difficult and ethically impossible. But even precise

41

empirical support of the kind which would greatly simplify the marking off of target groups for disease control and/or health interventions that maximize inputs in the development process do not exist. Effects on labor quantity and productivity, family stability and security, noting both the positive and negative aspects of demographic change, are as precise as we can get.

The most cost-effective health programs are those to control infectious diseases; by this is meant that the ratio of cost per death prevented, or cost per illness avoided, is lower for infectious disease control than for control of other health problems.

Finally, we know from evidence adduced from econometric studies of Engels Curves that as the proportion out of disposable income spent on food declines, the single most important new element of consumption added to the consumption basket is health care and health services. This suggests wider measurement issues for evaluating disease control and eradication schemes.

In conclusion, the following modalities for disease control and/or eradication and health intervention suggest a wider scope for assessing their economic impacts:

(a) vertical/disease control, surveillance or eradication programs (e.g. T.B., schisto, malaria, oncho, etc.);
(b) health care services provision and delivery with a wide variety of modes of delivery (i.e. rural health workers, clinics, immunization);
(c) health services delivery as part of general community development activities (i.e. immunization, parasite control, MCH);
(d) activities undertaken community-wide, which include selected parts of (1) disease control, (2) preventive services such as sanitation and immunization and (3) limited target group direct services delivery activities such as family planning, MCH, nutrition action and health education.

A wider set of health modes, including any or all of the above, will also bear directly (i.e. in the short or intermediate-run) or indirectly (i.e. after some time lags) upon activities affecting parameters of economic development. Most of these interdependences with health intersect with agriculture, water supply, and transportation (roads, etc.).

Decades of emphasis on economic growth as the key to alleviating the poverty, disease and helplessness of people living in developing countries has proved to do just the opposite: the daily lives of people, their material and social well-being are in many instances worse after economic growth than they were before. This has proved especially true in rural areas. Economic growth must not be at the expense of making only a few people better off and worse off. Redistribution of assets and social consumption must come first and economic growth in the future must have the capacity for equitable growth. This is the model, which should condition our thinking and our policies for health in the developing world.

The role of health is a crucial component for making the lives of people better. But health services and health resources are as inequitably distributed around the world, as are income and wealth. A conscious effort to assist countries in the redistribution of these services and resources ought to be a fundamental goal of those international and multilateral agencies active in health as well as national governments themselves. No amount of aid from the outside world can overcome the health problems of the poor without the serious and dedicated commitment of national governments. But governments and donors must appreciate that to improve health means more than just providing clinics and doctors, i.e. more health services. It implies better nutrition and more food; this means that what happens in agricultural production and distribution systems in countries is as much a health as an income concern. It also means safe water and clean and decent housing and other environmental sanitation elements. These, too, are health just as much as they are production concerns. Health and social development are so intertwined that one is part of the other even if one cannot analytically isolate the sources of causality. In the developing world, malnutrition, infection, poverty, disease, the birth rate and the maldistribution of income, wealth and social consumption are all part of the same social system: one is linked with the other and the whole is greater than the sum of its parts. It is difficult conceive of policies in health that will not affect all the parts and in turn be affected. Development as such can no longer be piecemeal and policies for increasing income must square with policies for improving equity.

REFERENCES

Weisbrod B. A., Andreano, R., and et al. *Disease and Development: The Impact of Parasitic Disease in St. Lucia*, Chap. 1. University of Wisconsin Press, Madison, 1973.

(A) *Micro studies*
Brohult *J. et al.* The working capacity of Liberian males: a comparison between urban and rural population in relation to malaria. *Annals trop. Med. Parasit.* 73, 487-494, 1981.

Collins K. *J. et al.* Physiological performance and work capacity of Sudanese cane cutters with schistosoma mansoni infection. *Am. J. trop. Med. Hyg.* 25, 410-421, 1976.

Ejezie G. C., and Ade-Serrano, M. A. Schistosoma haematobium in ajara community of badagry, Nigeria: a study on prevalence, intensity and morbidity from infection among primary school children. *Trop. Geogr. Med.* 33, 175-180, 1981.

Omer A. H. S. and el din Ahmed N. Assessment of physical performance and lung function in schistosoma mansoni infection. *E. Afr. med. J.* 51, 217-222, 1974.

(B) *Macro studies*

Cohen *J.* E. Benefits of eliminating mortality attributed to schistosomiasis in Zanzibar. *Soc. Sci. Med.* 8, 383-398, 1974.

Latham L., Latham M. and Basta S. S. *The Nutritional and Economic Implications* of *Ascaris Infection in Kenya.* World Bank Staff Working Paper No. 271, World Bank, Washington, DC, 1977.

(C) *Models of disease transmission*

Dietz K., Molineaux L. and Thomas A. A malaria model tested in the African savannah. Bull. *Wld Hlth Org.* 50, 347-357,1974.

Verma B. L., Ray S. K. and Srivastava R. N. Stochastic approach to the estimation of infective force and malaria parasite incidence rate in infants from longitudinal data. *J. Communic. Dis.* 12, 118-125, 1980.

(D) *Background data populations and water contact habits*

Bella *H. et al.* Migrant workers and schistosomiasis in the Gezira, Sudan. *Trans. R. Soc. trop. Med. Hyg.* 74, 36-39, 1980.

Kloos H. and Lemma A. The epidemiology of schistosoma mansoni infection in Tensae Berhan: human water contact patterns. *Ethiop. med.* J. 18, 91-98, 1980.

Polderman A. M. Transmission dynamics of endemic schistosomiasis. *Trop. Geogr. Med.* 31, 465-475, 1979.

Tayo M. A., Push R. N. and Bradley A. K. Malumfashi endemic diseases research project XI: water contact activities in the schistosomiasis study areas. *Annls trop. Med. Parasit.* 74, 347-354, 1980.

(E) *Studies of prevalence rates*

Bray R. S. and Anderson M. J. Falciparum malaria and pregnancy. *Tras. Soc. trop. Med. Hyg.* 73,427-431, 1979.

Koura M., Upatham E. S. and Ahmed M. D. Prevalence of schistosoma haematobium in Koryole and Merca districts of the Somali Democratic resrpublic. *Annls trop. Med. Parasit.* 75, 53-61, 1981.

St. Urchler D. *et al.* Intestinal parasitoses in eight Liberian settlements: prevalences and community anti-Helminthis chemotherapy. *Tropen. Parasit.* 31, 87-93, 1980.

Shiff C. J. *et al.* Seasonal patterns in the transmission of schistosoma haematobium in Rhodesia, and its control by winter applications of molluscicide. *Trans. R. Soc. trop. Med. Hyg.* 73, 375-380, 1979.

Taticheff S., Abdulahi Y. and Haile-Meskal F. Intestinal parasite infection in preschoool children in Addis Ababa. *Ethiop. med. J.* 19, 35-40, 1981.

Wenlock R. W. Age variation in prevalence of parasitic diseases in rural communities. *Med. J. Zamhia* 12, 13-16, 1978.

(F) *Results and costs of control programs*

Duke B. O. L. and Moore P. J. The use of a molluscicide in conjunction with chemotherapy to control schistosoma haematobium at the Barombi lace foci in Cameroon, III: conclusions and cost. *Tropen. Parasit.* 27, 505-508, 1976.

Hedman P. et al. A pocket of controlled malaria in a holodenemic region of West Africa. *Annls trop. Med. Parasit.* 73, 317-325, 1979.

Highton R. B. and Coudry A. W. The cost evaluation of mollusciciding operations in five irrigation schemes in Kenya. *E. Afr. med. J.* 51, 180-193, 1974.

Ralph Andreano

THE RECENT HISTORY OF PARASITIC DISEASE IN CHINA: THE CASE OF SCHISTOSOMIASIS, SOME PUBLIC HEALTH AND ECONOMIC ASPECTS[27]

Abstract: This paper examines the extent to which the prevalence of schistosomiasis may have increased during the period 1958-1964. Certain hypotheses are examined, mainly dealing with irrigation and water conservancy construction. The probable economic and demographic effects of schistosomiasis are also examined. The article concludes that schistosomiasis prevalence probably did increase, but that the economic-demographic effects of this were probably minimal.

The reopening of contacts between the West and the People's Republic of China has generated enormous interest among western scholars in the vastness and complexity of the social experiment under way in China. Chinese medicine, particularly the apparent success of acupuncture, and the level and quality of health services generally, have greatly interested observers in the West because of our own present difficulties with the cost and quality of health services. On another front, the Chinese experience of large public health projects is of enormous interest both to the West and to Third World countries. Much of the Third World is plagued with ravaging diseases, especially parasitic diseases, and the progress in China in controlling and eradicating such diseases is therefore of great relevance to all underdeveloped nations. In 1958 it was reported (1) that in nine years the People's Republic of China had made "unprecedented achievements in the eradication of the five major parasites [schistosomiasis, malaria, kala-azar, filariasis, and hookworm]..." There was widespread belief in western medical circles that the progress of the first nine years was sustained and that during the 1960s China had effectively brought under control the public health problems caused by these major parasitic diseases.[28]

---

[27]This article was originally published in the *International Journal of Health Services*, Volume 6, Number 1, 1976.

[28]Chen (2) reports that cholera, plague, and smallpox were also eradicated, and says that the incidence rate from malaria was less than 3 percent, that filariasis was practically eradicated from 38 districts and municipalities with 2.6 million patients cured, and that the number of kala-azar patients dropped from 350,000 to 10,000 within ten years. Although he notes that hookworm infection was still widespread, he says that up to 4 million persons (out of a total estimated infected population of 10 million) were cured of schistosomiasis and that many areas were now entirely free of the disease.

A recent survey (3) of schistosomiasis control efforts in China, however, although finding much to commend in the efforts of the Chinese, was nonetheless uncertain as to the present status of the disease. Reports on Chinese health conditions from returning visitors to China (4, 5) also fail to mention schistosomiasis as having been eradicated or, indeed, in a manageable control phase. It may well be that the ultimate goal of total eradication has sensibly been revised in favor of effective control of the rate of prevalence of the disease in already infected provinces. Whatever the actual case may be, it does seem likely that, in 1975, schistosomiasis is still a serious public health problem in China, much as it is in many other parts of the Third World.

Schistosomiasis has become in the eyes of most public health experts the most important disease in the world, rivaling only malaria, in terms of its potential for disrupting the daily lives of people and for adversely affecting the economies of nations. Estimates of the world's population infected with one or more of the strains of schistosomiasis range from 120 to 200 million persons. Populations at risk of infection, however, may be as much as 350 to 400 million, or roughly 10 to 15 percent of the total world population (6). The population infected and those at high risk of infection are located overwhelmingly in the poor parts of the world, in Asia, Africa, the Middle East, and Latin America.

Public health workers have alleged the economic losses due to schistosomiasis. To be staggeringly high these losses are attributed to reduced worker productivity, the reduced performance of schoolchildren, output and family income losses in communities, and, to a lesser degree, mortality costs for premature deaths of young children and adults. Few economists, however, have attempted to deal with these economic impacts and the results to date of those who have, as assessed by Cummins (7), suggest that the economic impact of schistosomiasis may be overemphasized by public health researchers, or it is taking forms which have thus far eluded the technical skills of the economist.

There is no reason to doubt that accomplishments in controlling the disease between 1949 and 1958 were real. Reports in Chinese medical journals indicate that a great deal of research was under way on the disease, that extensive efforts were made to kill snails by filling ditches and canals, and that public health efforts in rural areas were greatly stepped up, all of which suggests that progress in controlling, if not eradicating, the disease was considered a fundamental social goal. Some sort of milestone thus may have been reached in 1958, as claimed that year in the *Chinese Medical Journal (8)*.

What makes the Chinese case so interesting, however, is the integration of social theory and policy in the fight against disease. To transform a nation wracked with so many varieties of disease into one with a healthy, viable population is an accomplishment that requires more than factor inputs such as doctors, hospitals, and medicine. In the case of parasitic disease, especially schistosomiasis, the medical inputs may in fact be much less important than the change in values and attitudes toward work, living style, and social habits. Schistosomiasis is interrelated with a particular pattern of life among a rural population and, short of an effective and cheap drug; the only way to keep the disease under control is to bring about drastic changes in the values and habits of the people.

It is probable that during the 1950s, in the flush of victory of the Revolution and with the enormous energy and effort expended in all ways in China, there were great successes in the treatment and control of schistosomiasis. That view seems to have been accepted in the West, and there is little reason to doubt its validity (2).

DID THE PREVALENCE RATE OF SCHISTOSOMIASIS INCREASE AFTER 1958?

It is probable that from a high water mark reached in 1958 the prevalence rate did increase, but we can only suggest this was so on the basis of limited and inferential evidence (9). In 1966 there was a call for another national conference on the disease (10), the first called since 1958, and there were fewer reports of districts and villages being "cleared" of snails[29] (an example of such a report from 1968 is reference 11). In 1970 still another national conference was called. Moreover, greater ideological training and instruction in Chairman Mao's views on the need to eradicate schistosomiasis and how to do it appears to have been intensified in the late 1960s, perhaps as a result of the Cultural Revolution. "Thirty thousand barefoot doctors," as one report (12) put it, were told to pay heed to Chairman Mao's teaching to "get mobilized, pay attention to hygiene, reduce disease, improve health conditions..." As this report went on further,

> Elimination of schistosomiasis is a "protracted war," which requires a special force armed with Mao Tse-Tung's thought and having revolutionary spirit of a high degree. At present, a special force of mass schistosomiasis prevention with poor and lower-middle peasants and their children as the mainstay who are not detached from production has been set up in the outskirts of Shanghai. According to incomplete statistics, in nine *hsien,* there are more than 30,000 "schistosomiasis

---

[29]On the tenth anniversary of the publication of Chairman Mao's poem "Farewell to the God of Plague," the district the poem celebrated for its victory over schistosorniasis, Yukiang County in Kiangsi Province, reported the great progress made since 1958, but nowhere in the report did it claim that the county was free of schistosomiasis infection. In 1969 a number of reports appeared concerning efforts made in Shanghai and the success achieved. Elimination of the disease was not claimed (12).

prevention" workers, night-soil caretakers and "bare-footed doctors." They get together with the broad masses to play the role of the backbone in the movement for schistosomiasis prevention.

Perhaps one would be misled to interpret this kind of indirect evidence as an indication of anything being amiss. But the urgency of this rhetoric, together with the appearance in the international press of reports that a major schistosomiasis problem still existed in China, while not conclusive evidence, does suggest a picture far different than that portrayed in the West a decade earlier.

The burden of our claim, however, that the prevalence rate increased, or at least was not substantially reduced, during the 1960s, rests on an inferred link between irrigation and water conservancy construction and the spread of the disease. Schistosomiasis is a water contact disease: the propagation of the life cycle of the carrier snail and the human or animal host is intimately linked to water contacts. Water conservancy projects, irrigation, and power dam construction may have done as much in the past decade to spread schistosomiasis infection as any other human action. The Aswan Dam, power dams in Africa, and irrigation construction in Brazil, the Philippines, and elsewhere in the Third World countries all have been implicated in the growing proportions of populations infected with schistosomiasis or at greater risk of infection with schistosomiasis (13, 14).

During the Great Leap Forward in China (roughly 1958-1964), an important emphasis was placed on water conservancy, power dams, and irrigation construction. Quantitative evidence on the magnitude of these efforts is hard to come by. But an important part of the story has been carefully reconstructed by Chao (15). The limited quantitative information available does suggest that the number of irrigation construction and water conservancy projects grew during the first years of the Great Leap Forward, especially in the schistosomiasis provinces, where greater proportions of cultivated acres were under irrigation than elsewhere in China.[30] These points are illustrated in Tables 1 and 2.

Chao, in his recent work Agricultural Production in Communist China, 1949-1965 (15), points out two additional factors concerning the construction of irrigation facilities, which could support the view we are suggesting. The first factor that Chao notes is a change in the pattern of irrigation during 1959-1962. Prior to this period the most commonly used irrigation method in the rice regions made use of the water pond, which combined both water lift and gravity. Water was lifted from ponds into relatively short distribution channels where gravity

---

[30]It should be noted that irrigation increased in Northern China as well, and at rates comparable to those in southern provinces. There, however, the actual area irrigated was a smaller proportion of total cropland than in the south and the irrigation method used was to redirect the underground water flow through well drilling.

then carried the water to the adjoining rice fields. The ponds also were receptacles for surface run-off water and drainage from the rice paddies. Each pond, therefore, was in a sense a geographically localized irrigation system, which would largely tend to localize schistosomiasis infections to the population immediately surrounding the irrigation system. The new irrigation construction in 1958 to 1959, however, was on a much larger scale, and carried well beyond these localized ponds. By using gravity, it permitted irrigation of greater areas of rice land. Not only did the distribution channels have to be larger than previously, but also they were now interconnected to form an irrigation network, which covered a greatly expanded geographic area.

The potential for spreading schistosomiasis infection to previously "disease-free" parts of the population would appear to have been enhanced as a result of these developments in irrigation practice and construction. The one variable that might invalidate this theory would be if the snail population, used to the turbid, stagnant ponds, could not survive in water with a greater rate of flow or of different temperature. That is, if irrigation increases the speed of water flow or lowers the water temperature, does this "kill" the snail population? Research on this question is sparse but the evidence to date suggests that, at least at the speed of water flow and temperature commonly found in irrigation, water dams, and water conservancy construction in comparable areas in the West, a significantly large proportion of the snail population still manages to survive (16)

Table 1

Irrigated areas in schistosomiasis-infected regions of China (10,000 mou)a

Province	1957	1958	Rate of Increase 1957-1958	1959
			%	
Kiangsu	3,830	5,491	(43.4)	4,390
Honan	4,300	10,000	(132.6)	—b
Anhwei	3,400	5,500	(61.8)	6,100
Chekiang	2,500	2,670	(6.8)	—
Hupeh	2,800	2,970	(6.1)	—
Kiangsi	2,900	3,440	(18.6)	3,522
Fukien	1,480	1,804	(21.9)	—
Hunan	—	—	—	—
Kwangtung	2,090	3,590	(71.8)	4,400
Kweichow	793	1,690	(113.1)	—
Yunnan	1,230	1,500	(22.0)	2,238
Kwangsi Chuang	2,496	3,696	(48.1)	2,478
Shanghai Municipality	—	—	—	—

aSource, Social Science Research Council, Provincial Agricultural Statistics for Communist *China, Committee* on the Economy of China, Ithaca, New York, 1969. Figures for 1957, 1958, and 1959 taken from Table 1-A, p. 1 (Anhwei); Table 2-A, p. 11 (Chekiang); Table 3-A, p. 21 (Fukien); Table 5-A, p. 40 (Honan); Table 7-A, p. 60 (Hunan); Table 8-A, p. 70 (Hupeh); Table 11-A, p. 100 (Kiangsi); Table 12-A, p. 110 (Kiangsu); Table 14-A, p. 130 (Kwangsi); Table 15-A, p. 139 (Kwangtung); Table 16-A p. 149 (Kweichow); and Table 24-A, p. 227 (Yunnan).
bDash signifies data not available.

The second factor Chao suggests is the change in the cropping system, which occurred simultaneously with the expansion of irrigation networks in the rice regions. Previously, two different crops a year were grown in a large part of the rice region. Rice was grown using rainwater, which had been stored in ponds and other receptacles during the rainy season, and after the rice crop was harvested a different winter dry-land crop was planted. The availability of year-round water supplies in the new irrigation networks saw farmers in the rice regions shift to two continuous crops of paddy rice. This change in the cropping system suddenly increased problems of pest control. The previous system of having two alternate crops, it appeared, maintained a sort of ecologic balance by not permitting sufficient breeding time for pests of either crop to become a major problem. There have been reports, Chao notes, that continuous rice crops create a more favorable environment for breeding of pyralididae, a variety of moth, which attacks the rice plant. It is not too far-fetched to speculate that the continuous cropping of rice paddies has also permitted the snails to survive and reproduce over longer time periods than was true in pre-1958 China (15). Moreover, because the new cropping system has provided the opportunity for a longer work year, it has probably also increased the risk of infection for agricultural workers.

Table 2

Irrigated areas as a percentage of total cultivated area in schistosomiasis-infected regions of China in 1958 (10,000 mou)[a]

Province	Cultivated Area	Irrigated Area	Ratio
			%
Kiangsu	8,304	5,491	66.1
Honan	13,600	10,000	73.5
Anhwei	8,733	5,500	63.0
Chekiang	3,140	2,670	85.0
Hupeh	6,800	2,970	43.7
Kiangsi	—[b]	3,440	—
Fukien	2,219	1,804	81.3
Hunan	5,313	—	—
Kwangtung	5,800	3,590	61.9
Kweichow	3,136	1,690	53.9
Yunnan	4,110	1,500	36.5
Kwangsi Chuang	3,846	3,696	96.1
Whole nation	161,680	107,000	66.2

[a]Source, Social Science Research Council, Provincial Agricultural Statistics for Communist China, Committee on the Economy of China, Ithaca, New York, 1969. Figures for cultivated and irrigated areas taken from Table 1-A, p. 1 (Anhwei); Table 2-A, p. 11 (Chekiang); Table 3-A, p. 21 (Fukien); Table 5-A, p. 40 (Honan); Table 7-A, p. 60 (Hunan); Table 8-A, p. 70 (Hupeh); Table 11-A, p. 100 (Kiangsi); Table 12-A, p. 110 (Kiangsu); Table 14-A, p. 130 (Kwangsi); Table 15-A, p. 139 (Kwangtung); Table 16-A, p. 149 (Kweichow); and Table 24-A, p. 227 (Yunnan).

[b] Dash signifies data not available.

THE ECONOMIC IMPACT OF SCHISTOSOMIASIS

Is it likely that there were significant economic-demographic effects if the prevalence rate for schistosomiasis did increase during the 1960s? There is little doubt that, in the minds of party leaders, and especially of Chairman Mao, schistosomiasis has had a profound demographic and economic impact in China. Statements in the 1950s, and the renewed attack on schistosomiasis in the 1960s and at present, all suggest that the cost of the disease is not simply the human suffering involved but also a loss in the productivity of workers, the lessened fertility of women, and the diminished alertness and attentiveness of schoolchildren. That is, just as western economists have come to treat expenditures on health as both consumption and investment in augmenting the quantity and quality of human capital, so has Chairman Mao. But, of course, the Maoist view goes well beyond the western concept of "human capital." As recently as August 1969, the relationship between schistosomiasis and agricultural production, for example, was explicitly noted (12). In one provincial report after another for earlier years, especially in the 1950s, a linkage between the health of workers and their productivity in agriculture and "party" duties, as well as the effects of schistosomiasis on the fertility of women and the performance of schoolchildren, were well recognized. One statement (17), which seems typical of the perceived relationship between health and productivity is as follows:

> Health work must proceed with a view to developing production; it should be closely integrated with and serve production. Under the unified leadership of the party committees, production and health work must be closely coordinated and planned. The more intense the production, the more attention must we pay to health work; the better the health work is done, the higher will be the production level. This, in a nutshell, is the dialectic unity in the relationship between production and health.

One report in 1960 (18) reported "on the average, the disease causes a 40 percent loss in the patients' capacity to work..." The Chinese literature, sparse though it is, also reports purported economic benefits from schistosomiasis control, treatment, and eradication. Four farming cooperatives in Hunan Province, for example, reported a gain in total population between 1955 and 1957 of about 15 percent, an increase in rice production of 10.8 percent, and a gain in the total work points of from 19 to 44 percent over the same years, after schistosomiasis was believed to have been eradicated (1). In Rentun Village in Shanghai a population increase of 31.3 percent during 1949-1958 was attributed to schistosomiasis control as was a doubling of the labor force and a threefold increase in average yield per mou of rice land (19). Over the same period a report from Jiashan County, Chekiang Province also reported a threefold increase in the labor force and a 150 percent rise in individual income of brigade members. "Women for years childless," this report also noted, "are now proud mothers" (11).

One does not know what to make of these reports. In view of work done elsewhere on schistosomiasis and its presumed economic effects, it does not seem likely that these reported demographic and economic effects could be attributable to a reduction of schistosomiasis alone. As Jordan and Webbe (16) have commented: "Convincing evidence that schistosomiasis is invariably a serious public health problem is lacking, and the importance attached to it will vary from place to place in relation to other diseases and the socio-economic conditions prevailing." Only a few studies have attempted to isolate the demographic and economic impact of health variables and/or specific diseases (20-22). One study on *Schistosomiasis mansoni* found no appreciable effects on the performance of schoolchildren, their height and weight, the fertility of women, or the productivity of adult rural and urban workers (20). One does not know what to make, therefore, of a reported morbidity rate of either 40 percent, as noted earlier, or of two others reported for 10 villages in Kiangsu Province and for the Tianning Peoples Commune in Chekiang Province. In Kiangsu Province morbidity rate of 35 to 40 percent was reported for the period 1945-1955 and 26.6 percent for 1957 (23). In Jiashan County at the time of liberation, it was noted that 76 percent of those infected "were unable to work" (11).

Nonetheless, there are perhaps two good reasons for thinking that schistosomiasis could have substantial demographic and economic effects in China.

The first reason is that schistosomiasis in China also affects animals, particularly work animals. It was reported in 1959 (24) that 2.5 million oxen were infected with schistosomiasis. What proportion of the total oxen population this figure represents is not known. Studies in the Philippines (cited in reference 16) show that certain domestic animals were capable of transmitting the cycle of infection even if human transmissions were controlled. Dogs and cows were both found to be most effective in transmitting high-infected egg counts in their feces. High prevalence rates were also found in cats, water buffalo, pigs, horses, sheep, goats, wild mice, and rats. Two work animals, the ox and the water buffalo, were proved to be highly susceptible to schistosomiasis infection. A survey made in August 1957 (25, 26) for 10 hsien of Kiangsu Province, in which 11,000 water buffalo and oxen were examined, reported infection rates of 10.73 and 40.13 percent, respectively. This same study also reported on the correlation of human and animal infection rates in Kiangsu and Hunan Provinces. Animal and human infection rates were nearly identical in all the cases examined. This suggests a strong linkage between place of work (in the paddies) and infection for both humans and animals.

The potential impact of animal infection on humans might be as follows: (a) continued transmission of the disease cycle and greater chances for human reinfection than when only humans are the reservoir hosts; (b) large prevalence and infection rates of animals possibly causing serious deterioration of the nutritional value of the population's food supply in the case of animals used for food; (c) morbidity of animals used in agricultural production, particularly the water buffalo, reducing the efficiency of capital used by farmers and potentially lowering acreage yield per. capita.

The second reason is the severity of S. *japonicum* infections, the main type of schistosomiasis infection found in China, compared with other varieties of schistosomiasis. There are no comparative studies of demographic or productivity effects from the different varieties of schistosomiasis, but by piecing together studies done on S. *japonicum* and S. *mansoni* (16, 27, 28) we can suggest that S. *japonicum is* more likely both to produce serious physiologic complications and to have a higher intensity of infection (at comparable egg counts). From these indications it does seem that the likelihood exists that S. *japonicum will* have greater economic impact than studies in the West, largely on S. *mansoni,* would suggest.

Of course, this is pure conjecture. The data simply are not available to perform any kind of a reasonable test, which could isolate the demographic and economic effects of schistosomiasis from the many other factors that affect population, output, and productivity changes. Nevertheless, a few pieces of potentially useful information are available, and we shall attempt to see what these data might indicate in the way of a positive relationship between schistosomiasis and important demographic-economic effects. It should be emphasized, however, that the most important piece of information, which would be necessary to causally link schistosomiasis and demographic-economic factors, is the intensity of infection of the population. That is to say, we do not know, quantitatively, how "sick" the people are and whether or not being, "sick" in some clinical-physiologic sense will affect their performance at work and in non-work-related activities. At present there is no way from experience obtained elsewhere to infer intensity of infection. Thus, the evidence we present below presumes that if a population is affected with schistosomiasis its performance and behavior will be altered. If we are not able to determine any aggregate effects, it does not mean that population growth or labor productivity were unaffected by schistosomiasis. Rather it means we cannot determine it from the data and model specification employed. And even if a positive association is "proved" not to exist between schistosomiasis and economic development variables, it does not really mean that the population's behavior and performance in non-work, non-reproduction capacities are affected.

What we propose to do is look first at some possible demographic effects in the twelve major schistosomiasis provinces. We shall then look at the possibility that schistosomiasis had output and labor productivity effects in the rural-agricultural sector of these twelve provinces.

DEMOGRAPHIC EFFECTS OF SCHISTOSOMIASIS

Table 3 gives the populations for 1953, 1957, and 1964 of the schistosomiasis infected provinces and Table 4 the percentage changes in the growth of population for the twelve provinces compared to the overall nation. If schistosomiasis had been successfully eradicated or brought under control in the 1950s, a strong hypothesis would predict that rates of growth (ignoring lags) in these disease-infected areas would exceed growth elsewhere, all other things being equal. As shown in Table 4, five provinces grew less than the nation did and seven grew more. The highest growth change occurred in Kweichow and Fukien. Fukien is a coastal province along the Taiwan Strait, and the population increase could well be associated with an increase in the armed forces. Also, between 1953 and 1957 demarcation lines of individual provinces were changed and perhaps these changes account for population changes rather than do real rates of natural increase. And, of course, national population policy effects may also be intertwined with these observed population changes.

If, as we suggest, the prevalence rate increased between 1957 and 1964 (again ignoring lags), a strong hypothesis would predict that the population growth of the schistosomiasis provinces, all other things being equal, would be significantly less than in non-schistosomiasis provinces.

For the period 1957-1964, six of the provinces had higher rates of growth than the country as a whole (though this determination depends somewhat on what population figure is used for the whole nation). These provinces were: Chekiang, Kiangsi, Fukien, Yunnan, Kwangsi Chuang, and Kwangtung. Yunnan and Kwangsi Chuang are both border provinces, and their growth changes during this period might be the result of a deliberate population relocation policy or of comparatively rapid industrialization. Also, as indicated above, Fukien's population changes are probably associated with a military build-up. This leaves the provinces of Chekiang, Kwangtung, and Kiangsi, the figures for which are quite interesting for our purposes. If, in fact, higher infection and prevalence rates followed higher rates of irrigation construction, and presuming that schistosomiasis does have demographic effects, one would expect lower rates of growth in higher irrigation areas than in lower irrigation ones. Referring back to the figures on irrigation construction given in Table 1, we see that both Chekiang and Kiangsu had less than average amounts of water conservancy and irrigation construction during the Great Leap Forward. This may have been due to topographic factors in both provinces, but it is just possible that because of lower irrigation construction these two provinces may have escaped any gains in increased infections in the early 1960s and continued to enjoy some relative equilibrium in schistosomiasis eradication and treatment work, with a concomitantly large population result.

Table 3

Population of schistosomiasis-infected regions of China from 1953 to 1964 (in 1,000 persons)[a]

Province	1953	1957	1964
Kiangsu	41,252	45,230	47,000
Honan	44,215	48,670	50,000
Anhwei	30,633	33,560	35,000
Chekiang	22,866	25,280	31,000
Hupeh	27,790	30,790	32,000
Kiangsi	16,773	18,610	22,000
Fukien	13,143	14,650	17,000
Hunan	33,227	36,220	38,000
Kwangtung	36,740	37,960	42,000
Kweichow	15,037	16,890	17,000
Yunnan	17,473	19,100	23,000
Kwangsi Chuang	17,591	19,390	24,000
Shanghai Municipality	—	—	—
Total infected areas	316,740	346,350	378,000
Population, whole nation[b]	587,960	646,530	713,400
Infected areas as % of whole nation[b]	53.9	53.6	53.0

[a]Sources, Huang Yu-chuan, Latest figures on population of Communist China, *China Monthly*, No. 56, p. 15, November 1, 1968; N. R. Chen, *Chinese Economic Statistics*, p. 124, Aldine Publishing Company, Chicago, 1967; Letter to author from John Aird, June 22, 1971.

[b]These figures exclude Taiwan and overseas Chinese, and are for year-end.

OUTPUT AND LABOR PRODUCTIVITY EFFECTS OF SCHISTOSOMIASIS

The limited amount of information available can also be used to see whether or not any light can be shed on the possible link between an increase in the prevalence rate of schistosomiasis after 1958 and the output of agriculture and the productivity of workers in the schistosomiasis provinces.

Relative Yield of Rice Land

If schistosomiasis infections do have important negative effects on agricultural output and productivity, we can postulate that yields of rice-the principal crop of the twelve provinces-should have declined relative to other crops, all other things being equal. Similarly, if schistosomiasis prevalence was reduced and there were positive productivity effects, we should expect relative yields of rice lands to increase. Table 5 gives little evidence to support our expectations, i.e. that between 1952 and 1957 the relative yields rose and that between 1957 and 1965 they fell. In fact, as shown in the table, the unit yield of rice land relative to all food grains rose only slightly from 1952 to 1957, and from 1957 to 1965, instead of falling, it rose by 7.3 percentage points. Stability in the relative yield of rice land is perhaps the most plausible interpretation one could give for the data in Table 5. Any labor productivity effects (positive or negative) that may have existed could have been offset by a large and complex number of other factors (such as climate, fertilizer inputs, etc.) that determine the yield of rice.

Ralph Andreano

Table 4

Growth of population in schistosomiasis-infected regions of China from 1953 to 1964°

Province	Percentage Change	
	1953-1957	1957-1964
Kiangsu	9.6	3.9
Honan	10.0	2.7
Anhwei	9.6	4.3
Chekiang	10.6	22.6
Hupeh	10.8	3.9
Kiangsi	10.6	18.2
Fukien	11.5	16.0
Hunan	9.0	4.9
Kwangtung	3.3	10.6
Kweichow	12.3	0.7
Yunnan	9.3	20.4
Kwangsi Chuang	10.2	23.8
Shanghai Municipality	—	—
Population, whole nationb	10.0	10.3

[a]Compiled from data in Table 3. b These figures exclude Taiwan and students outside of China.

Output Per Worker

Data on estimated average output per worker for the twelve-schistosomiasis provinces between 1954-1957 also suggests that if schistosomiasis control was producing positive effects on labor productivity, it is simply not discernible from a whole array of other competing and offsetting effects. Table 6 shows the output per worker for all food grains for the twelve provinces. If these data are to be believed, they show a marked fall in average output per worker for every province except Kweichow and for the whole country. The appropriate prediction, if schistosomiasis had large productivity effects, would be for either a rise or no change in average output per worker. On the other hand, if schistosomiasis does have large negative labor productivity effects (the magnitude of these effects would, of course, become benefits, all other things equal, if the disease were eradicated) the appropriate prediction is for a fall in both the average and marginal product of labor.

Table 5

Comparative yield of rice land in China, 1952-1971[a]

Year	Crop Acreage (1,000 mou)			Output (1,000 short tons)			Unit Yield: Rice Land Relative to Land under Other Food Grains (Percentage Points)
	Rice	All Food Grains	Rice as % of All Food Grains	Rice	All Food Grains	Rice as % of All Food Grains	
1952	425,734	1,684,491	25.3	68,450	154,400	44.3	175.1
1957	483,617	1,813,273	26.7	86,800	185,500	46.8	175.3
1965	—	—	23.0	114,126	—	42.0	182.6
1970	—	—	—	—	240	—	—
1971	—	—	—	—	246	—	—

[a]Sources, for 1952 and 1957 data, N. R. Chen, Chinese Economic Statistics, pp. 287 and 338, Aldine Publishing Company, Chicago, 1967; for 1965 data, People's Daily, February 7, 1966; for 1970 and 1971 data, T. Durdin, China discloses figures on grain output, New York Times, p. 12, April 2, 1972.

[b]Rice output figure for 1966, from an estimate by the hood and Agriculture Organization of the United Nations, cited in U.S. Bureau of the Census, Statistical Abstract of the United States, p. 818, U.S. Government Printing Office, Washington, D.C., 1970.

The point is therefore that, for the type of economy that China had during the 1950s, total output could be maintained because of the large elasticity of supply for labor, but that, at the same time, disease could still have effects on average and marginal products. If we reject the notion that substantial improvements, producing positive benefits, occurred in treatment and control of schistosomiasis during the 1950s, the picture seen in Table 6, with a fall in average product per worker, is consistent both with there being disease effects on labor productivity and with a growth in total output of food grains. However, during the 1950s grain output fell, and the inputs of labor rose at a much faster rate than did all other agricultural inputs (fertilizer, tractors, draft animals, etc.). To be sure, other factors such as natural disasters and the weather are also important explanatory considerations. But perhaps disease effects on labor productivity were indeed strong and the measure of success achieved in controlling schistosomiasis during the 1950s was overestimated.

Population-Irrigation-Rice Yield Effects

The limited evidence discussed thus far is not strong enough to support the two basic disease hypotheses under discussion, i.e. that (a) between 1953 and 1958 the prevalence rate of schistosomiasis declined; and that (b) after 1958 the prevalence rate rose. The demographic-economic impacts occur inversely for each hypothesis. But, as we have already discussed for demographic, labor productivity, and output impacts, we have at least two effects to consider: (a) productivity and output gains from improved irrigation; and (b) a rise in the birth rate because productivity and output gains increase family income. Working against these two effects are the disease effects. If schistosomiasis is eradicated (assuming that the disease does have negative productivity and output effects) this, too, could increase labor productivity, rice yields, and output per man. Similarly, if schistosomiasis does have negative effects on birth rates, its elimination would bring about an increase in population through changes in birth rates. Conversely, if schistosomiasis prevalence increases, the effects would work in the opposite, i.e., negative, direction. What we cannot know, from the limited data available, therefore, is the separate impact of these potentially offsetting effects, or whether or not disease effects are swamping non-disease effects on labor productivity, output, and population changes in the schistosomiasis provinces.

Ralph Andreano

Table 6

Output per worker in food grains in twelve Chinese provinces in 1954 and 1957, in catties[a,b]

Province	1954	1957
Anhwei	3,000	2,000
Chekiang	3,000	1,000
Fukien	3,000	1,000
Hunan	3,000	1,000
Kiangsi	4,000	2,000
Honan	4,000	1,000
Hupeh	4,000	2,000
Kiangsu	3,000	1,000
Kwangsi Chuang	4,000	1,000
Kwangtung	4,000	1,000
Kweichow	1,000	4,000
Yunnan	4,000	1,000
Whole country[c]	3,000	1,000
	[1,500]	[1,200]

[a]Derived from data on total output of food grains in reference 15, and from labor force data in N. R. Chen, *Chinese Economic Statistics*, Table 11.2, p. 474, Aldine Publishing Company, Chicago, 1967.
[b]One catty equals 1.1 pounds.
[c]The bracketed whole country figures refer to output estimates by Chao (15) for 1954 divided by a 1952 total agricultural labor force estimate of Chen; for 1957, a 1957 Chao output estimate was divided by a 1958 Chao labor force estimate.

64

Because of this difficult dilemma of identification, it would be best to pool all the information we have for the 1953 to 1958 period, and to see if the hypothesis that the prevalence rate improved (declined) during this period could be put to a somewhat more rigorous test.

The evidence we are going to pool is the change in population growth (x) between 1953 and 1958, the proportion of cultivable land under irrigation in 1958 (y), the rate of growth of new irrigation construction during 1957-1958 (z), the average yield of rice in 1958 for each province (w), and the percentage of the sown area in each province in rice production (s). What we will do with these pooled data is to put the relative changes in ranked form for each province and compute Spearman coefficients of rank correlation. The data on average output per worker are not included in the pooled information because these data are based on our own estimates and there is not enough variation to warrant a precise ranking.

If we accept the hypothesis that there was an improvement in schistosomiasis infection between 1953 and 1958, we should expect positive signs and high values for r_s between xy, xz, xw, and wz. That is, there should be a high positive correlation between rank in irrigated land and change in population for each province (xy). Similarly, rice yield rank (w) and irrigation rank (y) would be negatively correlated if the impact of schistosomiasis on productivity swamps the effect of irrigation on productivity, or positively correlated if the reverse were true. The computed rank correlation coefficients are as follows:

(1) $r_{xy} =$ -0.03   (4) $r_{wz} =$ -0.43
(2) $r_{xz} =$ -0.31   (5) $r_{wy} =$ 0.13
(3) $r_{xw} =$ 0.30   (6) $r_{xs} =$ -0.41

$$(7)\ r_{ws} = 0.52$$

With the exception of r_{xw}, which is not strong enough to support the hypothesis, the coefficients r_{xy}, r_{xz}, r_{wz}, and r_{xs} in sign and magnitude require a rejection of the hypothesis. Moreover, the finding that r_{xz} is less than r_{xy} may suggest that the negative effects of schistosomiasis on population growth after 1958 could be swamping all other effects; for it is beyond 1958 that the big push in water conservancy, power dams, and irrigation construction occurred on a much larger scale than was true between 1954 and 1957. Similarly, the high and negative coefficient of rice yield (w) against the rate of change in irrigation (z) suggests that negative disease effects may also have been dominating positive productivity effects from new irrigation. Though positive, the low value of r_{uy}-the average yield on rice land against the proportion of cultivable land under irrigation-may suggests that the positive effects of irrigation on output were being constrained by negative disease effects. Indeed, r_{at}'s being greater than r_{yty} seems also to support this explanation and to provide strong support to the idea that total output could be maintained, even if disease productivity effects were large, by adding more labor to existing land under rice cultivation. The interpretation of r_{ya}'s is that yields (per man, per unit of land) are high and positively correlated with the amount of sown area in each province under rice cultivation.

While admittedly this evidence is hardly conclusive, it does suggest that between 1953 and 1958 the probable degree of improvement in schistosomiasis infection was less than was supposed. For the post-1958 period we are given to conjecture. For example, if rwz continued to hold-i.e. average rice yields were negatively correlated with the rate of increase in irrigation construction-and rws remained positive, one might be observing for the post-1958 period the maintenance of total rice output but with larger labor/land combinations required because of negative labor productivity effects due to an increase in the prevalence rate of schistosomiasis. While one does not wish to push this line of reasoning too far, if the relationships that appeared to exist between the demographic-economic variables and disease effects during the 1950s continued to dominate Chinese experience in the 1960s, there would seem to be cause for concern, as apparently there has been and continues to be, regarding the economy-wide effects and the individual human suffering caused by the spread of schistosomiasis infection in China.

Acknowledgments

The author gratefully acknowledges the helpful comments of his colleague Kang Chao, the excellent research assistance provided by Jane Yu-Li, and the support of the University of Wisconsin's Health Economics Research Center.

REFERENCES

1. All China Conference on Parasitic Diseases. *Chinese Medical Journal* 77(6): 519-581, 1958.
2. Chen, W. Y. Medicine and public health. *China Quarterly* (6): 158-159, 1961.
3. Cheng, T.H. Schfstosomiasis in Mainland China: A review of research and control programs since 1949. *Am. J. Trop. Med. Hyg.* 20(1): 26-53, 1971.
4. Special Issue on China. Health Policy Advisory Council Bulletin, No. 47, December 1972.
5. Liang, M. H., Eichling, P. S., Fine, L. J., and Annas, G. J. Chinese health care: Determinants of the system. *Am. J. Public Health* 63(2): 102-110, 1973.

6. Wright, W. H. Schistosomiasis as a world problem. *Bull. N. Y. Acad. Med.* 44(3): 301-316, 1968.
7. Cummins G. Economic Implications of Schistosomiasis. Paper delivered in Symposium on the Future of Schistosomiasis Control. Tulane University, New Orleans, February 1972.
8. Outstanding achievements in health work in *1958* ("Health Bulletin"). *Chinese Medical Journal* 77(6): 582-586, 1958.
9. Worth, R. M. Health trends in China since the Great Leap Forward. *China Quarterly* 22: 181-189, 1965.
10. National Conference on speed-up of anti-schistosomiasis campaign in China. *Chinas Medicine* (1): 85-86, 1966.
11. As Chairman Mao directs, we follow: How schistosomiasis in Jiashan County was wiped out by "people's war." *China's Medicine* (10): 605, 1968.
12. U.S. Consulate General, Hong Kong. Survey of Chinese Mainland Publications, No. 4481, August 12, 1969.
13. Carter, L. J. Development in the poor nations. *Science* 163(3871): 1046-1048, 1969.
14. Carley, W. M. Science loses ground in war against disease in impoverished lands. *Wall Street Journal*, pp. 1 and 33, April 14, 1970.
15. Chao, K. Agricultural Production in Communist China, 1949-1965. University of Wisconsin Press, Madison, 1970.
16. Jordan P., and Webbe, G. *Human Schistosomiasis*, p. 169. Charles C Thomas, Springfield, 111, 1969.
17. Yun-Pei, H. Advance the great work of protecting the people's health. *Chinese Medical Journal* 80(5): 409, 1960.
18. Yang, L. An end to plague! *Peking Review* 5:20, February 2, 1960.
19. Struggle against schistosomiasis. China's Medicine 11: 669-672, 1968.
20. Weisbrod, B. A., Andreano, R. L., Baldwin, R. E., Epstein, E. H., and Kelley, A. *Disease and Economic Development: Impact of Parasitic Diseases in St. Lucia.* University of Wisconsin Press, Madison, 1973.
21. Barlow, R. *The Economics of Malaria Eradication.* University of Michigan Press, Ann Arbor, 1963.
22. Malenbaum, W. Health and productivity in poor areas. In *Empirical Studies in Health Economics*, edited by H. E. Klarman, pp. 31-54. Johns Hopkins Press, Baltimore, 1970.
23. Shang-Ying, H., Huei-Sheng, L., Ya-Fang, L., Ch'un-Sheng, C., Po-Yu, K., and Chia-Fu, Y. Reports of antischistosomiasis campaign in Meiyuan Hsiang, Wusih of Kiangsu Province. *Chinese Medical Journal* 77(6): 577, 1958.

24. Tsung-Chiang, H., Huei-Lan, C., Lien-Yin, H., and Hsin-Chih, W. Achievements in the fight against parasitic diseases in New China. *Chinese Medical Journal* 79(6): 514, 1959.

25. *Chinese Medical Journal* 77(6): 552-581, 1958.

26. *Chinese Agricultural Journal* 5: 20, 1958.

27. Hunter, G. W. 3rd, Frye, W. W., Clyde, J., and Artzwelder, S. W. *A Manual of Tropical Medicine*, Ed. 4., pp. 525-531. W. B. Saunders Company, London, 1966.

28. Jones, A. W. *Introduction to Parasitology*, pp. 118-132. Addison-Wesley Publishing Company, Reading, Mass., 1967.

SELECTION 6

THE WHO MALARIA PROGRAMME: A SYNTHETIC[31] REVIEW IN POLICY ANALYSIS[32]

OVERVIEW

Within the context of analysing alternative choices and examination of underlying processes, personalities and events, policy analysis has become a useful tool of management. By looking at how a policy has evolved, its rationale, especially it economic rationale, and its evolution and changes, decision makers and policy makers can learn how policies can or should be formulated and what factors influence the success or failure of policies. The present paper is an illustration of the policy choices and changes in the global malaria programme of WHO. As such it covers the time period from the evolution and adoption of the original policy of global eradication and its subsequent development into a malaria control strategy with emphasis on integration into primary health care systems. The perspective of the paper is from the viewpoint of WHO—as one of its major programme initiatives—and not from the perspective at the country level through obviously there is some unavoidable interchange and overlap between them.

In policy analysis studies, one typically starts with "the" policy: how did it evolve, why did it evolve, what factors and criteria were used to shape the policy adopted and why not some alternative one? What role did political forces play in shaping the adoption of this policy against other competing ones? Similarly, once a policy has been adopted, the classical policy analysis study, focuses on the forces working to make the policy succeed and those working against it. Such forces can be external events—i.e. changes in external conditions from what existed when the policy was adopted—or internal events, typically insufficient resources, or management, logistical, or shortcomings in rules and procedures necessary to successfully carry out a policy. Finally, in classical policy analysis one views how the original policy and its changes and evolution over time could fit into some rational, methodological, and consistent framework. This is not quite "what lessons have been learned", but more of an attempt to systematically structure the process by which policies get born, are shaped, and either succeed

---

[31]Synthetic, in the context of this report, means that no original research was conducted. Rather, published and unpublished sources of individuals in the Organization and its governing bodies form the raw material from which the account present here was drawn.
[32]Manuscript, March 19, 1990.

or fail. Another way of putting this is: were all the right questions asked before the policy was adopted?

The malaria programme of WHO is excellent material for an analysis of the sort suggested here. There was a major policy adopted with its attendant technology, underlying economic implications, and with substantial political support and in recognition of a major worldwide public health problem. Resources were allocated on the basis of the policy; events changed, external conditions changed, technology changed, and the basic economic parameters of the original policy also changed. After a time it was clear the original policy had to be changed and it was changed (simplistically put, the policy changed from eradication to control). What underlying combination of technology, economics, and politics produced the change? Again was the new policy based on a firmer set of parameters—especially economic ones than the original policy? Was the change endogenously produced (i.e. events outside the policy framework made the original policy irrelevant and dictated a change) or was the change in policy endogenously produced—i.e. those in charge of the policy saw it needed to be changed and pushed for the change.

In any survey of this sort one can, at best, only touch the highlights. Limitations of data, of written records, of how and what key participants thought and what analytical tools they used to support arguments, are often lacking. Inevitably then, a policy analysis study has its limitations not only with respect to the example under review, but also in regard to generalizations to other programmes and policies.

Still examples of the sort examined here serve a very useful purpose: they can be a showcase on methods of analysis, of highlighting the information and data deficiencies for policy formulation, and for illustrating the complex interaction of people, events and pressures that inevitably underlay any policy in any large organization. WHO is now, and was 25 years ago, a large, complex multi-service organization. Any major policy initiative that emerges in such an organization is the result of a complex set of forces, some internal to the organization, some from the rush of external events. At best, material of the sort presented here can only touch the surface.

The principal point to be stressed is that an examination of a major policy of WHO is meant to be a learning experience and not a critical exercise in assessing who or what should reap the rewards of success or the ignominy of failure. In complex organizations such as WHO, policies of the magnitude of malaria, though infrequent, are not rare. Hindsight is always easier than foresight. Yet if we are unwilling to learn from our past and unwilling to put our policies under the microscope of analysis, policies will continue to be formulated and resources allocated through a random rather than a rational process. In the case of the global policy of malaria one cannot discern "winners" and "losers".

70

In a remarkable series of papers (Najera, 1989, and Farid, 1980) who were first hand participants in the major malaria policies of the last 25 years have commented on nearly all the relevant aspects needed for a retrospective policy analysis. Similarly the Director General's report to the 22nd World Health Assembly (WHA) of the World Health Organization (WHO) ("Re-examination of the Global Strategy of Malaria Eradication") presents a thorough discussion of the evolution of the Global Malaria Eradication policy, and its subsequent successes and failures, and the rationale for a change in emphasis from eradication to control. Similarly, the reports of the Expert Committee on Malaria commencing in 1947 (first) through the 18th (1985) and the dozens of WHA and Executive Board (EB) resolutions, give a fairly comprehensive framework for tracing the evolution and changes in global malaria policies.[33]

There are usually three characteristics common to the adoption of major policies—especially in large international human service agencies such as WHO. First, the problem to which the policy is geared towards must be "great", "significant" or in the case of a health agency of "major importance to public health". Malaria as a worldwide problem certainly fits the grade in terms of importance. Not only was malaria a major public health problem worldwide but also it was recognized as such by all the key players, decision makers, and technical experts, and politicians. A second attribute necessary for a policy to be readily adopted is that the timing must be right—public and in this case world opinion must be already headed in that direction. Again, malaria eradication had been done successfully in a few places. Many malariologists and other public health experts felt that current efforts—basically treating malarial infections as a disease control strategy—coupled with the post WWII surge of world humanitarian opinion towards the colonial areas of Africa, and Asia made the time and environment ripe for a major thrust—namely global eradication of malaria. The third element necessary for the successful adoption of a new policy is that one must put forth a convincing rationale for the policy. A rationale has at least five elements (see Table XX):

1. the expected benefits exceed the costs of maintaining the current policy
2. there must be some (hopefully) quantitative probability estimate of the policy's chance of succeeding
3. there must be some finite time period for the policy
4. the policy must contain a technically possible operational strategy—i.e. how the policy can be implemented and achieved, and
5. there must be some recognizable, clear measure of success.

---

[33]See references for dates, titles and authors of the papers noted above.

The rationale for the switch from malaria control to global malaria eradication met some but not all these elements. The argument for expected benefits against costs was made implicitly rather then explicitly and comparison of control and eradication strategies were, at least at the country level but also from a global standpoint, made without appropriate use of some social rate of discount.[34] Further there was some underestimate of the infrastructure capability of countries basically to shift from control to eradication. There was also a belief that eradication was a race between known vector control technologies and the growing drug resistance of the mosquito vectors: time was of the essence. Finally, while no formal probability of success was widely promulgated, the inference of success was drawn from some limited country examples where eradication had shown implicitly some substantial benefits against cost (mostly North and South America, Europe). Whatever else, however, there was a sufficient number of elements present to make malaria eradication a policy just waiting to be adopted: it had the ring of authenticity.

But there is another dimension to this story. WHO, through its Governing Bodies and Expert Committees, promulgated a policy—malaria eradication—for which it, in fact, had very little control over. WHO as an international human services organization does not, per se, control sufficient resources to implement such a policy. WHO's outputs are the leveraging of its resources with those of other agencies and donors (which it did with initially great success for malaria), the dissemination of information, rules, procedures, and standards (which it also did, and the technical assistance for country programmes, for training of skilled workers, for technical advice on planning, management, logistics, etc. for national programs, and for supporting (and in some cases, initiating) research and development in support of the policy. But the ultimate success or failure of malaria eradication rested in the country programmes: WHO policies pushed countries to adoption of malaria eradication as a goal, but WHO governing bodies and Expert Committees did not have the power of success or failure in their hands. If one sees the process from this point of view, it becomes crucial for WHO, when it makes global policy statements; to be sure the statements are grounded in technical and economic rationality. Countries will follow, as they did with malaria eradication, the policies countries promote for adoption through WHO and its governing Bodies. It is important, therefore, that (as) major shifts in resources (result from) WHO promulgated policies, (that) the formulation of these policies conform to some rational process: is this the best available policy compared to alternatives? What are the expected benefits? Are these greater than the costs? What are likely to be some unintended but predictable events that could happen? Is the technology underlying the policy sound, able to withstand rigorous scientific standards? WHO cannot, because of the nature of its

---

[34]Cohen (1972).

constitutional make-up, innocently proclaim world policy without being prepared to answer questions of the sort posed above.

Once malaria eradication was adopted as WHO policy (1955) the diffusion and adoption of the policy by Member States was rapid and the necessary but not sufficient conditions that fuel the rapid diffusion of a policy, as listed in Table XX, neatly fit the case of malaria eradication; countries, donors, international institutions were ready to receive such a policy. The receptive elements were in place. However, as the malaria eradication policy worked its way through Member States acceptance, elements that could lead to its death were already evident. Some of these key elements are noted in Table XX; these are generic but all the participants to the malaria eradication policy who have written about it tend to emphasize one or the other of the elements noted in Table XX that led to the death of malaria eradication as a global policy.

Out of the death of a policy come the elements for a rebirth, a recasting and ultimately a finer, sharper, version of the original policy (see Table XX). This, of course, happened with malaria and the litany of reasons—economic, managerial, technical, etc.—exposed in the report of the Director General (DG) of WHO in 1969 ("Re-examination of the Global Strategy of Malaria Eradication") rather neatly parallels the generic elements of Table XX.

As we note in Table XX, the seeds for the death of a policy are implanted in the way the life of the policy is started. The report of the DG to the 22nd WHA (1969), after a careful assessment of which factors seemed essential for a successful malaria eradication and which ones did not, carefully, but firmly, buried the policy of malaria eradication in favour of one that worked "towards eradication" and depended on the particular epidemiological, health, and economic and social characteristics of the country. In listing the factors needed for success, the report noted the following:

1. *The methods*—interruption of transmission by insecticide spraying still valid where populations are stable but must be adjusted for migration: "the areas cleared of malaria are constantly exposed to the risk of importation of cases; the prolongation of programmes far beyond their original time schedule strains the national resources" (p. 118)
2. *The resources*
   a. National resources: "the overall financial position when malaria eradication was started was more favourable than it is today." (p. 118) Also, "there has also been a change of priorities in some developing countries, in view of the many other demands for funds for social and economic development." (p. 118)
   b. The international resources: "Here again, changes in the priorities of assistance from the international agencies have occurred during

recent years, and the contributions to the programme...have diminished." (p. 119)

c. The capacity to maintain achieved eradication: "there has been a tendency to integrate the malaria eradication service within the general health services in the later stages of the eradication programme without regard to maturity of development of the rural health services. This has resulted in deterioration of the services provided by both elements." (p. 119)

One of the leaders in the malaria eradication policy, Soper, is quoted by Farid (p. 16 1980) and follow-up comments by other major players (especially Bruce-Chwatt (Farad, 1980, p. 23). A statement by Bruce-Chwatt, also sums up the rationale for malaria eradication policy: "...critics think that the overall benefits [from malaria eradication] could have been obtained by other means and that the costs of the global programme were far too high in relation to its results." (in Farid, 1980, p. 23). Also, "...there was reasonable hope that a concerted and relatively short [10 years] universal campaign might eliminate the disease from the very large areas before...insecticide resistance spread all over the world." (in Farid, 1980, p. 23). Finally, "it has become fashionable to put much of the blame for the present situation in WHO...But the fact is that not much change can be expected until the relevant governments demonstrate their own interest and concern..." (in Farid, 1980, p. 24). And finally, several conclusions drawn by Najera seemed to summarize the state of affairs with the policy of malaria eradication: "there was a basic contradiction between the justification of the programme as a case against the development of resistance and the need for careful planning...and the establishment of an organization of such degree of perfection...clearly beyond the capabilities of most highly endemic countries" (Najera, 28 March 1989, p. 9). And again: "Progressively throughout the sixties a feeling was developing that the malaria eradication global programme could not succeed in a foreseeable future...although it was possible to reduce and even interrupt malaria transmission by insecticide spraying the large areas, it was very difficult, if not impossible, to establish effective surveillance in the absence of a solid health infrastructure." (Najera, 28 March, 1989, p. 10).

The report of the DG at the 22nd WHA was a fairly devastating comment on the first ten years of malaria eradication. And the new strategy proposed—now called the revised global strategy—is elaborated in the 15th Expert Committee Report (1970) as recognizing the need for malaria control as a routine activity of health services. But, after a review of the past, the Committee reaffirms the principles of malaria eradication. It is yet another decade (1978/79) before an Expert Committee (17th, 1979) and WHA and EB resolutions fully recognize the need for an articulated, malaria control—rather than global eradication—policy. The 17th Expert Committee Report enumerated the components of a control strategy. Finally in 1985, WHA Resolution Number 38.24 comes full circle from the global eradication policy of some 30 years earlier to pronounce that malaria control should be developed as an integral part of the national primary health care system. The tools of today's policy emphasize use of all appropriate technologies—drugs, vector control, research or vaccines, etc.—and these are memorialized in the 18th (1985) report of the Expert Committee and in WHA Resolution Number 38.24[35]

HOW DID MONEY FLOW?

In the global war to eradicate malaria, where did the money flow? As already noted, WHO's money, its Regular Budget, is used for: standards, norms, training, technical assistance, information and data, research and development. But one of the major outputs of WHO and its Governing Bodies is—international health policy. Sometimes the policy is micro level—health legislation, for example— sometimes it is macro or global—malaria eradication, smallpox eradication, the Global Programme on AIDS. When WHO articulates a global policy it is stating for the world the importance and hence the priority that should be attached to something, usually of worldwide significance for world health. Such policies permit WHO to leverage its resources—to attract other donors and agencies to contribute funds towards the implementation of the policy (i.e. country activities) and to WHO itself to help finance its work in support of the policy. The essence of policy analysis is to see how and where resources flow with announced policy and how the resources get used to advance the policy. In the case of malaria eradication—a clear example of a macro policy—WHO initially committed its Regular Budget to this priority and was successful, initially, in leveraging other resources from donors in support of the policy. At the height of the shift from control to global eradication, WHO expenditures on malaria from its budget in 1958-1959 peaked at nearly 30 percent of its total expenditures on all programs, a more than doubling from the pre-1959 years where the control strategy was the dominant policy. Nearly all of these funds were from the Regular Budget. But from this high point, malaria was never again such a major priority spending from the Regular Budget. In real terms (expressed in 1979 U.S. $) from all sources the resources for the global policy rose dramatically from 1957 to 1967, consistent with the adherence to the policy i.e. putting money where you say it should be put. But as a proportion of WHO budgetary expenditures, the high points were 1958, 1959: from that point onwards malaria becomes a declining fraction of the WHO budget, by 1970 becoming less than 10 percent of the total.

---

[35]All of the above from "Abstract" of Expert Committee, WHA and EB resolutions on malaria, 1947-1985.

There are two single year spurts (in 1975 the proportion doubles from 6 percent to 13 percent), but is halved again in 1976 and then nearly doubled again (from 6-11 percent) in 1977. In recent years as a proportion of the WHO Regular Budget expenditures on malaria have ranged between 4-5 percent of the total.

One must remember that the preceding description of the flow of funds refers to those under WHO control and to support WHO's role as coordinator of the global eradication programme. In such capacity WHO provided guidelines, information and data, technical and expert assistance to country eradication programmes, and a good deal of the technical and material infrastructure for organization, planning, and management activities. The bulk of the resources spent on malaria eradication came primarily from country sources heavily supplemented by the international donor community notably United Nation's Children's Emergency Fund (UNICEF), United States Agency for International Development (USAIDS) and the United Nation's Development Program (UNDP).

The question is: whether, given the level of WHO resources committed to malaria eradication, there was something lacking that if done could have made the policy succeed? That seems doubtful, given the epidemiological, technical and economic factors that were to doom the policy of global eradication from the very beginning. Other priorities -some with higher probability of success than maleria eradication. Still the products and services WHO provided in its role as coordinator were not neutral with respect to the possible success or failure of the policy of malaria eradication. As Farid (1980, p. 15) scathingly remarked: "Experts sitting in WHO headquarters in Geneva whose job was to coordinate the global programme, began to interfere, advising when to stop spraying and how to utilize the malaria funds, failing to leave the matter in the hands of those on the spot who knew about the local malaria situation. The reports of independent assessment teams...were shelved if they did not agree with the government's own views of policies or their own epidemiological criteria, which did not correspond to those developed by WHO Expert Committees on Malaria" (Farid, 1980, p. 15).

INSIGHTS FROM THE POLICY EXPERIENCE

How does an organization such as WHO decides what its priorities should be? How does an organization come to promulgate a policy of worldwide significance such as malaria eradication, Health For All, AIDS, policy emerge from some methodologically rational procedures? There is a wonderfully revealing paragraph in a paper by Najera (MAP 25.4, 1989, p. 2) which sums up the forces that were building toward the policy of global malaria eradication. "The idea of malaria eradication", he stated,

"Which had been postulated as early as 1916, gained currency after the war, as malaria epidemics had ravaged the devastated malarious areas of Southern Europe and DDT had shown to be extremely effective...The Expert Committee on Malaria...in their first five reports adopted a cautious attitude and indicated concern with the increasing reports of technical problems and of some disappointing results of the use of DDT, particularly in Africa. Nevertheless the appeal of malaria eradication became irresistible, as the impending DDT resistance was seen as a stimulus for a race to achieve eradication before its development. In 1954 the Pan American Sanitary Conference adopted a continental plan for the eradication of malaria from the Americas, which was extended to the World, in 1955, by the World Health Assembly."*

Such a policy statement by WHO and its governing bodies was to have profound significance as country after country switched its antimalarial campaign from control of the disease to its eradication. The policy was to affect resource flows and shifts from other uses to a new use: malaria eradication as a policy moved to the head of the priority list.

From the point of view of the analysis of public policy, as already noted earlier in this report, it is possible to understand what convergence of forces could lead to such momentous policy statements. (A similar set of circumstances could be said to have led to the Alma-Ata declaration). But any major change in policy has implicit and explicit resource allocation implications: in large complex service organizations the rational formulation of policy requires internal processes (or rules and procedures) so that all the right questions—at least those that can reasonably be contemplated—get asked and as many as possible answered.

In the Expert Committee reports at and around the time malaria eradication was put forward as world policy. There is not much, if any, discussion of the sort one would need for rational adoption of a policy. At the economic level of benefits and costs of malaria eradication compared to control the essence of the argument put forth was simple: it is better to commit to a 10-year capital investment which would yield eradication (total benefits higher?) than to continue annual resource costs for control (benefits lower?) which does not lead to eradication. One does not find a careful enumeration of the expected benefits or anticipated costs being realized. Najera (1989, p. 232) summarized the views of the 6th Expert Committee Report.

"The desirability of eradication over control, in the Committee's view, was justified by the social and economic value of eradication, the cost of which would represent a capital investment needing funds for only a limited time, and by the fear that insecticide resistance might impair the maintenance of control by means of residual insecticides."*

In other words, it was self evident that the benefits of eradication would exceed the benefits of control. That might have been true had there been a 100 percent probability of success over a 10 year period. But what about the costs? The only mentioned of cost is that "countries be able to afford their eradication programmes". But a careful enumeration of all the expected benefits-even if not all could be quantified—and, similarly an enumeration of all the costs could have provided a sounder and more rational basis for the choice of policies. Indeed as Cohen has noted, the original argument-put in a Benefit-Cost framework, had some logical flaws.

> "One of the arguments which has been advanced in favour of eradication, along with the technical ones, is although eradication is initially more costly it is cheaper in the long run because it is completed in a finite period of time (seven to ten years) whereas control goes on forever. It is, however, inadmissible to compare these two sets of outlays by simply adding up the projected annual costs of the two programmes over their expected lives; it is essential that the two expenditure flows be reduced to a common base to take into account the fact that, viewed from today, money next year is of lower value than money today..."

Cohen then points out that if an appropriate discount rate is selected so as to equate the resources flows of eradication and control in terms of present value, for some countries (and in retrospect for most countries) it was not obvious that the B/C ratio of eradication exceeded the B/C ratio for control. So, arguments of this sort, which might have classified classified the meaning of eradication as a policy were notably lacking; at the minimum such calculations should have been made at the country level. What is revealing, to a policy analyst so many years after the event, is that the rules, procedures, and policies of the Organization had no means by which such questions could be placed into debate. Expert Committees were dominated by technical people without benefit of the methodological insights that might have raised these questions had economists and other social scientists participated in the discussion.

At yet another level, also central to policy analysis, one looks in vain in the governing body and Expert Committee deliberations at the time malaria eradication is put forward as world policy for a discussion of the technical and longer term aspects of malaria eradication should it turn out to be successful. In the consideration of any policy not only must one enumerate (even if one cannot quantify everything) benefits and costs, one must also speculate on the conditions of sustainability should the policy actually succeed. As already noted, and repeatedly commented on in Expert Committee reports, countries from the start in shifting from control to eradication experienced problems (unexpected costs) from the attack, through the consolidation and maintenance-phases of the strategy. Could not these costs have been anticipated? Some were, of course, and were noted in Expert Committee documents. But there was no sustained debate about these issues at the time of the formulation neither of the malaria eradication policy nor during its first ten years of life. Finally, ten years after the policy is in operation, some conditions and observations for country success and failure are put forward. The basis of formulating policies that have a chance to succeed is that these conditions—which are really no more, no less than a list of potential benefits and costs—be set forth at the time and with as much knowledge as exists at the time. Some of the types of questions that might have been asked are:

1. What project (eradication) benefits (or output) could be sustained after funding ends if the policy is successful?
2. Who benefits from the programme's success? Has a constituency been built for the programme once the policy loses its priority?
3. What country policies threaten sustainability of the programme? How are these policies being mitigated? What alternative government policies would aid success and sustainability of the policy?
4. What organization, institutions, financial (i.e. management, technical expertise, cost recovery schemes, staffing and incentive structures) is being developed to continue project benefits once the policy recedes in importance? Can the management systems respond to changes, new technologies?
5. What provisions were made for recurrent costs including foreign exchange once the policy has succeeded?
6. Do projected benefits of continuing the policy justify the continued investment of resources compared to the opportunity costs and constraints and other health priorities?
7. What is an appropriate time period to ensure that the key conditions for sustainability will be substantially in place?

As was said at the beginning of this paper: hindsight is easier than foresight. It is easy at this time to look back at such a major policy as malaria eradication and fault it as a policy. That is really not the intent of this paper. It is not the malaria eradication policy that is at issue but rather the nature of policy formulation in a complex international service agency such as WHO. The integral operating procedures and rules of the Organization should have a process by which any policy—certainly one as major as was malaria eradication—is routinely analysed in some rational, methodologically pure manner: policy makers may still wish to pursue the policy even if it does not pass all the usual tests of rationality and efficient resource use. However, at least the road map will have been filled in and all the potential hazards noted. It bears repeating again and again, WHO does not have "products" in the typical sense of the term. It produces services: policies, research and development, technical assistance, training, guidelines, norms, standards, rules, technical information, etc. These services are produced in connection with the policy priorities of the Organization. A wider market of interests—the class of public health problems, the donor community, the Member States, sets these priorities. It is imperative that as the priorities become translated into global policies, WHO has the internal processes, able to subject such policies to some rational methods of choice before pronouncing new world policy. WHO's own resources, relative to the total, for malaria eradication were meagre; yet its promulgation of malaria eradication as world policy caused a dramatic shift in resources within countries, and between countries, through actions of the international donor and external assistance community. WHO's obligation is to make world policy—that is one of its constitutional functions—but such policies—because they always will have enormous influence on shifts in resource allocation—must be grounded, as much as possible, in some rational process of analysis.

REFERENCES-BIBLIOGRAPHY

Andreano, Ralph. 1983. "Economic issues in disease control and eradication." *Soc. Sci. Med.* 17 (24): 2027-2032.

Barlow, Robin, and Lisa M. Grobar. 1986. "Cost and benefits of controlling parasitic diseases." PHN Technical Note 85-17, Population, Health and Nutrition Department, World Bank, reissued January 1986.

Blumenfeld, Stewart N. 1985. "Operations Research Methods: A General Approach in Primary Health Care." PRICOR Monograph Series: Methods Paper 1, May 1985.

Carnevale, Pierre, and Jean Mouchet. *Prospects for malaria control*, pp 18/187.

Castro, Elssy Bonilla, and Karen Marie Mokate. *Malaria and its socioeconomic meanings: The study of Cunday in Colombia.*

Clyde, David F. 1987. "Recent Trends in the Epidemiology and Control of Malaria." *Epidemiology Reviews* 9: 219-243.

Conly, Gladys M. 1975. "The impact of malaria on economic development: a case study." Pan American Health Organization, Scientif Publication, no. 297.

CRED. 1989. "Sentinel Epidemiologic Surveillance in Bangladesh: Proposed Design and Operational Plan." CRED Working Document No. 78.

Drummond, M. F. 1987. *Principles of Economic Appraisal in Health Care.* Oxford Medical Publications.

Farid, M. A. 1980. "Le programme antipaludique—de l'euphorie à l'anarchie."*Forum Mondial de la Santé* 1 (1, 2): 9-39.

Gramiccia, G., and P. F. Beales. *The Recent History of Malaria Eradication.*

Grundy, F., and W. A. Reinke. 1973 "Health Practice Research and Formalized Managerial Methods." World Health Organization, Geneva.

Herrin, Alejandro, and Patricia L. Rosenfield. 1988. *Economics. Health and Tropical Diseases.* Papers, Summary, and Conclusions of the Meeting on the Economics of Tropical Disease, Manila, Philippines, 2-5 Sept., 1986 University of the Philippines, School of Economics.

Kondrashin, A. V., and N. L. Kalra. 1988. "Malaria as anthropo-ecosystem. Part I: General Concept.*" J. Com. Dis* 20 (1): 79-86.

Kondrashin, A. V., and N. L. Kalra. 1988. Malaria as anthropo-ecosystem. Part II: Diversity of Malaria Infection sub-system." *J. Com. Dis* 20 (4): 349-359.

Kondrashin, A. V., and N. L. Kalra. 1988. "Malaria as anthropo-ecosystem. Part III." *J. Com. Dis* 21 (1): 62-70.

Manson-Bahr, P. E. C., and F. I. C. Apted. 1982. "Malaria and Babesiosis." *Manson's Tropical Diseases*, 18th Edition. London: Baillere Tindall, 38-72.

Mills, A. J. 1987. "Economic study of malaria in Nepal: The cost-effectiveness of Malaria control strategies." Evaluation and Planning Centre, London school of Hygiene and Tropical Medicine.

Najera, J. A. "Malaria control—past, present and future." Offset Document; MAP/89.1

Najera, J. A. 1989. "Malaria and the work of WHO." *Bulletin of the World Health Organization* 67 (3): 229-243.

Najera, J. A. 1989. 'Malaria control: present situation and nedd for historical research." *WHO, MAP* 25.5.

Oberender, Peter, and Jochem Diesfeld. 1984. "Health Development in Africa: Introduction." *Soc. Sci. Med.* 17 (24): 1945-1946.

Organisation Mondiale De La Sante. 1988. "Acticités antipaludiques: les 40 dernière année: Programme d'action antipaludique." *Rapp. Trimest. Statist. Sant. Mond.*,41: 64-73.

Organisation Mondiale De La Sante. 1986. "Comité OMS d'experts du paludisme (dix-huitiéme rapport)." Série de Rapports Techniques, 735 Genéve: Organisation Mondiale de la Sante.

PAN American Health Organization. 1986. "Regional technical consultation of experts of malaria control." Brasilia, Brazil, 2-5 June.

PAN American Health Organization. 1988. "Status of malaria programs in the America." XXXVI Report, CD33/INF/2 (Eng.), 20 August.

Popkin, Barry M. 1982. "A Household Framework for Examining the Social and Economic Con Consequences of Tropical Diseases." *Soc. Sci. Med.* 16: 533-543.

Prescott, Nicolas M. 1979. "The Economics of Malaria Filariasis and Trypanosomiaasis." Magdalen College, University of Oxford.

Shapira Allan. 1989. "Chloroquine Resistant Malaria in Africa: The Challenge to Health Services." *Health Policy and Planning* 4 (1): 17-28. Oxford University Press.

World Health Organization. 1986. *WHO Expert Committee on Malaria* (Eighteenth Report). World Health Organization, Technical Report Series, 735.

World Health Organization. 1989. *WHO Expert Committee on Malaria* (Nineteenth Report). World Health Organization, 23 November.

World Health Organization. *Malaria, The Work of WHO 1986-1987.* Biennial Report, pp. 157-161.

Table XX
The Life, Death, and Rebirth of a Policy
(Necessary but not sufficient conditions)

Formulation of a Policy (Needed elements)	Transmission and Diffusion Of a Policy	Death Of A Policy	Rebirth Of A Policy
1. The problem must be great, significant, be recognized by key players and actors as such, experts, politicians, people/institutions with money i.e. if we do it this way (the policy) we will	1. The policy becomes accepted because a. People believe it, key actors give it credibility b. There is some prospect of "new" resources being available to do something you want to do but could not afford it.	1. The rationale as put forward was wrong, unrealistic, and technically unsound.	1. Measure of success put forward show it is not succeeding.
(1) Accomplish such and such (these are the benefits) if we do not do it his way—there will be consequences (the costs)	2. Policy becomes institutionalized, reinforced by hype, processes endemic to the proposers of the policy, etc.	2. Some of the key players become skeptical	2. Key players do not want to abandon something they have a vested interest in
(ii) There must be some quantifiable possibility that the policy will succeed—against all other existing and/or competing policies	3. The policy has the ring of authenticity to it—people looking for something like it, it articulates a feeling people already had.	3. The operational strategy was faulty, unworkable, unrealistic	3. The operational centers see the policy is not working—various reasons
(iii) There must be some finite time period for the policy; it must appear technically possible		4. Probability estimate for success proved too optimistic after field experience reveals problems.	4. The costs of maintaining the policy become disillusioning, become skeptical etc.
(iv) There must be an operational strategy for implementing the policy		5. The costs seem to be higher than anticipated—the benefits anticipated do not materialize fast enough	
(v) There must be some clear definition of success for the policy ("transmission" eradicated)			
3. The timing of the policy seems right—public opinion already needed in that direction			

SELECTION 7

ECONOMICS, HEALTH, AND TROPICAL DISEASE: A REVIEW[36]

Abstract—The paper examines individual diseases of the WHO Special Program in Tropical Disease Research (TDR). It focuses on the economic and social impact of research findings on the alternatives for intervention. It then moves away from individual diseases and looks at the broader impacts across all tropical diseases. The paper also weighs the potential and shortcomings of economic analysis in assessing various intervention approaches.

In conclusion, the paper stresses the significant role of economic analysis in future research on tropical diseases. Such research needs to use more tightly framed methodologies and more rigorously structured hypotheses. In this regard, hard economic analysis should be tempered by the insights of other social and medical scientists.

INTRODUCTION: ECONOMICS, HEALTH, AND DEVELOPMENT

Economists have long regarded work in health as a part of the theoretical and analytical work done under the rubric of human capital analysis, and they have made tremendous contributions to the analysis of health care issues, especially in industrialized societies. This paper is not, however, about health, health care, or the health sector in industrialized societies; it instead concerns those topics in the setting of the less developed, largely non-industrialized countries. It is about the relationship between investment in health and the advancement in levels of well-being. And in this arena the contributions of economic analysis and of the research of economists have been less powerful than one perceives to be the case in Western countries.

The linkages between health and economic development seem much more complex than comparable linkages in developed societies. There has been theorizing and much discussion in the literature regarding the causal links between health and economic development. A number of useful models have been produced and certain insights into the nature and direction of such linkages

---

[36]This paper was originally published in Alejandro Herrin and Patricia L. Rosenfield, (Editors), *Economics, Health, and Tropical Diseases*. (University of the Philippines, School of Economics) Manila, 1988.

Dr. Thomas Helminiak was a co-author of this page.

have emerged. Still, there is only primitive empirical knowledge concerning the subject, and the theorizing (beyond some obvious measurable truths) has not been reflected in empirical estimation of the linkages. This is primarily because of two almost insurmountable problems: (1) lack of a uniform, output-driven, measures of health, any (2) the causality between measures of health and measures of development. The light of economic analysis, so powerful in its illumination of health care policies and choices in the West, shines only dimly on the problems and policy choices in the Third World.

At least this is the conventional wisdom on the subject: the brand of economics we practice in the West has made (or can only make) marginal contributions to the complicated linkages between health (or disease) and development in the poor countries. We are not entirely sure that conventional wisdom is correct; we think it may not be, but the evidence to challenge it is fragmentary or incomplete. What seems to become clear from our paper is that the economist's mirror is powerful in reflecting the disease/development interchange, but that contributions to this literature have sometimes gone beyond the values and assumptions economists ordinarily make. Indeed, there is a larger social science at work, as we shall see in our discussion of research, but it seems to us that traditional economic analysis should be, but often is not, at the core of this social science. Economists always make assumptions, and we do have a value system that underlines these assumptions. Many economists trained in the Western vein take on values, and make assumptions, that free markets can work, that people do and will make rational choices, and that the interference with the free exercise of market behavior inhibits social choice and social welfare. Marxian, or neo-Marxian, analysis, of course, believes otherwise. Indeed it may be, though we do not agree, that Marxian economic analysis is a better fit than most Western economic analyses to the structural and basic conditions governing health and disease in the Third World. Our problem here is that the policy conclusions one derives from the Marxian perspective often require outright coercion by a central government, and we reject that as a common policy option.

A part of the intractable nature of the disease/development interaction and the limits of economic analysis may be due to the complexity and vast scope of this interaction. Health conditions as well as health resources are vastly different between the developed and underdeveloped world, as shown in the following simplified table.

In the present paper our ambitions are modest and we cannot stray too far from our focus, which is on the tropical diseases and what economic analysis has, or may have, to offer here. These diseases of the Special Programme for Tropical Disease Research are singled out because they are a focal point of a worldwide program and also because of the millions of people and the dozens of countries that are affected by these disease entities. In the international health community there are two themes (at least) that one must reckon with: (1) that represented by the Special Programme for TDR, and (2) the Health for All goals enunciated at Alma Ata. The current worldwide dilemma of diminishing or moderately increasing resources for health care and disease control in the Third World may make the contribution of economics more useful than ever. The poor countries will have to make do with less; and tropical disease control and/or eradication will have to compete for resources in a much tighter environment of resource availability than ever before [1]. While our perspective in this paper is on the tropical diseases, it is our intention to be sure that economic thinking on health research is informed by these wider opportunities for analysis.

Health and related socioeconomic indicators

	Least Developed Countries	Other Developing Countries	Developed Countries
Number of countries	31	89	37
Total population (millions)	283	3,001	1,131
Infant mortality rate (per 1000 liveborn)	160	94	19
Life expectancy (years)	45	60	72
Coverage by safe water supply	31%	41%	100%
Adult literacy rate	29%	55%	98%
GNP per capita	$170	$520	$6,230
Per capita public expenditure on health	$1.7	$6.5	$244
Public expenditure on health as % of GNP	1.0%	1.2%	3.9%
Population per doctor	17,000	2,700	520
Population per nurse	6,500	1,500	220
Population per health worker (Any type, including traditional birth attendant)	2,400	500	130

Note: Figures in the table are weighted averages, based upon estimates for 1980 or for the latest year for which data are available.
Source: American Public Health Association (1981).

For the most part work that is described as "economic" on tropical diseases has been dominated by cost-benefit analysis and cost effectiveness analysis. It is our view, however, that even in the developing world context, one can imagine research on tropical diseases that moves beyond these two frameworks. Research, though useful in itself, is meant to inform policy. The economics of households, and the economics of risk taking and avoidance, are two areas of microanalysis, which might be useful, and some studies have attempted this. At the macro level, theories of savings and investment and concepts from industrial organization are also other possible areas of application. And here several economists have made very helpful starts on such research. Still, the basic levels at which tropical diseases strike—rural settings, populations in poverty—make the application of powerful economic theorems seem not worthwhile. Somehow utility theory and preference functions seem inapplicable in describing the behavior of rural, diseased, mostly illiterate peasants. Rational choice making is a freedom enjoyed in industrial society; our question is whether or not the assumptions and values underlying this analysis have validity in the context of the poor countries. We think it does, but the research evidence and record, thus far, is mixed.

Economists and other social scientists have produced a sizable and growing research literature regarding tropical diseases. This literature has dealt with identification and evaluation of the economic and social effects of tropical diseases and the evaluation of the available strategies designed to mitigate such effects.

The fact, as pointed out by a number of writers, that a very small proportion of world resources is presently being devoted to the eradication or control of tropical diseases prompts the question of whether or not societies should devote more resources to eradicate or control these diseases. That is, in economic terms, should more disease intervention be produced, at the expense of producing less of something else?

While the "importance" of tropical diseases may be understood to be some function of the adverse consequences of these diseases to individuals and societies—the specification of these consequences has been highly imprecise and inadequate. Some observers have hypothesized that if the range and magnitudes of these adverse consequences were better understood, current allocations to tropical disease intervention would be appreciably expanded.

In (economic) principle, the case for increased (or decreased) allocations to tropical disease intervention will depend on the marginal return per unit of expenditure, on tropical disease intervention relative to that for allocations to other objectives. However, rigorous application of cost-benefit procedures to such intervention has been thwarted not only by the inability to specify and quantify the various possible benefits of intervention, but also by uncertainty as to how to evaluate these benefits in terms commensurable with the benefits of allocations to other objectives not related to tropical disease.

Outline of the paper

In this paper we first examine two broad areas of economic/ social science research for the individual diseases of the TDR programme: (1) their economic and social impact, and (2) a discussion of what the research tells us about the alternatives for intervention. This part of the paper is organized around a framework in which we list the possible types of effects. Research is then related to this classification scheme.

The next part of the paper moves away from the individual diseases and looks at the broader impacts across all tropical diseases. The research done by economists and other social scientists has a wider significance than what may be found from the research on any individual tropical disease. In this part of the paper we explore what has been done on disease impacts (for shorthand we describe these as impact studies) and assess what we have or can learn from this research when taken from the perspective of the economist's analytical insights. As we shall see, a lot of work has been done in the impact area, but much of it is faulted and wide gaps remain in research knowledge about disease impacts.

We next consider the work done on intervention approaches. Again, here, while work may, have been done on a single disease or subset of diseases, the basic research on intervention approaches has a wider significance. This is especially so as our perspective in this paper (especially in this part) is to weigh the potential and short comings of the role economic analysis may play in assessing various intervention approaches.

The final section of the paper sums up, as best as one can, what research by economists and other social and medical scientists tells us about disease impacts and intervention approaches. We conclude with some suggestions for other areas of research needed as well as the other dimensions of economic analysis that might be helpful to this research.

RESEARCH ON THE DISEASES OF THE TDR SPECIAL PROGRAMME

Introduction: typology on disease effects

Before examining research on the individual diseases, we first offer the economic and social impacts of tropical diseases. (It should be noted that our concern here is restricted to human effects.)

Health consumption effects. The most apparent (not necessarily the most important or most easily evaluated) effects of tropical disease are those that diminish the enjoyment—in economic terms, the consumption—of good health among affected persons. In this category we include not only the direct pain and suffering associated with tropical disease infection, but also the shortened enjoyment of life resulting from premature mortality, the grief of persons affected by either physical incapacity or the stigma of disease [2], grief related to impending early mortality, and the grief of relatives and friends of those affected by disease.

The existence of such effects is fairly evident, but we lack clear understanding of appropriate techniques to quantify them. Although there has been some effort to develop methodologies for capturing health consumption effects, empirical measurement has been minimal [3].

Social interaction and leisure effects. Social effects of tropical diseases include the stresses and constraints imposed on interactions between infected persons and other members of their households and communities [4]. Leisure time and recreation may also be reduced.

Short-term production effects. Most economic evaluations of the impact of tropical disease have focused on the quantification of production consequences. Short-term production effects include both market and nonmarket impacts. Among the former are effects on land and labor supply, and the actual expenditures made to provide treatment to those suffering from disease, as well as "avoidance" costs, representing the existing expenditures on persons for the purpose of forestalling these diseases [5]. These expenditures are considered as production effects, since if the diseases did not occur, the resources devoted to their treatment and avoidance could be directed to other production. Nonmarket production effects are those affecting production of commodities for home consumption and household services such as childrearing and household upkeep.

Determining the treatment and avoidance costs of tropical diseases has been largely regarded by economists as an accounting issue with relatively little research challenge and, hence, has received only subsidiary interest.

Most research attention in the area of production effects has involved the evaluation of factors of production—primarily labor and, in some instances, land. Evaluating the impact of disease on labor as a factor of production may include all of the following: (a) the temporary loss of labor days due to inability to work; (b) the permanent loss of labor supply days due to mortality; (c) reductions in the efficiency of labor days supplied due to debility. This area of evaluation, which describes the productive value of healthy human life and stresses the role of disease intervention programs as an investment in human productivity, has been termed the. "Human capital" approach.

Long-term production consumption effects. These include demographic effects on consumption, labor supply and capital formation demand for relative factor proportions; attitudes about risk; intellectual development; innovative behavior, etc. For example, those tropical diseases which have especially high transmission potential in certain land areas may reduce the supply of productive land, because the settlement and employment of land is discouraged. The long-term implications are obvious.

Some observers have inappropriately characterized the distinction between the health consumption and the production impacts of disease as representing, respectively, the "humanitarian" and "economic" approaches to the assessment of disease cost [6]. In fact, both the health consumption and the production categories represent economic costs and both have humanitarian implications. Economists have largely ignored the health consumption effects of disease not because these effects are in any sense "noneconomic," but rather—at least in large part—as a result of methodological uncertainty regarding how to evaluate such effects. It is also possible that information on production effects may have been in greater demand by advocates of increased funding for work on tropical disease. Evidence regarding production impacts of tropical diseases might be perceived to be more persuasive in the context of development-oriented government budgets (stressing investment for future versus current consumption).

A major point of the simple classification presented above is to distinguish the areas where empirical research has and has not been carried out for tropical diseases. Research conducted thus far has been predominantly restricted to effects on short-term, market sector production, with just a few studies touching upon some of the long-term production/consumption components. Little—if any—attention has been given to the areas of health consumption effects, social interaction and leisure effects, short-term nonmarket production effects and many of the hypothesized components of long-term production/consumption effects.

Research on the individual diseases

A summary, by individual tropical disease, of research progress in the interest areas just described follows [7].

Schistosomiasis

Description. Schistosomiasis is the broad term for a group of parasite infections caused by small worms (blood flukes) of the genus *Schistosoma.* The female worm produces large numbers of eggs, many of which are excreted; however, the nonexcreted eggs, which lodge in tissues of the body, may produce organ damage. When the *Schistosoma haematobium* species is the infecting parasite, the site of lodged eggs is the bladder and adjacent genito-urinary organs; when S. *mansoni* or S. *Japonicum is* involved; the intestine or liver is the site of lodged eggs. The intensity of infection (worm load) is considered an important factor in the determination of a wide range of symptoms, which may (depending on the invading species) include weakness, diarrhea, nausea, and loss of weight, difficulty in urinating, and liver and spleen enlargement. Infection of individuals occurs during exposure to the freshwater habitats of infected intermediate snail hosts—which, in turn, are infected when Schistosomone eggs are deposited in these waters from the excreted urine or feces (again depending on the species) of infected persons [8].

Health consumption effects. There is yet no methodology for economic evaluation of the various health consumption effects, which is either (a) operationally feasible, or (b) reasonably uncontroversial. At this stage one is left with statistical indicators of mortality and morbidity—which may require ingenuity for accurate estimation [9].

Morbidity (diminished enjoyment of healthy life). Beyond individually surveyed localities, statistics on the overall number of persons infected in most countries are highly imprecise. Generally, less is known about the number of cases of infection which have reached the stage where individuals are "sick" and where they or relatives and friends are experiencing health consumption effects. No evaluation studies are known to have been done in this area.

Mortality (terminated enjoyment of healthy life). Reports of both a WHO Scientific Group, meeting in 1965 [10] and a WHO Expert Committee, meeting in 1966 [11] expressed the belief that, at least in areas of high endemicity, appreciable mortality was associated with schistosomiasis. Currently it is estimated that schistosomiasis is associated with low direct mortality, but that its chronic pathological sequela of infection might underlie mortality attributed to other causes [12].

Two reviewed studies which attempted to measure the mortality effect (direct and indirect) of schistosomiasis failed to discern any effect [13]. A study by Weisbrod *et al.* [14], conducted in St. Lucia during 1967-69, included a mortality estimation component in its investigation of the impacts of schistosomiasis and four other parasitic infections. Multiple regression analysis of data from household surveys in two rural valleys, Cul-de-Sac and Roseau, supplemented by recorded general mortality information, found no significant relationship between the schistosomiasis prevalence levels of communities in the surveyed valleys and the mortality rates of these communities [15]. The authors acknowledged that infection intensity levels for the S. *mansoni* form, prevalent in St. Lucia, were only moderate [16]. Rugemalila, Asila, and Chimbe [17] investigated the mortality experience of 4,516 inhabitants of Bujashi, Tanzania, endemic for S. *haematobium,* seven years after a baseline study. The distribution of 238 deaths showed similar age and sex specific mortality rates among the 2,309 non-cases and 2,109 cases found excreting eggs at the baseline examination. Similar age and sex mortality rates were also found, both for the follow-up of those with and without urological sequela on the baseline exam and also for those cases, which were and were not treated with metrifonate. The findings were regarded to suggest that neither the disease nor its treatment affected the mortality of the studied population [18].

Social and leisure effects. No studies are known to have been done in this area.

Short-term production effects (market). Schistosomiasis studies are the most numerous among those investigating production impacts. Gwatkin has remarked, "the literature dealing with careful field research into the infection-productivity relationship is for all practical purposes little more than a literature about schistosomiasis and productivity" [19].

The schistosomiasis production studies have all attempted to evaluate the impact on actual or potential labor productivity—either through estimation of the disease's influence on labor supply and labor efficiency in actual working situations, or through attempted measurement of its influence on physiological work capacity. Impacts on effective land supply are not recognized for schistosomiasis. The schistosomiasis productivity impact studies have been essentially partial equilibrium. The subjects of the studies have been mostly agricultural estate workers.

The methodology of the earliest studies tended to be simplistic and was flawed by the use of a number of dubious assumptions. These included nonverified assertions of losses of productivity capacity for classes of infected workers and valuation of these losses at rates unlikely to represent actual marginal productivity. Authors pointing out such methodological weaknesses include, Weisbrod et al. [20], Prescott [21], and Gwatkin [22]. These early studies for the most part showed substantial productivity impacts due to schistosomiasis [22].

A subsequent series of studies sought to measure empirically the labor productivity impacts of schistosomiasis by comparing the work performance of infected versus uninfected employees. The results of these studies have been mixed. A cross-sectional study by Foster [23] on a Tanzanian sugar estate (1962-63) investigated the effect of schistosomiasis on worker days supplied and on productivity per day worked. No significant difference in either days supplied or daily productivity was found for infected versus uninfected canecutters; however, for irrigation workers—who may have had higher intensity infection levels—days supplied were significantly reduced. (Daily productivity was not tested for the irrigation workers).

Fenwick and Figenschou [24], in a later study (1968-69) on the same Tanzanian estate, examined the effect of schistosomiasis on earnings (reflecting the combined effect of days of work supplied and per worker daily productivity). They found significant earnings differences in a cross-sectional study; and in a time-series study the earnings of a group of infected workers receiving chemotherapy improved somewhat, relative to the earnings of the uninfected workers.

On the other hand, Gateff et al. [25] failed to obtain significant results for a series of hypotheses which measured both labor days supplied and productivity for sugar estate workers in Cameroon. The lack of significant findings for these hypotheses prevailed for both an initial comparison of infected. and uninfected workers and a subsequent comparison after the infected group were divided into a subgroup, which received chemotherapy and another, which received a placebo [26].

Two cross-sectional studies involving rural banana estate workers and female workers in an urban light manufacturing plant were carried out by Weisbrod et al. [14] in St. Lucia (1967-69). Worker productivity on the banana estate was investigated according to the following four hypotheses: (1) disease reduces weekly earnings; (2) disease causes workers to shift to physically less demanding jobs; (3) disease reduces productivity per day worked; (4) disease reduces the amount of labor time supplied per week. Multiple regression analyses were conducted, utilizing personal attribute data (based on a household survey and a work-site questionnaire); estate records on worker attendance, physical output and earnings, and infection data—based on both presence and intensity (egg load) of infection.

The banana estate study found no significant effect of schistosomiasis infection on weekly earnings for either males or females. However, schistosomiasis was found to be associated with lower daily productivity for males, though this effect appeared to be offset by greater average days worked per week by infected workers [27]. The latter result suggests that infected male workers compensated for their reduced daily productivity by working relatively more days in order to maintain earnings.

No significant production effects were found for the females in the urban plant in St. Lucia [14].

A follow-up study on the St. Lucian banana estate by Weisbrod and Helminiak [28] two years later, to examine whether increased duration of infection might increase the measured productivity effect, produced no significant impact findings. However, this study relied on the infection results of the original study, thus assuming that significant changes in infection status had not occurred for the infected and uninfected groups of workers. Again, as noted earlier, infection intensity in St. Lucia was only moderate. Thus the possibility exists that the physiological reserve threshold level—beyond which productivity impacts result—though not exceeded in St. Lucia, might be exceeded in areas of higher infection intensity.

A study by Barbosa and Pereira de Costa [29], employing a three-stage clinical gradient for infected workers on a Brazilian sugar estate, again produced mixed findings. No significant earnings differences were found in an initial retrospective study; however, in a subsequent prospective study, cane-cutters in the third stage of the gradient—"hepatosplenic schistosomiasis"—were found to have 35.1 percent less productivity (earnings) than those in the first stage of the gradient—"intestinal form, with or without intestinal symptoms."

A separate series of studies, mostly involving Sudanese sugarcane workers, attempted to measure the physiological *capacity* of persons with schistosomiasis vs. those without, according to laboratory tests. These studies [30, 31, 32, 33] described more fully in a later section, also offer mixed findings. Their results give some indication that persons with high intensity infection (generally interpreted on the basis of greater egg loads in their feces or urine) will have a reduction in their working capacities.

Short-term production effects (nonmarket). No studies are known to have been done in this area.

Long-term production/consumption effects. The only studies found that concern these factors are the few mortality and fertility studies (demographic effect elements) plus research on the relationship between schistosomiasis and academic performance (a possible input to long-term labor productivity, plus, perhaps, to intellectual development). The negative findings of Weisbrod et al. [14] for two rural valleys of St. Lucia, and of Rugemalila [17] for Bujashi, Tanzania, regarding estimation of the mortality effect of schistosomiasis, were noted above, in the section on health consumption effects. The Weisbrod study also attempted to estimate the fertility effect of schistosomiasis, again using multiple regression analysis and household survey data for the same two St. Lucian valleys used in the, mortality analysis. Again, no significant relationship was found between schistosomiasis infection and fertility [34].

Academic performance was also investigated by the Weisbrod study for a hypothesized negative association with schistosomiasis. Two sets of data were analyzed: (1) scores on a standardized reading test, as an index of scholastic performance, as well as infection and other attribute data, collected through an island-wide survey of 13-14 year-old schoolchildren; (2) class rank and attendance at school for 9-14 year-old children enrolled in school in a rural area of high prevalence, Babonneau, along with infection and height and weight data for the children, obtained from a separate data set. The only statistically significant result from the multiple regression analyses performed was a finding of *lower* absenteeism among schistosomiasis-infected students at the Babonneau School. The authors speculated that the contrary association between absenteeism and S. *mansoni* infection might result from the fact that infected children were not sufficiently well to assist in the fields on harvest days, but were able to attend school [35].

Intervention approach evaluation. The fact that the transmission cycle for schistosomiasis is dependent on interaction between individuals and the freshwater habitats of the intermediate hosts of the snail indicates a need for (a) better understanding of the economic and social activities of persons which promote this interaction, and the possibilities for efficiently altering relevant behavioral aspects [36]; and (b) attention to the implications of development projects which may enlarge the water habitats of the snail host and thereby extend transmission potential [37].

To advance the methodology for operationalizing cost-effectiveness analysis for schistosomiasis (as well as other tropical diseases) economists have, as we mentioned earlier, joined the debate over appropriate measures of effectiveness and have enhanced the state of mathematical modeling for schistosomiasis, extending the ability to predict the dynamic consequences of alternative control approaches [38].

Summary. Of the various effects, significant research attention has been given only to the area of short-term market production. The dubious methodology of many of these studies limits the sample of results in which one can have any confidence, and caution is obviously required in drawing conclusions from this small sample of studies. They might be considered to indicate that schistosomiasis, at least where infection intensity is not high, has only modest effects on short-term market-oriented production. Even this finding might be debated, however, since (1) the results are generally based on narrow, possibly unrepresentative groups of workers—arguably biased towards the selection of less severely diseased individuals; (2) the focus on market-oriented production ignores the possibility of adjustments which involve diminished nonmarket production; (3) with only a few geographic areas represented, it is not certain how representative these areas are relative to the many areas of the world in which schistosomiasis is prevalent; and (4) the short-term nature of the studies does not allow potentially significant long-term effects to be reckoned with.

Little is also known about health consumption effects (although there are some indications that the mortality component of this effect may be low for schistosomiasis) or social and leisure effects.

The research efforts of economists and other social scientists in the area of intervention approach evaluation, though at an early stage, appear—in contrast to the efforts at impact measurement to be yielding answers which are somewhat less ambiguous and which seem more likely to affect operational decision-making.

Malaria

Description. Malaria is an infectious parasitic disease, transmitted by female mosquitoes of various species of the anopheline genus. Characteristic symptoms include periodic fever and chills, anemia, and various complications due to the involvement of certain organs. Infection due to the *Plasmodium falciparum* parasite species—considered to be the most serious form of malaria—tends to be associated with a high fatality rate among persons lacking immunity. Individuals who survive acute stages of the disease may be weakened and, in the chronic form, be more susceptible to other diseases [39].

Health consumption effects. The state of research efforts here resembles that of schistosomiasis. The impression, however, is that the mortality and morbidity

95

components of this class of effects may be somewhat greater for malaria than for schistosomiasis. Still, there is uncertainty about the true mortality effect of malaria, because deaths of weakened persons with chronic malaria are sometimes attributed to other causes. Newman, as described in a later section, demonstrated for Sri Lanka and Guyana a methodology for estimating the true mortality effect of malaria; his methodology is retrospective, however, following a successful eradication campaign [40].

Social and leisure effects. No study seems directly to examine social or leisure effects for malaria. Conly's Paraguay study, described in the next section, infers the existence of such effects through its evidence of intrahousehold substitutions.

Short-term production effects. As an acute disease, with relatively dramatic effects, malaria has been commonly assumed to have significant impacts on production. However, as with schistosomiasis, many of the studies providing estimates of production effects have poor empirical grounding.

The impact of malaria has been considered to involve negative influences on both labor and land productive factors; but none of the studies reviewed examines limitations on effective land supply; all focus on labor supply and efficiency effects. Unlike those of schistosomiasis, very few field studies have been done to directly measure output losses due to malaria. A number of studies have been based on questionnaire surveys of households. These studies include problems of reliability regarding respondents' self-diagnosis of malaria and their estimations of labor time lost owing to malaria episodes. Other studies, employing national statistics, use questionable assumptions about the actual number of days of labor lost per malaria case and the valuation of this lost labor [41].

The dominant field study, by Conly [42], has attempted to measure directly the production impact of malaria. In Conly's study, 69 farming families in eastern Paraguay were divided into three groups, based on whether they were much, moderately or little affected by malaria; and data on their farming activities were collected through the completion of fifteen forms during repeat visits over a period of twenty months [43]. Conly's study is richly descriptive of the diverse possible impacts of the disease and the coping patterns of households, but some uncertainties exist in interpreting the study for actual impact costs of malaria among the affected households. While the 12 "much malaria" families appear to have been substantially influenced, Prescott [44] has observed that the role of malaria is somewhat in doubt, since Conly did not analyze the share of malaria in total disability days. Unlike most other production impact studies, Conly's was not restricted to production for market, including both cash and noncash agricultural production of families. The study suggests, though the quantitative effect is not clear, that malaria-affected families stressed the production of their cash crops [45]. As noted previously, Conly's evidence on intrafamily adjustments—to attempt to maintain agricultural production when some family members had malaria—suggests the possibility that other production within the household may have been sacrificed, although specific information on this was not reported.

A recent study by Bonilla de Castro [46] assessed the production effects of malaria in Cunday, Colombia. It specified a mathematical model and, as units of analysis, utilized both households and individuals, among which four groups were recognized: students, salary or wageworkers, family helpers, and independent workers. Although the statistical results are unclear, it seems that no significant production effects were found. The study refers to absenteeism among the various groups due to malaria. It indicates that, along the lines of Conly's findings, the work of absent members was always taken over by nonsalaried family members, "who increase their work load in order to replace the ill worker, as well as to continue to carry out their own activities" [47]. The author suggests that the lack of significant production effects might be due to the fact that the form of malaria in the study area was *Plasmodiuin uiuax,* noted to be a mild strain [48].

A study by Brohult et al. [49] used bicycle ergometry to analyze the influence of malaria on physical capacity. It compared adult Liberian farmers living in holo-endemic rural areas, where malaria is ubiquitous, with mining company work; living in mesoendemic areas, where the population is partly protected: It concluded that physical performance was not influenced by malaria, since the measurement of working capacity was not lower in either the holo-endemic groups or in subjects with positive malaria smears. The comparison methodology of two distinctly different occupational groups raises some concern, however.

Long-term production/consumption effects. The dominant contributions here are the excellent studies by Barlow [50]. He estimated the long-run effects of malaria eradication in Sri Lanka, using a detailed general equilibrium model of the national economy and Newman's demographic estimates. Barlow's model, which takes into account the effects on capital formation as well as labor productivity, simulated per capita income in Sri Lanka during the 30 years following eradication, assuming eradication had not occurred, and compared the results with the actual observed values with eradication.

His model includes the assumptions, among others, that capital formation is directly determined by the amount of public and private savings, and that, labor inputs are expanded by eradication effects on the working-age population (via mortality and fertility impacts) and by decreased morbidity and debility among the work force. The results of the simulation showed that the positive productivity effect of the increased labor input due to eradication dominated in the short run (about the first eight years). Subsequently, however, the contribution of eradication was estimated to produce a greater growth in population than in income. This result occurred because eradication expanded the total population more rapidly than the work force and caused public non-investment expenditure to grow faster than taxes, resulting in reduced capital formation. Consequently, over the long term, per capita income was found to be lower (by about 6 percent by year 31 following adoption of eradication) with eradication than without [51].

Unfortunately, there have been no other long-term analyses for malaria in other geographical settings, and generalization of Barlow's statistical findings to other areas would clearly be untenable.

Intervention approach evaluation. Only one study has been reviewed in this area, though there are undoubtedly many other contributions by economists and other social scientists. (Authors Note 2001: The World Health Organization now has a special program called Roll Back Malaria which is an attempt to contain the major re-emergence of Malaria in the 1990's. Also the paper, Selection 6 in the present volume, is also a retrospective of the WHO Malaria Eradication effort).

Banguero [52] presented a methodology for the analysis of social, economic, and health determinants of malaria incidence in Colombia. A model for multiple regression analysis of malaria determinants was designed and tested with Colombian data. Among the variables found to be significant were demographic factors (sex, age, and number of persons in the household), occupational status, wage income, source of water and waste disposal, and certain preventive measures that were employed.

Summary. The studies by Barlow and Conly both represent excellent methodological advances in the study of the impact of tropical disease generally, as well as for malaria specifically. Nevertheless, we remain woefully ignorant of the social and economic effects of malaria in those countries of the world where it is still prevalent. The results of Barlow and Conly are valuable for their suggestions of future research efforts, but they cannot be generalized in simple fashion to other malarious regions.

Filariasis

Description. Filariasis is a general disease term, which applies to various forms of filarial parasitic infection. Prominent forms include Bancroftian and Brugian filariasis, transmitted by mosquitoes and producing attacks of fever, inflammation of the lymphatic system, a bronchial-asthmatic condition and, potentially, the dramatically disfiguring disease known as elephantiasis; Onchocerciasis (river blindness), transmitted by blackflies of the genus Simulian (associated with fast-flowing water) and producing uncontrollable itching as well as possible skin and vision disorders, with eventual blindness; Loiasis, transmitted by the red-fly Chrysops and producing itching and swelling in various parts of the body, including the eye; Dracontiasis (guinea-worm infection) transmitted by ingestion of water containing the crustacean Cyclops and producing localized inflamed sores which often involve the joints [53].

Health consumption effects and social and leisure effects. Given the dramatic nature of a number of the conditions associated with some forms of filaxiasis (especially disfigurement and vision impairment), exceptional health consumption and social effects seem likely for those so affected. However, no evaluations by economists or other social scientists are known to have been done in these areas.

Short-term production effects (market). Most of the studies that have been done in this area involve onchocerciasis. This may be because blindness, which May result from onchocerciasis, constitutes a particularly dramatic and unequivocal limitation. Evaluations of the production impact of onchocerciasis have involved both labor output effects and limitations on the effective supply of land. Labor productivity is expected to be affected primarily. through instances of blindness—reducing the amount of labor supplied—and through the diminished labor efficiency of those whose vision is impaired but who continue to work. Effective land supply is widely hypothesized to be affected by the discouragement, caused by the disease, of utilization of agricultural land near the watercourses, which are the breeding sites for the onchocerciasis vector.

A sampling of studies seeking to evaluate the production impact of onchocerciasis includes the following.

Waddy [54] described onchocerciasis in Africa, providing an essentially anecdotal account of the production impact of the disease. He cites a community in northern Ghana where, in 1948, nearly 20 percent of the men over 30 were blind: "Males in this age-group should be the mainstay of the community's labor force and it is unnecessary to stress the economic effects of blindness on this scale" [55]. Waddy also observes that since onchocerciasis does not itself shorten life, the economically unproductive blind have to be maintained. He suggests that the depopulation of river valleys may be the most serious economic effect of onchocerciasis, noting that a population-density map of the densely, inhabited area around the Red and White Volta rivers clearly showed the retreat of population from the rivers [56].

Williams [57] attempted to provide quantitative estimates of the economic benefits of onchocerciasis control in Ghana. He included as benefits the expected effects of onchocerciasis eradication on increased labor output, increased cultivation of new lands, and increased cattle production. His estimates, however, are admittedly based on guesses and assumptions. No eradication cost estimates was included in the study.

Bradley [58], in a Nigerian field study, also stressed the role of onchocerciasis in depopulating river basin areas. He determined that village desertion in the area studied was caused by several interconnected factors, of which onchocerciasis was only one—though perhaps the most important. Bradley also observed that while onchocerciasis was responsible for some out-movement, its principal effect seemed to be in deterring in-movement. His study does not attempt to evaluate the magnitude of economic losses due to the depopulation effect.

Evaluation of the other forms of filariasis has been relatively few. Kessel [59] offers a series of anecdotal reports on the production impact of filariasis, mentioning (based on a personal communication from Wilson) a rubber plantation that employed 600 laborers and experienced 150 attacks of filarial fever or lymphangitis a year, each attack lasting about three days [60].

Camacho [61] estimated a benefit-cost ratio for a filariasis control program in Sorsogon Province, Philippines. Productivity losses were calculated according to a series of questionable assumptions (including the prevalence, rate for workers, the number of attacks per year per infected worker, the average duration of the attacks, marginal product of lost work time equal to the minimum agricultural wage, etc.) without empirical verification.

Belcher et al. [62] studied the impact of guinea-worm disease on agricultural labor productivity in Southern Ghana. The methodology for the impact measurement was limited to the conduct of "a detailed interview...in 20 households in which the male head had been incapacitated by guinea-worm infection during the year." The interview included questions regarding length of disability, types of agricultural activity missed, and whether alternate labor sources had been used [63]. Besides the questionable reliability of this collection of information, its conclusions are rather vague: e.g., "untreated farmers were completely disabled for over five weeks and few households succeeded in finding alternate labor sources so that a major crop was lost. The cost of guinea-worm disease in a self-employed Ghanian farmer is not easy to measure but is clearly more than a month of laborer's fees" [64].

The questionnaire replies in the Belcher study indicated that families with incapacitated working members sought to shift work to healthier members, though the opportunities for such shifting, among the studied households, apparently were quite limited.

Long-term production/consumption effects. No work is known to have been done here.

Intervention approach evaluation. In a retrospective analysis of a control program for onchocerciasis in the Farako focus of Mali, Prescott [65] cites the need for improved cost information and especially for a mathematical transmission model capable of predicting the long-run effectiveness of alternative control techniques.

Prescott, Prost, and LeBerre [66] used the Onchocerciasis Control Program (OCP) in West Africa for an illustration of cost effectiveness weighting issues. The cost-effectiveness of the OCP was compared to that for measles immunization in Ivory Coast and Zambia according to four different choices of effectiveness measure. Onchocerciasis control was found less efficient according to three measures: per year of healthy life added, per productive year of healthy life added, and per discounted year of healthy life added. Onchocerciasis control was, however, found more efficient when the effectiveness measure used was per discounted year of productive healthy life added. This study illustrates the sensitivity of cost effectiveness results to the choice of measure.

Summary. Although a number of studies have dealt with measurement of short-term production effects (mostly for onchocerciasis), this methodology does not allow even tentative conclusions regarding short-term production effects for any of the filariases, and no study results were available for any of the other impact areas. Though only two studies were reviewed in the intervention evaluation area, it seems that useful methodological contributions are being made here.

African trypanosomiasis and Chagas' disease

Description. African trypanosomiasis (sleeping sickness) is transmitted by infected tsetse flies and produces fever, headache, joint pains, and—in progressive forms—lesions involving the brain, heart, and small blood vessels, leading to psychosis, somnolence, and coma. The disease has both a chronic and an acute form, transmitted by separate species of the trypanosome parasite.

Chagas' disease, the American variant of the trypanosome infection, is transmitted by bugs involving various species of *Triatoma* (also, rarely, by blood transfusion from infected donors). The disease may produce fever, malaise, swelling, diarrhea, and anemia, with possible 'mortality in the acute stage. During the chronic stage, severe heart damage and sudden mortality may occur. Transmission is commonly associated with poor housing and hygiene conditions, which provide a suitable environment for the triatomine bugs [67].

Health consumption effects, social and leisure effects. The severe symptoms and mortality associated with these diseases obviously have significant health consumption effects, although no evaluation by economists or other social scientists are known to have been done in these areas.

Short-term production effects (market). African trypanosomiasis is understood to have production impacts both through its influence on labor output and through its discouragement of land utilization in areas where the tsetse fly vector is widespread. Land supply effects have not been attributed to Chagas' disease.

Economists and other social scientists seem to have conducted few, if any, evaluation studies of the production effects of either African trypanosomiasis or Chagas' disease. Most of the impact estimates are anecdotal.

Wilson *et al.* [68], referring to African trypanosomiasis, state: "Not only does disease cause considerable human suffering, varying degrees of mortality and serious loss of efficiency wherever it occurs, but whole units of population may require to be moved out of infected areas with the consequent disruption of all human activity." They note that where one or more tsetse-fly species is prevalent, livestock is absent. Also: "A heavy expenditure of money and effort is necessary to provide the necessary drug-therapy to keep the disease in check." They conclude, "if tsetse flies could be controlled, the cattle production in Africa could be increased by 125,000,000 heads, or more than doubled with a consequent increase in the national—incomes and improvement in diet" [69]. The basis for the estimate is not indicated.

Concerning Chagas' disease, a WHO Study Group [70] commented: "Although no special evaluation of the economic harm caused by Chagas' disease has been made, existing data show that it must be very considerable. In the first place, the incapacitating symptoms of the chronic forms of the disease generally develop in the second half of life when the individual is making his greatest contribution to society. Secondly, the disease is found principally in rural areas where those affected are often rendered incapable of the heavy physical work demanded of them" [71].

Intervention approach evaluation. Limited attention has been given to the economic and social aspects of transmission.

Apted et al. [72] have identified some of the occupations, which carry increased risk of trypanosomiasis infection. For men, these include hunting and especially fishing. Female occupations at risk are collection of both firewood and mushrooms.

Davies [73], studying the factors influencing trypanosomiasis in Botswana, noted that due to the fact that most of the traveling and hunting was done by men, giving them greater tsetse contact, the disease was largely acquired by adult males. He also observed that the groups, which were more dependent on cattle, tended to live away from tsetse-belt areas, which was not the practice of those groups that did not own cattle.

As mentioned above, poor housing conditions are linked to transmission of Chagas' disease. The triatomine bug vector finds excellent shelter and breeding places in "dirty poorly lit houses, built of adobe, mud or cane, with numerous cracks in the walls or partitions and with a large number of accumulated household objects" [74].

Summary. Studies reviewed concerning African trypanosomiasis and Chagas' disease depends mainly on anecdotal information for impact estimates. No economists or other social scientists were involved in any of the evaluations of these diseases.

Leishmaniasis

Description. The leishmaniases are a heterogeneous group of different diseases, transmitted by the bites of sandflies, producing a wide variety of symptoms. Effects may range from trivial, self-healing sores to irreparable disfiguring lesions. In visceral leishmaniasis, or kala-azar, effects include irregular fever, increasing enlargement of the liver and spleen, anemia, progressive wasting and without treatment—probable death within two years [75].

Health consumption effects, social and leisure effects. No studies by economists or other social scientists are known to have been done in this area.

Short-term production effects. In the past, some leishmaniasis disease forms may have had significant effects on land supply as well as labor output. Moskovskij and Duhanina [76] refer to Sen Gupta's statement that previous epidemics of kala-azar caused large tracts of agricultural land in India to lie fallow, owing to migration of populations. The authors note that while these epidemics apparently no longer menace India, the possibility of new mass epidemics in other developing countries may remain a threat [77].

No empirical evaluations seem to have been conducted.

Intervention approach evaluation. Saf janova [78] noted that the economic activities of mankind are of great importance in determining the epidemiological situation for leishmaniasis foci. The author stresses that careful recording and analysis of these factors, as they develop, are essential for leishmaniasis control.

Leprosy

Description. Leprosy is a chronic communicable disease, believed to be transmitted through prolonged skin-to-skin contact with an infectious person, via a bacillus agent. The disease has a number of forms, ranging from benign to malign, and a wide spectrum of clinical effects. It is most commonly associated with skin lesions, as well as deformities and mutilations, which result from nerve damage [79].

Health consumption effects, social and leisure effects. According to a WHO study group: "The implications of M. leprae infection for morbidity and mortality are still not clearly defined. It is believed that only a minority of infections may present any clinical manifestations...Leprosy is not generally considered to be a fatal disease, but there are several studies indicating that death rates are higher among leprosy patients than among non-affected individuals in the same population" [80]. Given the strong personal prejudice associated with the disease, considerable social as well as health consumption (grief) effects resulting from that prejudice appear certain to exist, although no empirical studies of them have been reviewed.

Production effects. No studies on either short-term or long-term production effects are known.

Intervention approach evaluation. Mutatkar [81] states that social prejudices and ignorance about the disease are considered to constitute major hindrances to control. He also stressed the need for cost-effectiveness studies to evaluate alternative approaches to leprosy control [82]. No empirical studies were reviewed.

Summary. No studies were reviewed for any of the evaluation areas.

Conclusion

We still know distressingly little about the overall economic effects (health consumption, social and leisure, production) of tropical diseases. Among the studies containing some degree of sophistication and rigor, we so far have limited findings for schistosomiasis and malaria alone. The schistosomiasis studies largely concern the area of short-term market-oriented production, with some work on longer-term production/consumption factors (mortality and fertility, academic performance). For malaria, sophisticated studies of production effects are few, though Conly's Paraguay study encompasses some elements of nonmarket, in addition to market, production. We also have some innovative work on long-term demographic effects of malaria in two countries, and long-term production/consumption effects for one of these countries (in each case, the information is retrospective after eradication).

For the other tropical diseases, virtually no systematic studies have been conducted in any of the economic effect areas. For schistosomiasis and malaria, no studies have been done to evaluate health consumption and social effects. Even the findings on short-term production effects for schistosomiasis (the focus of most of the small number of more sophisticated studies) can be questioned. While the results are, in any case, somewhat mixed, one can argue that the production effect findings are limited by, e.g., their biased sampling of worker categories (relative to typicality of disease severity), by the lack of representativeness of the geographic areas in terms of infection intensity and disease severity, and by the restricted focus on market production, ignoring possible trade-offs from household and other nonmarket activity.

Most of these shortcomings in the study of short-term production effects could, in principle, be remedied by carefully designed studies representing a range of infection intensities, geographic areas, and types of employment, and nonmarket as well as market activity. With improved epidemiological information, it may be possible to develop predictive estimates of the demographic effects of these diseases for various areas.

On the other hand, the analysis of health consumption and social interaction effects requires further methodological development. A major concern is whether it is possible to establish meaningful, noncontroversial numeraires for quantifying various aspects of health consumption and social effects. Then, there is the problem of whether or not it is possible to achieve acceptable aggregation of these numeraires within the health consumption and social effect categories. Finally, assuming such aggregation is obtained within these categories, can these categories be further aggregated with each other and with production effect measurement?

While such aggregation is certain to be difficult and controversial, the alternative is to require resource decision-makers to comprehend and sum up (mentally aggregate) the diverse individual effects. The first step in this area will probably require additional information from epidemiologists on prevalence and intensity of infection for the tropical diseases, followed by the cooperation of epidemiologists and economists in the development of numeraires for health consumption and social effect evaluation [83].

We are still left with the problem of how to measure many of the subtle, synergistic; often long-term effects of tropical diseases—including those affecting innovation, risk-taking, and how life is perceived. It has been speculated that these aspects may represent the more important effects of tropical diseases, but we do not really know how to go about measuring them.

It seems evident that hard thought should be given to whether researchers investigating tropical disease effects should continue to examine such limited areas of impact as short-term market production. At this point, it appears that emphasis ought to be placed on the development of methodologies for including nonmarket (especially household) production, health consumption, social and, to the extent possible, longer-term effects of tropical diseases.

Work in the second broad research area reviewed, evaluation of intervention alternatives, is more promising. Though it is in its early stages, and does not lack problems of methodology and disputed findings, the efforts of economists and other social scientists seem to have advanced the possibilities for determining efficient selection from alternative disease intervention strategies. Continued efforts in this area appear highly worthwhile.

EVALUATING THE IMPACTS OF TROPICAL DISEASE

The preceding review of social and economic research on the six tropical diseases of the Special Programme indicates, that despite the considerable attention given to evaluation of the impacts of the diseases, much of the work to date has been methodologically flawed or constrained in such ways as to limit the conclusions one can draw. Given the prevalence of these problems throughout the studies, we regard it useful to review these deficiencies here.

Evaluation issues

We have identified the following problems associated with impact evaluation studies of tropical diseases.

Assuming production losses. A few of the earlier labor productivity studies merely assigned, without empirical evidence, assumed losses of productive' capacity to workers infected with tropical diseases. These assumptions of production losses have generally failed to be supported by other empirical studies [84].

Different disease states. A number of difficulties arise in connection with differentiating between persons with different disease states [85]:

a. An infected person is not necessarily a diseased (functionally impaired) person; and the extent (state) of severity may vary greatly among those with a given tropical disease infection.
b. Available diagnostic measures for some of the diseases imperfectly distinguish the states of severity of the disease, or even sometimes between those who are and are not infected.
c. The measures of infection intensity that are sometimes relied on may not have a linear relationship with disease severity.
d. Studies of schistosomiasis in particular have been criticized for dealing with areas of low disease severity overall, as well as for failing sufficiently to' distinguish between disease severity 'states within the areas selected.

The problem of discrimination of severity state has largely been the result of diagnostic deficiency rather than study design. Studies done in low-severity areas may not offer results that are valid for areas of higher severity, nor would findings from high-severity areas be valid for low-severity areas. (As discussed later, the extent to which results can be extrapolated between geographic areas is debatable, even given comparable severity levels, owing to variation in factors influencing activity responses to severity states.) Further, disease severity levels in certain geographic locations. may change naturally over time, increasing or decreasing, either because infection levels in individuals change owing to evolving or altered transmission dynamics, or because disease severity advances with continued exposure of an individual to a given level of infection intensity, or, perhaps, because of developing immunity responses in infected persons [86].

Naturally, it is critical for a study to include a reasonably typical range of severity states of a disease (recognizing possible variation by age, sex, and site) in the community studied. It may also be desirable, to consider whether and by what amounts disease prevalence and severity levels appear to be increasing or decreasing under the existing environmental and socioeconomic circumstances of the community.

Limitations on activity. Persons may also experience nonlinear activity effects under varying levels of disease severity. It has been hypothesized that people have certain (limited) physiological reserves, which, within ranges of disease severity, allow those having a tropical disease to maintain customary levels of work and other activity [8?]. Beyond some threshold level, for when either the severity of the given disease increases or some new disease is superimposed, these physiological reserves may no longer be able to compensate and activities will be affected. Individuals also might be affected during shorter periods of high activity, when their reserves are stressed. It has therefore been argued that failure to recognize the "using up" of physiological reserves because of tropical disease infection may understate the cost of disease.

The amount of physiological reserves before disease infection may vary among persons in different locations, depending on inherited—health stocks (perhaps reflecting nutritional or genetic influences), or other, earlier health problems.

The physiological reserve hypothesis appears plausible and also seems consistent with evidence of the nonlinear relationship of effects and infection intensity. On the other hand, it is not well understood (1) to what extent there is a cost in using up otherwise unused reserves; (2) in what proportion of cases there is a cost because the reserves at some point are exhausted (i.e., activity is reduced), either because of (a) high infection intensity of the given tropical disease alone, (b) intermittent activity stresses, or (c) combination with another disease.

For the issue of effects on production and social activity perhaps only the instances in which reserves are exhausted are relevant. Study requirements would then include (as they should in any case) assessing disease impacts across a reasonably typical range of activity, including a typical (relative to the community the results intend to describe) range of disease severity states, both with respect to different levels of infection intensity of the particular disease and with respect to the interaction with other causes of ill health in the community. Still, study results may be limited to the particular state of disease severity at a site at a given time, not easily allowing for evolving disease severity patterns over time.

A series of studies concerning schistosomiasis in East Africa (with some overlap among the researchers involved in the separate studies) have sought to investigate the impact of disease on physiological capacity through controlled laboratory tests, as opposed to observation of productivity differences under actual working conditions. These studies have yielded varying results: Davies [30] found that schistosomiasis infection produced no effect in the physiological responses to exercise by 40 children using a stationary bicycle ergometer. Omer

107

and Ahmed [31], however, found significant differences in the responses to a stepping test for infected and uninfected Sudanese male nurses. But Collins et al. [32] again found no infection-related differences in physiological responses of 194 Sudanese sugar cane workers to a bicycle ergometer test [88]. Awad el Karim et al. [33] noted significant adverse physiological responses, again using a bicycle ergometer, among 19 severely Infected canal cleaners. The study—found no significant differences between those who were lightly infected and those who were uninfected (both groups consisting of villagers who were not involved in canal cleaning work). The results of this study are extremely interesting, indicating that physical capacity, in the instance of schistosomiasis, may only be affected at high levels of infection intensity; however, the extent to which actual activities are affected under such infection intensities remains uncertain.

Utilizing a rather different approach, Kvalsvig [89] observed the spontaneous activity of children attending two primary schools in Natal, finding that infected subjects tended to have higher activity levels than uninfected subjects [90]. There was, however, a fall in activity levels among individuals with high egg counts and among those with both S: *mansoni* and S. *haemotobium,* especially under hot, humid conditions, when the decline in activity was greater than that of the control subjects. The results were interpreted by the author as indicating that high-intensity infections may affect activity under more stressful conditions [91].

Brohult et al. [49], as discussed earlier, used bicycle ergometry to test the working capacity impact of malaria on Liberian men. They found no significant effect on physiological work capacity for the tested workers.

Representativeness of populations studied. Impact studies have tended to concentrate on workers employed on agricultural estates or other organized industries. Studies of such workers have been much easier to implement, given the organized work environments and available work records. However, the findings of such studies may be poorly representative of disease impacts for the general populations of these countries, which are usually dominated by peasant farmers. Two difficulties have been pointed out: (1) these estate and other organized workers might be associated with a natural selection process whereby those employed in these areas are less severely infected/diseased or have superior physiological reserves; (2) the work environments, type of work, or the compensation procedures associated with these employments may elicit atypical responses to the tropical disease state.

The first difficulty, suggesting the possibility of bias in disease severity representation, reemphasizes the need for studies to include a full range of disease severity states, taking into account their representation in the studied community. Possibilities for selection biases among any working group must be carefully evaluated. The second difficulty, regarding the possibility of biases in measured production activity responses according to employment, might either be treated as a hypothesis to be tested separately by comparing workers in various organized and non-organized work environments, or by simply making impact studies more comprehensive by including a typical range of employment activity. Study cost considerations may be an inhibiting factor, however.

Household work adjustments. Even among those who work primarily on their own farm plots, the impact of disease may be partially masked by intrahousehold adjustments in work assignments. It is possible that healthier household members may substitute for those who are suffering from a tropical disease in order to maintain work on the household farm plot.

For estimating production and social impact costs, we need to know what activities are sacrificed, if any, in connection with the intrahousehold adjustments. Do those who substitute temporarily delay other productive activities abandoned, or only? Or is production activity maintained at the expense of household chores, childcare, school attendance, community activities, or valued leisure—some of which might also have longer-term production impacts? Alternatively, adjustments might be made at relatively low cost, to the extent that they involve household members who are largely without duties during the substitution periods. (Even if no alternative duties are sacrificed costs will—still arise if the foregone leisure is valued.)

A number of researchers, including Popkin [92] have advocated the development of a broader framework for examining tropical disease impacts, focusing on the household. The proposed framework would include all dynamics of the household, including market and home production, social interactions, and interchangeability between these activities. Popkin notes that the "New Home Economics" framework; at its most general level, offers a means of examining interrelated issues of household behavior. It emphasizes the value of time within the household and notes the importance of considering nonmarket aspects of behavior in assessing household welfare [93].

Since few studies focus on household responses to tropical diseases, the empirical evidence regarding intrahousehold adjustments is dominated by a single study, that of Conly [42] previously described, on the effect of malaria on farming families in eastern Paraguay. Conly's descriptive study suggests that other household members did tend to substitute for those who were ill to maintain certain areas of farming activity; however, among the families observed such substitution was not adequate to prevent production losses. This study did not provide details on the activities sacrificed by those who substituted for ill members of the household.

The previously described study of guinea worm disease in southern Ghana, by Belcher et al. [62], based on an interview of twenty households in which the male head had been "incapacitated" by guinea worm infection during the year, identified the shifting of farming chores to healthy family members as the first step toward minimizing work loss. The study indicates, however, that even among households with several adult men, the opportunities for such shifting may have been limited, since the other men were usually also affected. Housewives were noted to be heavily burdened with household chores and childcare and unable to do more than the lighter farm work [94].

Household agricultural adjustments. Households may also respond to disease by shifting the emphasis given or attention devoted to different crops, perhaps attempting to maintain cash crops, at the expense of neglecting noncash crops. The primary evidence regarding this hypothesis is provided again by Conly [42], who observed that the families affected by malaria devoted a larger proportion of available labor to the principal cash crops at the expense of food crops. This suggests that a study, which simply focused on the level of market production, might understate the impact of this tropical disease.

Deficient estimation of losses in labor production. In economies with appreciable unemployment, evaluation of labor productivity losses under the assumption that in the absence of tropical disease the lost labor time caused by it would be a net increment to employment will be likely to overstate the loss. On the other hand, the system of labor exchange in these countries may operate imperfectly; thus, labor productivity losses, even in labor surplus economies may not be well met by existing unemployed labor. Further, despite substantial average unemployment during the year, there may be periods of critical demand for labor during certain periods, such as when crops are planted and harvested [95]. Many studies have ignored the probability of obtaining net employment additions, corresponding to estimated labor. productivity losses, in the absence of the tropical disease, taking the above factors into account. Studies have also employed simplifying assumptions about the marginal productivity of labor supply losses due to tropical diseases. The use of measures of average product, legislated minimum wage, or even average agricultural wage may poorly represent the actual marginal product of the potential labor supply increment [96]. Another problem is that, even where the use of an existing wage reasonably represents the current marginal productivity of labor under the disease situation, the elimination of the disease, given a substantial labor supply effect, may well alter the marginal productivity of labor [97].

Deficient estimation of losses in land supply. Studies of the effect of tropical disease on land supply have usually not produced conclusive results. Mainly involving malaria, onchocerciasis and trypanosomiasis, their estimations of the inhibiting effects of these diseases on the settlement and employment of lands have been of highly uneven quality, being frequently conjectural and often based on controversial assumptions [98].

Prescott [99] has reviewed analyses of land supply effects of onchocerciasis and trypanosomiasis. He observes that onchocerciasis was only one of many causes of depopulation of river valleys where onchocerciasis transmission occurred [100].

In his estimates of possible land supply effects from onchocerciasis eradication in northern and upper Ghana, Williams [57] notes that any movement to new land would probably begin four to five years after the start of an eradication program and would not become substantial until eight to ten years after initiation of the program [101].

Barlow [84] pointed out that the output increases determined by health improvements through resource relocations have generally been exaggerated, since estimations have usually not adequately recognized the offsetting decrease in the areas from which the human and financial resources migrate [102].

Uncertainty effect of disease. In addition to short-run adjustments in response to immediate disease impact, individuals and households may make long-run adjustments. The added uncertainty due to threat of disease may, for example, lead to adoption of work activity patterns that involve less economic risk should disease occur, but which have a lower return than the activities that would be selected in the absence of disease threat.

To the extent that hypothesized long-run adjustments affect all members of a community, including those who do and do not have the disease during a study period, these adjustments will be especially difficult to identify, measure, and evaluate.

Regarding adaptation patterns associated with threat of disease, Conly [42] inferred that the threat of malaria among farm families in eastern Paraguay contributed to the growing of manioc, which was apparently regarded as a sort of insurance crop, since it withstands considerable neglect, does not need to be harvested at any particular time, and can be left growing until a family finds harvesting convenient [103].

Deficiency of short-term estimations. The short-run, partial equilibrium approach of most studies may overlook a number of other significant effects of tropical disease. Gwatkin [19] writes: "Many of the channels through which improved health might be expected to influence output are long ones. This applies especially to changes in the relationship among factors of production: one cannot expect quickly to produce more technological innovation or more entrepreneurial behavior by simply curing a couple of bouts of diarrhea. It is quite unlikely that people who have been chronically ill since birth and have adopted a lifestyle consistent with their debilitated condition can be rehabilitated and made effective workers immediately" [104]. And Rosenfield [2] notes: "Large-scale, plantation agriculture has been observed to have replaced labourers with machines in order to guarantee a supply of essential effort because reliance on workers placed crops in substantial jeopardy" [105]. From a household perspective, it has been suggested that a major effect of tropical diseases may be a reduction in families' qualitative investment in their children [106]. On the other hand, Barlow points out that societal saving may be inversely correlated with the dependency burden, which will tend to be reduced by the existence of disease [107].

Long-run impacts of tropical disease on intellectual development and innovative activity remain largely speculative, although some studies [108] have sought to measure the short-run impact of disease on academic performance [109].

Stevens [110] conjectures that the long-run impacts of impaired health status are more important than those observed in the short run. However, researchers have found it to be extremely difficult to provide empirical evidence on the presumed long-run adverse impacts of tropical disease.

Still another partial equilibrium difficulty, emphasized by Andreano [111], is that the prices that exist in developing countries reflect the existing distribution of income and wealth. To control or eradicate tropical diseases will affect this distribution. If the benefits of control or eradication are calculated on the basis of the existing distribution, they may be different—perhaps lower—than those that would be calculated according to the post-eradication or control distribution [112].

Deficiency of estimation of demographic effects. A particular shortcoming of the partial equilibrium, short-run approach of most studies, which may give substantially, misleading results, is to disregard demographic and capital formation effects of tropical diseases [113]. The control of a disease may affect population growth through a reduction in mortality associated with the disease, as well as through an increase in fertility. Consequent long-term demographic effects may influence per capita income through the increased size of the population among which, the total product (which may be enhanced by factor supply and productivity effects) is to be distributed, as well as through influences on capital formation which are determined by the demographic effects.

Official statistics often provide extremely poor information regarding the contribution of tropical diseases to mortality, owing to the presumed frequent indirect influence of these diseases on death and as Newman observes, the existence of deep ambiguities in the term "cause of death" [114]. Official records, of course, provide no direct information on the fertility impact of tropical diseases.

A study by Newman [40] on the demographic effects of malaria eradication in Sri Lanka and Guyana succeeded in splitting the post-eradication crude rate of natural increase in the population into two segments: autonomous increase, and that resulting from the eradication of malaria. Newman attributed 60 percent of the acceleration in Sri Lanka's population growth to malaria eradication, 40 percent, in the case of Guyana. This estimation demonstrated the existence of the suspected multiple ratio between the actual and official mortality impact of malaria and offered quantification of this ratio for these two countries.

Newman provided an extremely valuable statistical and methodological advance in estimating the demographic impact of tropical disease. Nevertheless, Prescott, noting the significant difference in the demographic effects of malaria control found by Newman for Sri Lanka and Guyana [115];—observed that Newman's procedure, involving comparison of autonomous and observed changes in demographic indices, is not relevant to the problem of predicting future demographic effects of malaria control. The demographic effect will differ between countries and will have a wide margin of error [116].

As described in a previous section, using simulation modeling and Newman's demographic estimates for Sri Lanka, Barlow explicated the dynamic influence of the labor supply and capital formation effects of malaria eradication in Sri Lanka and, in turn, the long-term influence of these effects on Sri Lanka's per capita income [50].

Gwatkin [19] comments that mortality and fertility rates have fallen substantially since the period on which the Newman and Barlow studies were based. Consequently, further declines in mortality would not be likely to exert a similar constraint on economic expansion [117].

The effort by Weisbrod et al. [14] to estimate the true mortality and natality impacts of tropical disease has been described in an earlier section. In this study, regression analyses using household survey data for two St. Lucian valleys failed to find any association between schistosomiasis and either mortality or natality [118].

Multiple disease effects. Where persons are commonly infected with multiple diseases, evaluating the separate impacts of individual tropical diseases is methodologically and statistically difficult. On the other hand, efficient interventions may apply to more than a single disease [119] and the interactive impact of the combination of diseases controlled is not likely to equal the sum of individual disease impacts assessed separately. Given the existence of hypothesized synergistic effects between diseases, the evaluation of individual diseases regarded in—isolation will understate their actual impacts when they occur, as is usually the case, in combination with other diseases.

Dual causality. The fact that the activity of individuals may not only be affected by tropical diseases but may also influence the likelihood and intensity of disease infection for these persons can easily introduce biases into studies which fail to take this dual causality into account. It has been suggested that persons who are naturally more active may, in some instances, experience greater frequency of contact with tropical disease vectors and thus become more highly infected than those who are less active. Similarly, where disease transmission is linked with some employment activity, those who have been engaged in the activity longest, and thus are the most experienced, may also have the highest infection levels [120]: Failure to recognize and specify these relationships may lead to underestimation of actual impacts.

Conclusion

It is clear from this review that a wide variety of effects have received at least some research attention. It is not clear that economists' contributions have had any greater power or significance than the work of other scientists, yet there does seem to be a trend in recent work by economists that draws from a larger part of the framework of economic analysis than classical cost-benefit research. Viewing disease impacts in a household production/consumption framework looks very promising. Our review has shown a heavy emphasis on limited areas of impact, especially short-term market production. A household framework would make expansion of nonmarket effects more revealing. And from the perspective of the economist, the disease impact studies, with few exceptions, have not grappled with the possible longer-term impacts on such things as risk taking, innovation, and life perceptions that affect personal savings, life outlook, and the willingness to invest in human capital of all kinds. It is our belief that modeling longer-term disease impacts has some promise and could offer a useful blending of what economists have to offer with what our fellow medical scientists believe.

EVALUATING TROPICAL DISEASE INTERVENTIONS

Productivity impact studies alone may increase our understanding of the significance of tropical diseases in a community, extending our appreciation beyond quantitative evidence or whatever intuitive sense may exist concerning health consumption loss and social impairments as a result of the diseases. However, without analyses of the costs of disease intervention [121] and the epidemiological effects of the control measures, nothing can really be said as to (1) whether or not it is actually worthwhile to allocate scarce resources to controlling a disease; or (2) which control approach, given the existence of technical alternatives, ought to be selected from an economic efficiency perspective. It is quite possible that whether or not it is deemed worthwhile to allocate control resources will depend on the individual control approach considered. It may therefore appear more straightforward to ask, first, which is the most efficient control approach, and then whether this approach is worthwhile. However, many countries are already deciding to allocate resources for tropical disease intervention before they have completed cost benefit analyses. Consequently, cost-effectiveness studies alone can be valuable.

Evaluation issues

Following are some of the issues concerning evaluation of control approaches by economists and other social scientists.

The time horizon. Many of the earlier impact studies were based on the implicit assumption of immediate and complete eradication as the single intervention option. The inference was that total disease impact costs represented (immediate) intervention benefits. More' recent studies have emphasized that either eradication or control interventions will result in a gradual transition between disease states within the target community.

Depending on the specific time pattern of the disease state transition—and, more specifically, the time pattern for alleviation of production, health consumption, and social impacts—as a result of an intervention program, different present-value assessments of the benefit of the intervention will result. Thus, in addition to knowing by what amount a given disease state and its associated impacts will be reduced, it is also important to know when these reductions will be realized, as well as the amount and timing of intervention expenditure. It is possible that one intervention may generate superior aggregate reductions (per expenditure unit) in disease impacts, but may be considered inferior to another intervention that generates somewhat smaller reductions (per expenditure unit) but in a shorter time period.

Information on the impact of control measures on disease epidemiology and the cost pattern of the control measure is therefore necessary for both cost-benefit and cost-effectiveness studies. Cost effectiveness studies, requiring only the measurement of physical benefits (production, health consumption, or social) generated by disease interventions, are somewhat easier to undertake than cost benefit studies in which analysts are faced with the methodologically difficult problem of assigning monetary valuations to the physical benefits.

The measurement unit. While cost-effectiveness studies eliminate the need for monetary valuation of the benefits of control approaches, they still require assessment of the various benefits of individual interventions according to some standardized (at least within a benefit class, if not across benefit classes) measurement unit(s). This is necessary since the different intervention approaches, which are to be compared, will undoubtedly produce different quantitative effects of the various health impacts of the tropical disease [122]. A major factor in selecting effectiveness measures has been the ease of obtaining reliable information meeting the requirements of these measures. Given that separate, alternative interventions are likely to produce different impact patterns with respect both to categories of health (mortality and morbidity) and health effect on activity, it would be desirable to include the broader span of relevant health impacts in the evaluation.

115

However, efforts to aggregate the different categories of disease impact on health are subject to considerable controversy, especially because of the need to incorporate judgments on the appropriate weighting, of the separate impact categories [123]. Where the interest of the study is in extending the boundaries of research knowledge regarding the separate areas of disease impact, there may be reason for separate description of the impact categories [124].

On the other hand, officials who are currently making decisions on allocation of resources are forced, on the basis of whatever little information may be readily known to them, to determine weighted aggregations of health impacts, possibly through some poorly structured process. Prescott remarked: "the question is not whether but how aggregate health benefits should be integrated with aggregate income benefits in the appraisal of health programs" [125].

The different effectiveness measures used take into consideration various aspects: number of lives saved; increase in healthy days of life; increase in the number of persons protected against a specific disease; or reduction in the number of cases (or prevalence rate) of a specific disease [126]. In commenting on these measures, Barlow observed [126] that "number of lives saved" is generally regarded as a rather narrow rule, especially with respect to diseases whose principal impact may be on morbidity. The measure based on the number of persons protected is also unsatisfactory because it may be ambiguous as to the contribution of an intervention to "protection."

Reduction in number of cases of a disease is the measure perhaps most commonly employed. A variant of the latter measure, reduction in number of case-years of disease, seems more informative, however. Analysts who use this measure include Rosenfield, for schistosomiasis [37] and Prescott, for onchocerciasis [65].

"Increase in number of healthy days of life" is an appealing effectiveness measure in accounting for different patterns of mortality and morbidity alleviation associated with various interventions. The measure was, advanced by the Ghana Health Assessment Project Team [127] and Morrow [128] and has also been used by, among others Prost and Prescott [129] for onchocerciasis, Prescott [130] for schistosomiasis, and Prescott, Prost, and Le Berre [66] for onchocerciasis.

The "days of healthy life added" measure suggests better capability of representing the range of health impacts of a disease than the measure involving number of cases (or case-years) prevented. Accordingly, as employed by the Ghana Health Assessment Project Team, the former measure is amenable—though not without controversy—to comparing interventions across a number of different diseases. In Ghana this measure was used to evaluate the comparative impact of 48 disease problems, in assessing priorities [127, 128].

The "days of healthy life lost" statistic, as used by the Ghana Team, is subject to a. number of measurement problems that can significantly affect the comparative results. As admitted by the team's researchers, the data required for the estimations are not available from routine sources, requiring resort to consensus. Also, the approach attributed mortality and sickness to single diseases, whereas a combination of diseases may well be involved. Further, other social and economic consequences of diseases are implicitly assumed to be proportional to the health index components (incidence, disability and case fatality rate) [131].

Another proposed effectiveness measure, which has some intuitive appeal, is that of added "quality-adjusted life years." However, this measure seems also to involve considerable measurement problems. Further, as Thompson and Fortess [132] point out, it is hard to specify just what life quality is. Probably because of these difficulties, this measure has not been used to any great extent.

In addition to the issue of the weighting of health impact categories, the use of specific aggregative measures has been criticized for omitting for giving a zero weighting to) certain classes of disease-intervention benefits. Berman [133], for example, complains that a multifaceted problem cannot be solved in an acceptable way by any single decision criterion [134].

There also exist problems of accounting for when the impacts are alleviated by an intervention and which population groups benefit from the impact alleviation. The use of discounting procedures to reduce credit for the alleviation of impacts occurring comparatively late relative to those that occur quickly, is generally accepted [135].

More controversial is whether there should be age-preference weighting, to give greater credit, for example, to productive healthy years than to those years, which are associated with non-productive ages. A similar issue is whether disability years (where consumption requirements continue) should be accorded greater weight (i.e. considered a more costly impact) than premature death years [66, 136].

Another factor in weighting benefits is to take into account the impact of the intervention on social objectives of income distribution by recognizing the extent to which given impact alleviations benefit the wealthy vs. the poor [137].

As a resource allocation tool, the assigned weights should, as Feldstein notes, "reflect the value judgments of the responsible government official...The process of assigning weight is obviously difficult, but it is also clearly unavoidable. Any rational method of choosing among programmes must reflect such a set of relative values even if these are never made explicit" [138,139].

The economic and social context of disease transmission. In seeking optimal intervention strategies, social scientists have begun to stress the importance of understanding the role of economic and social influences on tropical disease transmission [140]. These influences may include the economic and social environment in which people live as well as behavioral aspects—the day-to-day economic and social activities of individuals, which bring them into contact with disease transmission processes. Recognizing people's beliefs and attitudes about diseases and about various approaches for preventing or controlling diseases may be necessary for the design and implementation of successful control programs [141]. It can also be useful to investigate the possibility of eliciting community participation in control efforts and the implications of such participation for control program effectiveness [142].

Effects of development projects. It is now widely recognized that major development projects, especially those involving water resources, as well as the settlement of new lands may have significant adverse consequences for tropical disease transmission. Economists and other social scientists, besides evaluating the potential tropical disease consequences of such projects, may help us understand whether (1) efficient means can be found for modifying these projects to limit their adverse influences on disease transmission; or (2) separate compensatory control projects should be added to the planning of the disease-contributing project [143].

The use of mathematical models. The need for improved predictive information on the dynamic impact of alternative interventions on transmission has led some economists to join in the mathematical modeling of tropical disease transmission. The modeling efforts, thus far restricted to schistosomiasis, have sought in particular to recognize the human behavioral aspects of transmission and to allow predictions of (a) the impact of water resource projects on transmission; and (b) the cost-effectiveness of alternative interventions.

Rosenfield has led modeling research to investigate the impact of water resource projects on transmission. A schistosomiasis transmission model originally developed by Rosenfield, Smith, and Wolman [37], based on data from a pilot irrigation project in Iran, was later modified by Rosenfield [37] on the basis of St. Lucia data to take account of human behavioral aspects in transmission. The later model was used by Rosenfield to evaluate the cost-effectiveness of four alternative control strategies in St. Lucia. The output of the model is age-specific prevalence rate, allowing the estimate of case years of infection prevented by the alternative control strategies. As. noted by Prescott [130], this output measure does not provide information on the amount of morbidity and mortality associated with the prevented case years.

Bekele and Golladay [38] have recently provided a significant advance in mathematical modeling in their development of a model, also for schistosomiasis, which they characterize as "phenomenological." The model allows each of its terms to be revised in each time period as a function of both natural processes and control activities. This model permits the identification of dynamically efficient strategies of control according to an optimal selection of control activities. Model output, however, is still based on prevalence rather than morbidity and mortality.

Valuing costs. The actual measurement of the costs of interventions against tropical disease requires particular care, especially in developing countries where market prices may not well represent opportunity costs. Where controlled exchange rates and other price distortions are present, the use of shadow prices may be called for. Rosenfield, Golladay, and Davidson [144] note that inadequacies of accounting and monitoring systems may force investigators to develop their own cost estimations. Kaewsonthi [122] emphasizes those outsiders conducting cost and performance studies of any disease control program face great difficulties in really understanding systems and procedures and collecting information to measure what occurs in practice. Further, intercountry comparisons will be difficult because of different budgeting and accounting systems, different views on costs, and different structures of the organizations responsible for the disease control programs [145].

Conclusion

This review indicates the promising contribution of economic analysis to research on tropical diseases. Perhaps because the problems have more definitive parameters, traditional economic analysis has been (and can be) very helpful in formulating resource allocation strategies. Our caution here is that economists take the time and effort to learn what medical scientists know before formulating analyses of intervention approaches. The conventional tools of economists seem, nevertheless, to have sufficient application in this area for us to urge their continuance as a research priority.

THE FUTURE: SOME CONCLUDING COMMENTS

This paper has covered a complexity of issues and analyses, but its contribution and message are fairly simple. They can be summarized as follows.

1. There has been an extraordinary amount of research on tropical diseases; a lot of it is flawed, but a lot of it has real potential for policy.
2. The traditional discipline of economics used in the research we covered has scratched only a part of what the power of economic analysis might offer.
3. There are still areas of great policy significance about which little or no research has been done or is underway.
4. The next generation of research on tropical diseases (and health in general) in Third World countries must use more tightly framed methodologies and more rigorously structured hypotheses. In this, economic analysis can be helpful beyond the boundaries of classical

cost-benefit analysis, which to date has dominated intervention studies, and the economics of market production, which has dominated impact studies.

5. The best research—i.e., research that has the best chance of affecting policy that in turn improves levels of well-being—will require hard economic analysis. But such analysis must be tempered by the insights of other social and medical scientists. The simplicity of economic models and underlying values and assumptions can inhibit analysis and at the same time make that analysis yet more powerful. Research on disease questions must strike a balance between good research, important questions, and applicable methodologies.

Finally, it is our view that to make progress beyond what has been reviewed and examined here will require a generation of economists and social scientists indigenous to Third World countries. The problems as, posed by economists and medical scientists from the industrialized countries are often short of the mark, especially when one views the policy intervention potential of such research. We also feel, quite strongly, that because field information is so difficult, costly, and time consuming to collect, a proper role, which WHO could support, would be the assembling of a computerized data bank from studies done around the world. While data from one country setting do not transfer so easily to another, it is still true that some central questions 'can cut across in useful ways. A computerized data bank available to researchers for training as well as original research purposes could lower the cost of such research in Third World countries and make possible a larger number of scientists willing to take part in research on health and tropical disease questions.

Acknowledgement—The fine review by Anne Mills and Margaret Thomas, *Economic Evaluation of Health Programmes in Developing Countries (Eva*luation and Planning Center, London School of Hygiene and Tropical Medicine, 1984) was very helpful in our attempt to locate studies relevant to this paper.

REFERENCES

1. See Andreano R.L. World economic conditions and health for all. World Health Forum, *WHO*, Geneva, forthcoming.
2. Concerning the person afflicted by disease, epidemiology distinguishes between infection, involving the invasion of a person by a disease organism, and the disease state, involving damage to the person as a result of the invasion. Epidemiologists also refer to intensity of infection, involving the number of invading organisms and the severity of disease,

reflecting the extent of damage done by the disease organism. In referring to the effects or consequences of disease, we imply the existence of some impairment (physiological, psychological, emotional, social, etc.) that ultimately results from the disease organism. The selection of subjects for a study by researchers may include persons in the "disease" category who, while infected, have low infection intensity and/or low disease severity and/pr low (or no) impairment. It is also possible that very low levels of impairment due to a disease may not be measurable. For a further elaboration of this issue, see Rosenfield P.L., Golladay F. and Davidson R.K. The economics of parasitic disease: research priorities. *Soc. Sci. Med.* 19, No. 10, 1117-1126, 1984.

3.   Evaluation according to "willingness to pay" (WTP) has been advocated by some. This approach would, in principle, capture individual preferences concerning the value placed on alternative states of health. (Lost earnings as well as health enjoyment effects of disease would be reflected.) See Dunlop D.W. Theoretical and empirical issues in benefit identification, measurement and valuation related to parasitic disease control in poor countries. *Soc. Sci. Med.* 19, No. 10, 1036, 1984 for a discussion of the WTP concept and attempts to operationalize it. Carrin C. Economic evaluation of health care interventions: a review of alternative methods. *Soc. Sci. Med.* 19, No. 10, 1016-1017, 1984 points to some of the problems in accurately determining WTP which has led researchers to seek alternative methods. Some of the other methodologies that have been explored to obtain valuations of health (implicit private valuations, risk-compensating wage differentials, and explicit public valuations) are briefly summarized by Prescott N. and Warford J. Economic appraisal in the health sector. In *The Economics of Health in Developing Countries* (Edited by Lee K. and Mills A). Pp. 136-137. Oxford University Press, Oxford, 1983 though these approaches may be more suitable for developed than for developing countries.

4.   The need for research attention in this area has been emphasized by Rosenfield P.L., Widstrand C, C. and Ruderman A.P. How tropical diseases impede social and economic development of rural communities: a research agenda. *Rural Africana* 8-9 (Fall-winter), 12-14, 1980.

5.   Some studies categorize treatment and avoidance expenditures as "direct" costs of disease, and the losses related to factor input effects as "indirect" costs. In other studies, however, the labeling of these categories is reversed. The terms are probably not particularly useful in any case and, given their inconsistent application, may as well be avoided.

6.   This review retains usage of the somewhat redundant phrase "economic and social effects," although "social effects" are also a matter of economic cost.

7.   Given time and other research resource limitations, it is likely that numerous relevant studies have been missed by this review.

8.   This description is drawn from a number of sources, but particularly from WHO. Report of the second scientific working group on social and economic research: guidelines to assess the social and economic consequences of the tropical diseases. TDR/SER-SWG (2)/80.3, 37-39,1980.

9.   While mortality represents an unambiguous impairment, degrees of morbidity require specification. The Second Scientific Working Group on Social and Economic Research proposed a classification system denoting levels and accurateness of impairment; See WHO [8], pp. 10-16. It is not yet clear, however, whether such classifications may provide a basis for economic evaluation of health consumption effects.

10. WHO. Measurement of the public health importance of bilharziasis. Report of a WHO Scientific Group, WHO Technical Report Series No. 349, pp. 44-45, WHO, Geneva, 1967.

11. WHO. Epidemiology and control of schistosomiasis. Report of a WHO Expert Committee, WHO Technical Report Series No. 372, p. 12, WHO, Geneva, 1967.

12. See WHO [8], p. 38.

13. Given the various concerns, described earlier, regarding methodological problems, as well as likely geographical specificity for many—if not all study findings reviewed here, these findings should, of course be regarded cautiously.

14. Weisbrod B.A., Andreano R.L., Baldwin R.E., Epstein E.H., and Kelley A.C. *Disease and Economic Development: The Impact* of *Parasitic Diseases in St. Lucia.* University of Wisconsin Press, Madison, 1973.

15. See [14], pp. 109-113.

16. The fact that a study does not deal with an area of "high" infection intensity, does not, of course, diminish its value. Naturally, findings of appreciable disease effects obtained from high infection-intensity areas could no more be suggested to be relevant to areas of lower infection intensity than can findings of low disease effects, from low or moderate infection-intensity areas be suggested to be relevant to areas of higher infection intensity. Given the enormous difficulty of selecting a single area, which perfectly typifies all areas in infection intensity (lack of sufficient epidemiological information to specify what is "typical" and the likelihood of nonlinear relationships between infection, disease severity, and economic effects), one is left with selecting several different infection intensity areas, which collectively describe the range of infection intensity experience.

17. See Rugemalila J.B., Asila J., Chimbe A. *Schistosomiasis haematobium* and the mortality occurring in an endemic community at Bujashi, Tanzania, *Trop. Geog. Med.* 37, No. 2, 114-118, 1985.

18. A study by Cohen J.E. Some potential economic benefits of eliminating mortality attributed to schistosomiasis in Zanzibar. *Soc. Sci. Med.* 8, 389-390, 1974, using published data, estimated that the elimination of schistosomiasis in Zanzibar would have increased life expectancy at birth in 1960 by about 1.8 years and would have extended the life of the average male in 1960 by 2.3 years. Utilizing various assumptions, Cohen also estimated the production effect of this mortality. The author emphasizes, however, the inadequate nature of the data used.

19. See Gwatkin D.R. "Does better health produce greater wealth? A review of the evidence concerning health, nutrition, and output", unpublished A.I.D. document (August), p. 16, 1984.

20. See [14], p. 22.

21. See Prescott N.M. The economics of schistosomiasis and development. *World Development.* 7, 1-4, 1979

22. See [19]. p. 45.

23. See Foster R. "Schistosomiasis on an irrigated estate in East Africa: III. Effects of asymptomatic infection on health and industrial efficiency." *J. Trop. Med. Hyg.* 70 (August), 185-195, 1967.

24. See Fenwick A: and Figenschou B. M. The effect of *Schistosoma mansoni* on the productivity of canecutters on a sugar estate in Tanzania. Bull. Wld. Hlth. Org. 47, No. 5 (May), 567-572, 1972.

25. See Gateff C., Lemarinier G., Labusquiere R. and Nebout M. Influence de la bilharziose vesicale sur la rentabilite economique d'une population adult jeune du Cameroun. *Annales de la Societe Belge de Meaecin Tropical* 51, No. 3, 309-324, 1971.

26. The Gateff study was not reviewed directly. The discussion here is drawn from the comments of Gwatkin [19], pp. 48-49, and Prescott [21], pp. 6-7.

27. See Baldwin R.W. and Weisbrod B.A. Disease and labor productivity. *Economic Development and Cultural Change,* 22, No. 3 (April), 414-435, 1974.

28. See Weisbrod B.A. and Helminiak T.W. Parasitic diseases and agricultural labor productivity. *Economic Development and Cultural Change,* 25, No. 3 (April), 505-522, 1977.

29. See Barbosa F.S. and Pereira da Costa D.P. Incapacitating effects of *Schistosomiasis mansoni* on the productivity of sugar-cane cutters in north-eastern Brazil. *Am. J. Epid.* 114, No. 1, 102-111, 1981.

30. Davies C.T.M. Energy expenditure and physiological performance of Sudanese cane cutters. *Br. J ind. Med. 33,* 181-186, 1976.

31.   Omer A.H.S. and Ahmed N. el din. Assessment of physical performance and lung function in Schistosomiasis mansoni infection. *E. Afr: Med. J.* 51 (February), 217-222, 1974.

32.   Collins K.J. et al. Physiological performance and work capacity of Sudanese cane cutters with Schistosomiasis mansoni infection. *Am. J. trop. Med. Hyg.* 25, No. 3 (May), 410-421, 1976.

33.   Awad el Karim M.A. et al. Quantitative egg excretion and work capacity in a population infected with Schistosomiasis mansoni. *Am. J. trop. Med. Hyg.* 29, No. 1 (January), 54-61, 1980.

34.   See Andreano R.L. The recent history of parasitic disease in China: the case of schistosomiasis, some public health and economic aspects. *International Journal of Health Services 6,* No. 1, 53-68, 1976. This study investigated possible demographic effects for twelve schistosomiasis-infected provinces of China for the period 1953-64. The results do not significantly support a demographic effect for schistosomiasis in these provinces. The study was, however, dependent on speculative evidence regarding prevalence changes during the period, as well as other imperfect information from China.

35.   See [14], pp. 68-72. Weisbrod et al. include a review of other studies of the association between schistosomiasis and academic performance (pp. 68-70).

36.   Social scientists have begun to participate in elucidating some of the behavioral aspects of schistosomiasis transmission and the implications for control. See e.g. Dalton P.R. A sociological approach to the control of Schistosoma mansoni in St. Lucia. *Bull. Wld. Hlth. Org.* 54, 587-595, 1976.

37.   As described in a later section, these issues have been dealt with in Rosenfield P.L. The management of schistosomiasis. Research Paper R-16, Resources for the Future, Washington, D.C., 1979; and Rosenfield P.L., Smith R.A. and Wolman M.C. Development and verification of a schistosomiasis transmission model. *Am. J. Trop. Med. Hyg.* 26, No. 3, 505-516, 1977.

38.   The modeling research of Rosenfield [37], Rosenfield, Smith, and Wolman [37], and Bekele A. and Golladay F.L. An optimal approach to planning efficient strategies of schistosomiasis control. Unpublished World Bank document, November 1984, is discussed in a later section.

39.   This description is drawn principally from WHO [8].

40.   See Newman P. Malaria Eradication and population growth, with special reference to Ceylon. Bureau of Public Health Economics Research Series No. 10, School of Public Health, University of Michigan, Ann Arbor, 1965; Newman P. Malaria control and population growth, Journal *of* Development Studies 6, No. 2 (January h 133-158,1970.

41. Some of these studies have been reviewed in Prescott N.M. The economics of malaria, and trypanosomiasis. Paper prepared for UNDP/World Bank/WHO Special Programme for Research and Training in Tropical Diseases, WHO, Geneva, February 1979.
42. Conly G.N. The Impact of Malaria on Economic. Development: A Case Study. Pan American Health Organization, Scientific Publication No. 297, 1975.
43. As a result of the relatively high unit cost of conducting this descriptive study, the sample size of the study was rather small: There were 41 farms in the "little malaria" group, 16 in the "moderate malaria" group and 12 in the "much malaria" group. The author notes that the sample size did not allow the usual statistical tests to be applied informatively, but states that the interpretation of the findings "rests primarily on consistency among many small indicators which add up to a convincing picture of the effects of illness on these farm families" [42, p. 83]. The author also recognizes the problem created by the fact that the group used as a comparison standard, the 41 farms with "little malaria," was not, as would have been desirable, malaria-free [42, p. 87].
44. See [41], pp. 25-29.
45. See [42], p. 4.
46. Bonilla de Castro E. Development of research training project in socioeconomics of malaria eradication in Colombia, executive summary. Unpublished report to Special Programme for Research and Training in Tropical Diseases, WHO, Geneva, 1985.
47. See [46], p. 2.
48. See [46], p. 3.
49. Brohult J. et al The working capacity of Liberian males: a comparison between urban and rural populations in relation to malaria. *Annals of Tropical Medicine and Parasitology* 75, No. 5, 487-494, 1981.
50. See Barlow R. *The economic effects of malaria eradication,* Bureau of Public Health Economics, Research Series No. 15, School of Public Health, University of Michigan, Ann Arbor, 1968 (also in American Economic Review Papers and Proceedings 57 (May), 130-148, 1967); and Barlow R. and Davies C.W. Policy analysis with a disaggregated economic-demographic model. J. *Publ. Econ.* 3, 43-70, 1974.
51. See Barlow and Davies [50], p. 52.
52. Banguero H. Socioeconomic factors associated with malaria in Colombia. *Soc. Sci. Med.* 19, No. 10, 1099-1104, 1984.
53. This description is drawn principally from WHO [8, pp. 41-43] and Nelson G.S. Research as an aid to filariasis and onchocerciasis control. In Health Policies and Developing Countries (Edited by Clive Wood and Yvonne

Rue), pp. 167-172. Royal Society of Medicine, International Congress and Symposium Series No. 24, Grune and Stratton, New York, 1980.

54. See Waddy B.R. Prospects for the control of onchocerciasis in Africa. Bull. Wld. Hlth. Org. 40, 843-858, 1969.

55. See [54], p. 844.

56. See [54], p. 845.

57. Williams D. The probable economic effects of the eradication of onchocerciasis in Northern and Upper Ghana. Unpublished WHO document, PD/70.1, 1970.

58. Bradley A.K. Effects of onchocerciasis on settlement in the Middle Hawal Valley, Nigeria. *Trans. R. Soc. Trop. Med. Hyg.* 70, No. 3, 225-229, 1976.

59. Kessel J.P. Disabling effects and control of filariasis. Am. J. *Trop. Med. Hyg.* 6, 402-414, 1957.

60. See [59], p. 409.

61. Camacho V.M. Control of filariasis in the province of Sorsogon imperative to economic growth. *Philippine Journal of Public Health* 13, *Nos. 1* and 2 (July-March), 19-44, 1968-69.

62. Belcher D.W., Wurapa F.K., Ward W.B. and Lourie I.M. Guinea worm in Southern Ghana: its epidemiology and impact on agricultural productivity. *Am. J. Trop. Med. Hyg.* 24, No. 1, 243-249, 1975.

63. See [62], p. 244.

64. See [62], p. 248.

65. Prescott N.M. On the prediction of effectiveness in economic analysis of onchocerciasis control programmes, with reference to the Farako Focus, Republic of Mali. Magdalen College, University of Oxford, unpublished, 1980.

66. Prescott *N.,* Prost A. and LeBerre R. The economics of blindness prevention in Upper Volta under the onchocerciasis control program. *Soc. Sci. Med. 19,*No.10, 1051-1055, 1984.

67. This description is drawn from WHO [8], pp. 45-46, 49-51, and WHO. *Comparative Studies of American and African Trypanosomiasis.* Report of a WHO Scientific Group, WHO Technical Report Series No. 411, WHO, Geneva, 1969.

68. Wilson S.G., Morris K.R.S., Lewis I.J. and Krog E. The effects of trypanosomiasis on rural economy. Bull. Wld. HIM. *Org.* 28, 595-613,1963.

69. See [68], pp. 595-596, 611-612.

70. WHO. Chagas' *Disease,* Report of a Study Group, WHO Technical Report Series No. 202, WHO, Geneva, 1960.

71. See [70], p. 11.

72. Apted F.I.C., Ormerod W.E., Smyly D.P., Stronach B.W. and Szlamp E.L. A comparative study of the epidemiology and endemic Rhodesian sleeping

sickness in different parts of Africa. *J. Drop. Med. Hyg. 66* (January), 1-16, 1963.

73. Davies J.E. Sleeping sickness and the factors affecting it in Botswana. J. *Trop. Med. Hyg.* 85, 63-71, 1982.

74. Zeledon R. Epidemiology, modes of transmission and reservoir hosts of Chagas' disease. In *Trypanosomiasis and Leishmaniasis With Special Reference to Chagas' Disease*, pp. 51-85, Ciba Foundation Symposium 20 (new series), Associated Scientific Publishers, Amsterdam, 1974.

75. See [8]; pp. 53-54.

76. Moskovskij S.D. and Duhanina N.N. Epidemiology of the leishmaniases: general considerations. Bull. *Wld. Hlth Org.* 44, 529-534, 1971.

77. See [76], p. 529.

78. Saf'janova VM. Leishmaniasis control. Bull. Wld. *Hlth. Org.* 44, 561-566, 1971.

79. See [8], pp. 55-56.

80. WHO. *Epidemiology of Leprosy in Relation to Control,* Report of a WHO Study Group, WHO Technical Report Series No. 716, WHO, Geneva, 1985.

81. Mutatkar R.K. Social and economic aspects of leprosy. 1:JNDP/World Bank/WHO Special Programme for Research and Training in Tropical Diseases, unpublished WHO document, TDR/SER-LEP/KL/81.4, p. 5, 1981.

82. See [81], p. 13.

83. It is conceivable that a method (such as a workable willingness to pay approach) might be developed that would shortcut the requirement of further epidemiological information.

84. For a review of this issue in the area of schistosomiasis studies, see [14], p. 22 and [41], pp. 2-4. See also Barlow R. Health and economic development: a theoretical and empirical review. In *Research in Human Capital and Development* (Edited by Sirageldin 1.), pp. 45-75, Putnam Press, Greenwich, Conn., 1979.

85. The various aspects of this issue have been discussed by a number of authors. See, especially, Rosenfield P.L. Schistosomiasis transmission and control: the human context. IIASA Conference, The Management of Pest and Disease Systems, October 22-25, WHO document TDR/SER/(SC1/80.5), 1979; [2], pp. 1118-1119; and [21], p. 4.

86. Except for malaria, which may have little cumulative effect, the diseases of the TDR program are chronic and may produce gradual, cumulative damage ([2], p. 1118). Some researchers have conducted studies which follow up earlier studies at given sites to examine hypotheses of evolving severity over time. Weisbrod and Helminiak [28] followed up an earlier labor productivity study of schistosomiasis on a banana estate in St. Lucia,

conducted by Weisbrod et al. [14] two years earlier. Also, Fenwick and Figenschou [24] did a schistosomiasis study on a sugar estate in Tanzania investigated five years earlier by Foster [23]. The Fenwick and Figenschou analyses involved different dependent variables than the analyses of Foster, however, and so did not directly test the validity of the evolving severity hypothesis. (These studies are reviewed elsewhere in this paper.)

87. [14], p. 86; and Workshop on the development of guidelines to assess the social and economic consequences of the tropical diseases. UNDP/World Bank/WHO Special Programme for Research and Training in Tropical Diseases, October, TDR/SER/SWG(2)/80.3, 1980.

88. The subjects of the Collins et al. study were also observed under field working conditions, in addition to the laboratory testing. The infected workers were found to cut a statistically significant greater amount of cane than the uninfected workers. It was speculated that the infected workers had greater experience, which in turn was correlated with their exposure to infection.

89. Kvalsvig J.D. The effects of schistosomiasis on spontaneous play activity in black schoolchildren in endemic areas. Sa *Mediese Tydskrif,* July 11, 61-64, 1981.

90. Like Collins *et* al. (previous note), the author hypothesized that there was selective exposure to infection by more energetic children. (This hypothesis was preferred to the alternative hypothesis that infection determines higher activity levels. This preference was considered consistent with the accompanying evidence of decline in activity among those who were highly infected.)

91. See [88], p. 63.

92. Popkin B.M. A household framework for examining the social and economic consequences of tropical diseases. *Soc. Sci. Med.* 16, 533-541, 1982.

93. See [91], p. 538.

94. See [62], p. 248.

95. See Rosenfield (1984) as cited in [2], p. 1122.

96. See [21], pp.4-6.

97. See Dunlop, cited in [3], p. 1036. Other problems created by the use of partial equilibrium analysis are discussed in a later section.

98. Evaluations of results of the Onchocerciasis Control Programme in West Africa were not available for this review. It is possible that this major disease control effort may produce more conclusive results regarding the influence of onchocerciasis on effective land supply.

99. See [41], pp. 47-52.

100. See [41], p. 49.

101. See [57], p. 7.

102. See Barlow [84], pp. 68-59.
103. See [42], p. 94. Andreano has remarked: "the real developmental importance of control or eradication...will come from the synergistic effects in a dynamic sense on how life is perceived now, on attitudes toward family and home, and on the behavioral attributes of daily life...the removal of health as a daily, constant barrier around which life must take place will surely have impacts that transcend their sudden removal or reduction" (Andreano R.L. Economic impact studies on parasitic disease: a select review of research since 1973. In *International Congress* of *Parasitology Proceedings* 2, 86, 1982
104. See [19], pp. 10-11.
105. See Rosenfield, as cited in [2], p. 1123.
106. See Bekele and Golladay, cited in [38], p. 7. *This* represents an aspect of human capital theory. *Thus,* the possible reduction in care, attention and education received by children due to disease burdens of families is seen as diminished investment in their children, which will also diminish their children's future production/earnings capability.
107. See Barlow [84], p. 60.
108. See for example [14], pp. 68-72.
109. Attendance and performance of children in school, which may be influenced by tropical diseases, represent an input into "intellectual development. It is also possible that some tropical diseases might otherwise affect intellectual growth—either by directly interfering with the development of mental capacity during childhood or as a result of engendered apathy, diminishing the nurturing of mental capacity.
110. Stevens C.M. Health and economic development: longer run view. Soc. Sci. *Med.* 11, 809-820, 1977.
111. Andreano R.L. Economic issues in disease control and eradication. Soc. Sci. *Med.* 17, 2027-2032, 1983.
112. See [111], p. 2029.
113. Barlow [84] notes that the appropriateness of partial analysis depends on the size of the analyzed impact relative to the total system. Thus, where the labor supply impact is fairly small relative to the size of the labor force, a partial analysis may be adequate; however, where substantial labor supply impacts on the labor force are present, use of partial analysis will tend to give misleading results [84], p. 56. On the other hand, according to a more broadly defined view of partial analysis,—its use may also overlook the possibility of various trade-offs between observed market production and unobserved nonmarket production, or may ignore synergistic and other long-term consequences of tropical disease, thus biasing the measured production effect downward.
114. See [40], 1970, p.134.

115. While the postemedication acceleration in population growth for the two countries differed substantially, Newman has noted that in both Sri Lanka and Guyana eradication accounted for 0.7 of a percentage point of the subsequent crude rate of natural increase. See Newman P. Discussion of R. Barlow's paper, "The economic effects of malaria eradication." American Economic Review, Papers and Proceedings 57 (May), 155-157,1967.

116. See [41], p. 19. In a study of estimated lasses due to malaria mortality and morbidity in Thailand, Kuhner discusses (in a footnote) consideration of extrapolating the Newman findings to Thailand according to adjustments suggested by experienced malariologists. Due to the difficulty of obtaining "reasonable and scientifically founded coefficients," the Newman ratios were not applied. See Kuhner A. The impact of public health programs on economic development: report of a study of malaria in Thailand. International Journal of Health *Services* 1, No. 3, 285-292, 1971.

117. See [19], p. 25.

118. See [14], pp. 65-68.

119. See Prescott N. and de Ferranti D. The analysis and assessment of health programs. *Soc. Sci. Med.* 20, No. 12, p. 1238, 1985.

120. For illustrations of the model specification difficulties presented by this sort of dual causality, see the earlier discussion (in footnotes) of some of the results of the study by Collins et al. [32] and Kvalsvig [89].

121. A disease intervention might include: (1) eradication—the complete elimination of disease transmission; (2) control—reducing the level of transmission; (3) acting to constrain circumstances, which might enhance the likelihood of transmission. In this review the term "control" will be broadly used to indicate any of these intervention strategies.

122. Kaewsonthi has argued that comparisons to determine which of two or more approaches is most cast-effective is really valid only when (1) the processes are true alternatives (i.e., are not complementary), (2) the processes achieve the same percentage of effectiveness given the same target, and (3) conditions (existing cases, geographic factors, population density, migration) are the same for each approach. See Kaewsonthi S. Cost and performance appraisal of malaria surveillance and monitoring measures. Final report to Special Programme for Research and Training in Tropical Diseases, May 1983.

123. Multi-attribute problem analysis is suggested as a way of choosing among health projects where a number of attributes are involved, without having to weight the attributes and combine them into a single measure. For s discussion of the MPA methodology, see Carrin C. Economic Evaluation of *Health Care* in *Developing* Countries, pp. 102-111. St. Martin's Pres New York, 1984.

124. See "Workshop,, [87], p.10.

125. Prescott N.M. Comment on article by D.J. Bradley. *Epidemiology and Community Health* 33, No. 1 (March), 71-73, 1979.

126. Barlow R. Costs and benefits of controlling parasitic diseases. Center for Research on Economic Development, University of Michigan, unpublished, pp. 3-4, January 1985.

127. Ghana Health Assessment Project Team. A quantitative method of assessing the health impact of different diseases in less developed countries. *Int. J. Epid.* 10, No. 1, 73-80, 1981.

128. Morrow R.H. Jr. The application of a quantitative approach to the assessment of the relative importance of vector and soil transmitted diseases in Ghana. *Soc. Sci. Med.* 19, No. 10, 1039-1049,1984.

129. Prost A. and Prescott N. Cost-effectiveness of blindness prevention by the onchocerciasis control programme in Upper Volta. *Bull. Wld. Hlth. Org.* 62, No. 5, 795-802, 1984.

130. Prescott N.M. Evaluation of the economic impact of schistosomiasis and benefits of control: current views. Unpublished WHO document, SCH/ED/WP/84.47, 1984.

131. For an elaboration of some of these problems, see Carrin [123], pp, 99-101.

132. Thompson M.S. and Fortess E.E. Cost-effectiveness analysis in health program evaluation. *Evaluation Review* 4, No. 4 (August), 549-568, 1980.

133. Berman P.A. Selective primary health care: is efficient sufficient? *Soc. Sci. Med.* 16, No. 10, 1054-1059, 1982.

134. Similarly, Rosenfield, Golladay, and Davidson argue "a range of consequences needs to be described to indicate to the decision-maker the entire spectrum of such consequences, since there is not one generally agreed upon measure"([2], p. 1125).

135. The appropriate discount rate for weighting future vs. current benefits and costs of interventions is, however, subject to debate. To the extent that there is a disparity in the relative time patterns of intervention benefits and costs, the favored intervention may be sensitive to the discount rate that is chosen. Carrin [3], p. 1018, summarizes some of the issues regarding discount rate choice. While a popular method of dealing with selection of the appropriate discount rate is to offer estimations based on two or more rates, as a form of sensitivity analysis, Klarman feels that this method does not well serve decision-makers (Klarman H.E. The road to cost-effectiveness analysis. *Milbank Memorial Fund Quarterly of Health and Society* 60, No. 4, 585-603, 1982).

136. Abel-Smith argues strongly against such weighting. See Abel-Smith B. (with A. Leiserson). *Poverty, Development and Health Policy.* Public Health Papers No. 69, WHO, Geneva, 1978.

137. Squire L. and van der Tak G. Economic *Analysis of Projects. A* World Bank Publication, Johns Hopkins University Press, Baltimore, 1975.

138. Feldstein M.S., Piot M.A. and Sundaresan T.K. Resource allocation model for public health planning: a case study of tuberculosis control. *Bull, Wld. Hlth. Org. 48,* Supplement, Chapter 6, 75-78, 1973.

139. On this point, see also Stoddart C.L. Economic evaluation methods and health policy. *Evaluation and the Health Professions* 5, No. 4 (December), 393-414, 1982.

140. Rosenfield [85] has emphasized this. For related research in this area, see Banguero [52]; and Andreano R.L., Helminiak T.W. and Li J.Y. The world distribution of schistosomiasis: some quantitative economic comparisons. J. Trop. *Med. Hyg.* 77 (August), 170-176, 1974.

141. Among those who have done studies on this subject, see: Hongvivatana T. Illness behavior of patients at a malaria clinic in Bor Ploi District, Kanchanaburi Province, Department of Social Sciences, Faculty of Social Sciences and Humanities, Mahidol University, unpublished, February 1982; Hongvivatana T. Integrated vector control at a community level: socioeconomic and cultural aspects, unpublished WHO document, VBL/ECV/EC/82.16, 1982; Hongvivatana T., Leerapan P. and Smithisampan M. An observational study of DDT house spraying in a rural area of Thailand, *J. Trop. Med. Hyg.* 85, 245-250, 1982; Ogunmekan D.A. Control of malaria with special reference to socioeconomic factors, *Tropical Doctor* (October), 185-186, 1983.

142. Studies related to this issue have been done by Rajagopalan P.K. and Panicker K.N. Financial rewards ensure community involvement. *Wld. Hlth. For.* 6, 174-176, 1985; and Hongvivatana T. Knowledge, perception and behavior of malaria. Final report submitted to UNDP/World Bank/ WHO Special Programme for Research and Training in Tropical Diseases, unpublished, n.d.

143. Bradley observes that deteriorating health as a result of economic development is widespread. He notes that while health cost should be added to other costs of development, the matter has been handled in practice (if at all) by setting aside an arbitrary sum for the mitigation of undesirable effects. "The economics of health as a component of development has not been handled in a systematic manner, partly for the good reason that too many medical as well as economic uncertainties are involved" (See Bradley D.J. Prevention of disease in the tropics: questions in health economics. *Epidemiology and Community Health* 33, No. 1 (March), 66-73, 1979).

144. As cited in (2), p. 1123.

145. See [122], pp. 32-34.

SELECTION 8

THE PHENOMENON OF HEALTH CARE REFORM: U.S., EUROPE, ASIA, AND LATIN AMERICA[37]

INTRODUCTION

The worldwide effort to reform systems of health care finance and delivery gained urgency after the 1978 WHO Alma Ata meeting, commonly known as the "Health for All by the Year 2000" declaration. It was not so much that the Health for All declaration itself had policy impact on countries, but rather it focused world attention on how far short countries were (in the developing and developed worlds) in providing affordable and efficient health care delivery systems for their populations. World-wide disparities in access to services, a skewed distribution of health resources toward acute, hospital based care, and flawed, inefficient and unequitable finances for services were brought into focus by the Alma Ata declaration. A health sector policy paper by the World Bank (1987), a pioneering study of health care in Asia (1987) by the Asian Development Bank, a series of quantitatively sound analyses of the health care systems of industrial countries by *OECD*, and finally the landmark 1993 *World Development Report on Health*, all have since the Alma Ata declaration shaped our knowledge of health care systems, their problems and the need for reform. These studies have shown where systems have perhaps gone wrong, and what policies and programs which might, tend to make all health care systems both more efficient and equitable.

In all these studies some common themes have emerged and with a few exceptions these themes transcend the wealth and economic growth of countries, affecting both rich and poor, and fast or slow growing economies. At the risk of simplification let me summarize the most important findings and commonalities across all systems.

1. Rising public and professional expectation in what medicine can and should accomplish.
2. Changing patterns of disease, the emergence of new diseases (such as AIDS), and the reappearance of old diseases (e.g. malaria).

---

[37]Paper presented to CIEMEX-WEFA Meeting, "Macro-Economic Tendencies in Mexico: 1994-2000/Health and Social Security," Morales, Mexico 13th-15th July 1994.

133

3. Major demographic shifts: in rich countries, the aging of the population, in poor countries the preponderance of younger (perhaps bi-model) age groups mainly from population growth and the effectiveness of public health interventions.

4. Advances in Medical technology both in diagnostic equipment, but also in new therapies and interventions, and drugs.

5. Inefficiencies in delivery systems. Health care services are produced in systems that are basically inefficiently organized. There is usually little relationship between capacity of services and utilization of services. Consequently, hospitals, the central unit in the health care production system, have tended to dominate delivery systems. Primary care has come to be viewed as hospital rather than community oriented. Thus, to produce health services in virtually any type of a delivery system usually involves an inefficient and cumbersome, hence expensive, delivery and treatment system.

6. Inefficiency in Finance Systems. In any delivery system regardless of type, the method of financing services generates an inefficiency of incentives for use on providers, consumers, and even governments themselves. Removing barriers to payment for services (ala Sweden and U.K.) does not insure that the delivery system will operate efficiently or that the expenditures of the system will be contained at a socially acceptable level of quality. When utilization pushes against resources, price or non-price rationing is resorted to, and benefits are eliminated or restricted ("queuing" for elective survey, or denying treatment on the basis of age, are examples). In social insurance financed systems there is no coherent structure between payment for services and the value of services. And in fee-for-service insured systems, incentives are all biased against practicing cost-effective medicine.

7. Worldwide expenditures on health care have risen dramatically, and with but few exceptions, without a comparable increase in health performance. There have been some dramatic gains in Life Expectancy (LE), and Infant Mortality Rates (IMR) in the developing world in the past 15 years. But most authorities attribute these gains to improvements in public health (water supply, sanitation, immunization, nutrition) and not conventionally delivered health care services.

In summary all industrialized countries (and to a similar extent all developing countries) are facing grave issues in health services. The problem can be stated quite simply: in rich countries and poor the demand for health services is outstripping a country's capacity to pay for these services.

Demand for services is rising worldwide because of variety of factors as noted above: such as, population growth, new technology, new diseases, and changing preferences and attitudes. In many rich countries, demand and the cost of services is growing faster than a country's wealth. These problems and observations seem as true for health care systems that are mostly private and market driven (such as U.S.A.), purely publicly financed systems (such as U.K.) and for the in-between variety of mixed public/private systems as exist around the world including countries such as Mexico which rely heavily on social security funds to finance services.

It is useful to make a distinction a this point between how health services are financed and how they are delivered: the following diagram illustrates the possibilities. A system can be publically financed (through general or specific taxes, and/or general government revenues) and it can have services delivered privately with all facilities and providers not government employees. Alternatively a system can be privately financed (through payroll taxes, government contributions, etc.) and have services delivered in public or quasi-public institutions where all the inputs are under government employment and control. Two other options are: public finance and delivery, and private finance and private delivery [WHO 1993 (a)]. The presence of insurance—private or social—makes the most likely form a combination of both public and private financing and delivery. Key issues under any pure or mixed system is how revenues are collected to finance services and how providers and institutions are paid for delivery for services or if they have an internal system of pricing.

Financing	Delivery of Services

Public
   (Taxes, government Budget)
	Public/Quasi Private
	   (Government hospitals, Clinics, MD's salaried)

[Social Insurance] **Private/Quasi Public** Employment-based Insurance-(payroll taxes) (Co-insurance, deductibles)	[Social Insurance] **Private/Quasi Public** Private Hospitals, Clinics, Private Practice (Profit/not for Profit)

Payment Sources

FFS (fee for service)
Salaried
Capitation
Revenue Sources
Taxes, income, general, payroll
User charges
Copayments
Subsidies

In evaluating the performance of health care systems, economists use a number of concepts:

1. Efficiency
2. Equity
3. Health outcomes
4. Quality

As demand and utilization rise it is increasingly clear that most health care systems have large elements of inefficiency and waste. In public systems thought to be "free", large and costly queues and travel times do not allocate services as efficiently as prices and produce inequity and inefficiency. Incentives to economize on service use by consumers are minimal; incentives of service providers to produce care and services economically do not exist. In private systems waste and inefficiency arise out of the provision of services being driven by payment mechanisms such as fee-for-service. Inequities exist in all systems, however financed. In public systems the opportunity costs of different income groups ration services through waiting times and this produces inefficiencies and inequities. In private systems if you cannot pay for care, are unemployed, or are uninsured, your access to the health system is restricted if not excluded.

The health outcomes measured against spending do not correspond as one would hope. Many countries spend less than their wealth would indicate they could spend but get better performance [World Development Report 1993, p. 54]. In others the result is just the opposite. Quality of care is also a problem. In public systems there are few incentives to keep technology current, to be sure care is appropriate, and to have provision of drugs, diagnostics, and therapies in supply sufficient to meet demand. In other systems, technology drives the costs of the system and produces often a two-tier level of quality: high quality for those who can pay, and low quality for those who can't.

These issues—efficiency, equity, health performance, and quality—are at the core of how well or how badly a health care system functions and are our perspective for observing the phenomenon of health care reform. The rising tide of demand for more services worldwide runs up against these issues when questions arise about how health services are financed. In rich countries with private or mixed systems, health care costs have risen automatically and inequities have increased. In systems largely publicly financed (either through general taxation or from central government revenues and budgets) the rising demands have run up against budget constraints. The demand for services is rising faster than governments can or are willing to pay for them (or to increase taxes to pay for them). Consequently public systems produce large inequities as a result.

HEALTH CARE POLICIES

The worldwide response to these problems has varied but some common themes have emerged. Three themes have emerged:

1. To install in health care systems, more competition and market driven incentives.
2. More government regulation on such things as provider payments, new technology, budgets and prices.
3. More innovative sources of new finance such as user charges or cost recovery schemes, extensions of private, employment based insurance premiums or new forms of social insurance for health and extension of existing systems and finally other new taxes. In many countries a fourth theme is also apparent: decentralization of management (especially decentralization of Ministry of Health), responsibility in order to bring a better match of incentives for consumers and providers to seek and provide more cost-efficient services.

COMPETITION

New policies emphasizing market solutions are apparent in all types of health care systems. In private ones (such as U.S.A.) managed care (or capitation) such as HMO's (Health Maintenance Organization), PPO's (Preferred Provider organization), and health care networks are now widely used so as to create competition among providers and to put them at financial risk. In public systems (such as Netherlands and U.K.) internal competition between parts of the systems (say hospitals) by permitting patients to choose providers (and rewarding providers who meet these market tests) is now widely practiced. In some public systems shift-offs to a purely private delivery system are taking place both as a source of relief for government budgets and to create competition within the public system so as to improve quality and consumer acceptance (such shifts can also reduce waiting times as well).

REGULATION

Government regulation regarding provider payments, drug pricing, new technology, manpower mix and provision, price and/or budget controls is on the rise in all kinds of systems. It is generally and correctly believed that private systems, or those that are market driven, cannot insure equity. Things such as primary and public health (water supply, sanitation, immunizations, etc.) will be undersupplied. Consequently as health care systems move more toward market driven incentives, the need for governments to insure equity in access and provision increases. The basic issue of what government's role should be in health service provision is also highlighted by the issues surrounding increased use of government regulation [OECD 1992, p. 7-8]. Many economists believe governments should only be responsible for the things that private markets cannot produce; public goods, goods and services with positive externalities (and government regulation or taxation of goods with negative externalities) and other areas where private markets fail to produce what society believes in the desired or socially acceptable amount. But health care systems have elicited a wide variety of possible rationales for government intervention and regulation, which transcend traditional economist axioms.

NEW SOURCES OF FINANCE

The use of user charges has grown dramatically worldwide. Nearly every public system has some type of user charge or a cost recovery system [Gertler and van der Gaag, 1990]. Regrettably, these have not produced, in most instances, the hoped for dramatic additions to government health care budgets or restructured incentives. Some economists have also shown that user charges have (or can be) regressive thus further increasing inequity. Extensions of health insurance (either employment based or social insurance) have occurred in many countries. But with a few exceptions the success of these ventures in shifting costs for government budgets has been limited. Utilization of the private sector has met with some success in countries. Some countries have encouraged new forms of managed care in the private sector and have been able to shift some public revenues better by partitioning populations on ability to pay principles. Some countries have also succeeded in privatization of large parts of their formerly public services, especially inpatient hospitals. Decentralization of Ministry's of Health is underway nearly everywhere. In principle this is a desirable policy because it can create the correct incentives by which cost effective services can be delivered. It can also greatly improve consumer satisfaction with services as well. Decentralization does have the potential to improve efficiency, equity, and quality. But it is a hard thing to do and the successful cases of this being done worldwide are not large.

HEALTH CARE REFORMS IN EUROPE

Against this broader background of the forces fueling the reform of health care systems, let us survey what has been happening in Europe. The main problems (perhaps simplified) have been summarized by OECD (1992)[38] as:

- gaps in access to services and income protection when medical care is required
- unacceptably rapid increases in health expenditures
- concerns about inefficiency and poor performance.

In Europe one has a cross section of types of systems (as noted earlier) all of which involve third party payment. The variety of health system models found in Europe range from public contracts (compulsory or voluntary health insurance

---

[38]This OECD Report examines seven Europe countries: Belgium, France, Germany, Ireland, The Netherlands, Spain, and United Kingdom.

with direct payments to providers), compulsory health insurance, integrated models (where both the provision and insurance for the care is supplied by the same organization, e.g. a "sickness fund"), social health insurance (compulsory health insurance as part of social security system), to voluntary, indemnity type insurance, finance, and service delivery. Nearly all countries of Europe have introduced some major reform of their systems in the 1980's and 1990 's. The reforms were concentrated on containing costs (usually with the use of global budgets—i.e. a fixed sum allocated to be spent on health prospectively), improving incentives on providers and consumers for more costs-efficient use and provision of services, and some demands of competition involving consumer choice, managed care, reduction in some parts of government regulation of individual provider payments, and a variety of other mild reforms.

It is clear that the reforms currently underway in Europe are yet to be fully implemented so as to be evaluated. Global budgets have managed to put some lid on the rate of expenditure growth. But it should be remembered that these systems are high cost, even by comparison with the U.S. The recent OECD (1992) evaluation of seven countries suggests inequities and inefficiencies still persist and that reforms will have to be pushed for yet some time to overcome the basic problems as noted above.

HEALTH CARE REFORM IN ASIA

Asia has some of the fastest growing economies of the world and some of the poorest. It has nearly the same variety of health care systems as elsewhere in the world but with one exception. The private health care market has a larger presence there than in most other regions. But reform in health care is being pursued in Asia with the same vigor and for much the same reasons as elsewhere in the world. In the ADB (1987) study some fifteen Asian countries are looked at in detail ranging from Fiji to China to South Korea. The same problems as elsewhere affect Asian countries: rising expenditures, inefficiency and inequity, and in the poor countries coverage, managerial waste and inefficiency. What is perhaps different in Asia than elsewhere is that the reform efforts are almost all biased toward introducing greater market competition in systems, more extensive use of private and social health insurance to expand coverage, and policies to introduce more incentives into all aspects of the system, and a higher level of private payments. Still it is fair to say that in especially poor countries, such as the Philippines, where all these reform efforts are underway in some fashion or the other, and in richer places such as Malaysia, Thailand, and Indonesia, health care expenditures continue to rise, inefficiencies abound, and inequities of access and coverage still predominate. What perhaps distinguishes Asia from other parts of the world in their reform efforts is that the bias is toward market solutions, in some cases outright privatization of formerly public systems, and in greater reliance on health insurance, managed care, and capitated payment systems. It is still too early to say what results may be achieved but as of the moment health performance and coverage has improved somewhat, but the system still remains quite inequitable, somewhat inefficient, still biased toward curative care, and a long way from achieving value for money spent.

HEALTH REFORM IN THE U.S.

As the richest economy in the World, the U.S. also has the richest health care system as well where nearly 14 percent of GDP will be spent on health care. The U.S. is at a crucible moment with a seemingly strong momentum toward reform. President Clinton has introduced a major bill based on employer mandates, subsidies, a generous benefit package, program cut backs (Medicare and Medicaid) and some nominal tax increases, all geared toward expanding coverage (from current 85-87 percent levels to universal), containing system costs (through managed competition, premium caps, and perhaps ultimately global budgets), and improving efficiency. There are at least seven competing proposals before Congress in addition to Clinton's ranging from very limited and very gradual movement toward universal coverage financed through program reductions, increased out-of-pocket costs, government subsidies, to a so-called single payor (i.e. government) system where the Federal Government would collect all insurance premiums and dole those out on some basis (perhaps through states, or regional alliances, etc.). Everyone would be covered, some form of global budgeting would likely be included, and perhaps some additional taxes would be levied. The health care debate has become extremely politicized and it is very difficult to predict what, if anything, will emerge in the Congress that could be called health care reform. What is fueling the current impetus to reform in America is the perceived waste and inefficiency of the present system and its obvious inequities as measured by the percent of the population without insurance coverage. A telling statistic is that if the Clinton program were enacted without change and it worked as predicted by the year 2000 the percentage of GDP spent on health would be 17.3 percent as compared to the "no reform" scenario of 18.9 percent. So health care reform in America seems a long way off—there is no consensus on what to do, why it should be done, and what would work. Stay tuned.

HEALTH REFORM IN LATIN AMERICA

Health care systems in Latin America are dominated by large social security/health insurance systems. In Latin America as a whole the social security systems cover perhaps 60 percent of the population of the continent. In some countries more, in some less. The remaining coverage is from private insurance, and government systems financed through general taxation. A quotation from B. Abel-Smith (1985) best sums up the situation.

> It should be pointed out that in quite a number of Latin American countries, health insurance has generated formidable inequalities. There in inequalities in the benefits provided by different funds and within funds. There may be inequalities in the benefits provided between the employee and his dependents and between the benefits provided to different hierarchical groups of employees. But the major inequality is between the regularly employed mainly urban worker who has rights to mainly curative health services including high technology services, though there are often considerable bureaucratic obstacles to using them, and the urban poor without rights and the vast agricultural population who are not regularly employed and not only have no rights but also are without much in a way of local services. Doctors are drawn towards the urban areas under the social security programmes developed under Ministers of Labour while Ministries of Health are grossly under-financed and cannot recruit salaried doctors on any scale even for the high priority work of public health to combat the main killing diseases that affect these countries. The problem has long been recognized, but there are political obstacles in the way of radical solutions. (Page 959)

But like elsewhere reform efforts are underway in Latin America and they resemble much of what is happening elsewhere in the world. Privatizing (e.g. Chile), decentralizing systems of delivery (Brazil, Argentina), extending social security system coverage (Panama and Costa Rica), investing more in models of managed care, market driven incentives, and user charges (Bolivia) are all being implemented. Many countries are currently considering reform proposals of many shades and types. Mexico is certainly one of, them. All the systems in Latin America suffer from waste, inefficiency, bad management, and gross inequities especially toward the urban and rural poor. In Mexico your current system, as I understand it, has some 40 million people (out of 86 million) covered in the ordinary program of social security. Another 10 million are covered for primary care only ("Solidarity" Program), another ten million are covered by smaller social security institution systems and perhaps twenty-five million are uninsured and supposedly covered by the government facilities administered by the Ministry of Health. Recent studies [Lastiri, 1991] have also shown a vibrant and growing private health care system, which is widely used by people covered in one way or another by some of the other social security institutions and/or the MOH. I am not sure what the shape of reforms are under consideration in Mexico but the problems in need of reform seem obvious: unequal access and coverage, inefficiencies (especially in duplicative acute care coverage), consumer dissatisfaction with quality levels, and rising personal and governmental expenditures.

The World Bank places 1990 total health expenditures (in current exchange rates) at nearly $20 million or $132 per capita, and 4.2 percent of GDP. The Bank in the private sector places some 25-30% of total expenditures. This would place Mexico below Brazil (relative to GDP per capita) and close to the trend line for 60 countries ranked by the Bank in this manner. In other words Mexico's spending levels do not seem extravagant even though they have increased in recent years. It would seem that reform in Mexico ought not be difficult to pursue, say compared to the level of difficulty faced in America. There is a large social insurance net, and one could imagine this being extended, the role of the MOH being contracted to public health and public goods production, and a greater degree of subsidization for the poor and the uncovered. Some elements of the market could well be introduced into the social security system and management and payment system could be reformed. But it is not my place to even suggest what you should do.

SOME EXAMPLES OF REFORM

Surprisingly there are examples worldwide of successful reform. What these successes have in common is that they all started with an incisive analysis of the system problem, a clear reform model and attainable objectives, and sustained government policies and a will to accomplish the reforms. The successes also show that policy makers in most cases were able to negotiate the treacherous path between vested interest groups and local (or regional) political constitutes. Only a few points are noted in the following examples; each one is a detailed story in itself.

South Korea

From 1976 onwards Korea as a matter of national policy began to systematically extend coverage in a national health insurance system. The first stage of the compulsory social security program for medical care was in July 1977 and was applied to business firms with 500 or, more employees. More and more groups were added (recently including rural farm worker) so that coverage is approaching universal. The delivery system is basically private and is financed through general taxation, employer/employee contribution, extensive user charges, and local government taxes [Asian Development Bank 1987, p. 373]. Costs have risen in the system, but it is clear that many of the inequities observed in other systems are less prevalent in Korea.

Health Cards in Thailand

Thailand has introduced a rural health insurance program in 1984, which has proved to be both a unique and successful way to extend coverage to uninsured populations, extract more resources for public care, and improve efficiency at governmental clinics and hospitals. The system's ongoing and has been evaluated a number of times by outside scholars. The basic details are simple. Health cards are sold to rural households at affordable prices. These entitle the household to a fixed number of illness episodes treatable at government clinics and health posts to free MCH Care and certain immunizations. In emergency hospital referral a cardholder can pass through a "Green Channel" (i.e. avoids the waiting lines) for faster service. This simple health insurance scheme has a number of attractive features.

- it encourages use of MCH/EPI Services
- it increases use of sub-district health posts often by-passed.
- it reduces congestion and waiting time at hospitals
- it raises capital to finance other health service.
- it rewards provider performance through collection of fees.

On the whole the health card system has worked as planned and the system has been extended to many rural areas of Thailand [Asian Development Bank 1987, p. 87-88]. Currently some 1.3 million people (2.3 percent of population) are covered with average expenditure per head of 63 Bhat [Dow 1994, p. 13].

ProSalud in Bolivia

Since the middle 1980's, privatization of the Bolivian health system has had its ups and downs. Extensive use of user charges has been introduced and up to date results are mixed. One experiment in privatization is worth noting as it has also some of the incentive properties of the Health Card reform effort in Thailand. ProSalud is a private non-profit system, which charges almost the same fees, as does the Ministry of Public Health. The program is nearly 91 percent self-funded. Recent studies show that the system, used in just as yet a single area, has provided great consumer satisfaction with quality of services and has brought high levels of satisfaction to the providers who work in the system. The private physicians of Bolivia oppose the system because ProSalud seems to be directly competitive with their practices. Yet this is a case where competition (mostly government induced) is having a desirable impact on quality and efficiency. Replication of the Prosalud model to places of greater diversity such as La Paz, are underway [Ii 1993, pp. 88-89].

Global Budgeting in Germany

What has come to be called the public contract model[39] [OECD 1992, p. 9] has gained favor as a way that industrialized countries could contain costs. In the reconversion of health care systems in the formerly socialist countries of Central and Eastern Europe [WHO 1993 (b) and 1991(c)] the public contract approach is being followed. This model is also incorporated in parts of the Clinton health reform package. Basically a target expenditure level for the whole system is set prospectively, contracts between insurers and providers are then made on the basis of this target, and penalties and rewards are built-in between insurers and providers for staying within the expenditure caps. Evaluations of global budgeting are mixed: they seem to work for a while, but then break down. Germany, still an expensive system as measured by share of GDP to health (around 10 percent) seemed to weather rising expenditures levels in the 1980's by the public contract/global budgeting model [OECD, 1990, p. 30]. But in the early 1990's expenditures (especially drug costs) began to escalate and a sharper budgeting program had to be reestablished.

Overview of Examples

There is a lot underway in most countries in regard to health reform. Many fronts are and will have to be explored. What is clear is that what we call free market type reforms can work under most conditions. But alone they are not enough. Government policies and interventions can stimulate free market conditions but efficiency of health care systems and equity are yet to be attained on a universal basis.

---

[39]This model, as defined in [OECD 1992, p. 9] refers to "compulsory or voluntary health insurance which involves direct payments, under contract, from the insurers or third parties to the providers...In this model providers are often independent and contractual payments are often by capitation or fee for service."

THE WORLD BANK PRESCRIPTION FOR REFORM

The World Bank [World Development Report 1993] has put forward an aggressive and ambitious agenda for reform. Those dealing with low-income countries as well as rich countries are worth our attention. In some sense the Bank's prescriptions cut across all income groups. But those dealing with middle-income countries (where Mexico is placed) are worth some attention.

Middle-income countries, argues the Bank, need to focus on four key areas of policy reform:

(1) phasing out public subsidies to better-off groups
(2) extending insurance coverage more widely
(3) giving consumers a choice of insurer, and
(4) encouraging payment methods that control costs.

(1) Phasing Out Subsidies to Well-off Groups

The Bank singles out a number of countries on this score and Latin America in particular. These subsidies are sometimes obtained through loopholes in a country's tax code, direct subsidization to social insurance funds, and service upgrading (for ultimate recovery from the funds) to insured patients. "These subsidies", the Bank [World Development Report 1993, p. 161] notes, "...are widespread in Latin America, [and] mostly benefit the middle classes and are therefore regressive." If countries charged the full cost of services to insured patients for services not included in their coverage it would impose more financial discipline on social insurance funds and free-up government resources that could then be redirected toward the poor.

(2) Extension of Insurance

The Bank notes what countries such as Korea and Costa Rica have done in extending insurance coverage to previously uncovered populations such as the self-employed, farmers, the elderly, and the poor. Extension of coverage can remove the systemic inequities inherent in multi-tiered systems of health finance. The Bank also couples an essential package of insured services (those with high cost-effectiveness) with the extension to universal coverage.

(3) Consumer Choice

Competition among insurance funds (or among suppliers of a clearly stated prepaid package of benefits) improves quality and encourages efficiency. "And even where there is a little or no direct competition among insurance funds," the

Bank notes [World Development Report 1993, p. 161],..."multiple semi-independent insurance institutions may still have an advantage over a single large parastatal agency."

(4) Cost Containment

Here the Bank strongly recommends use of prepaid care, copayments, managed care, capitation payments and other forms of payment generally associated with market driven reforms. The Bank addresses a special concern for governments to improve the incentives created by social insurance.

The above is just a brief sketch of the Banks prescriptions for reform. But as mentioned earlier, the Bank notes that there are multiple routes to reform. The common elements all seem to focus on a reorganization of governmental roles, greater competition and consumer choice, and stronger incentives to economize on care through incentive structured payment and reimbursement systems. A final quotation seems poignant and telling:

> Everywhere health sector reform is a continuous and complex struggle. Neither governments nor free markets can by themselves allocate resources for health efficiently. As policy makers try to reach compromise, they must deal with powerful interest groups...and strong political constituencies...[World Development Report 1993, p. 165].

SUMMARY

It is clear that reform efforts of health care systems (both of delivery and finance) are underway world-wide in rich countries and in poor ones. The forces driving reform efforts are the poor performance of public systems, the high cost of all systems, the rising expectations of population for medical care, and for a variety of technologically induced changes. It is not clear that world-wide any country has yet succeeded in producing a health care system that is both efficient and equitable and is producing outstanding (or even acceptable) health outcomes. Costs are rising everywhere, governments are under pressure to do better, and no one wants to spend more public money, yet everybody seems dissatisfied with the status quo.

Ralph Andreano

SELECTION 9

NOTES ON HEALTH SECTOR REFORM[40]

ABSTRACT

This paper argues that the agenda for reform of the health sector first formed in 1978 in the Alma Ata Declaration and reinforced and expanded by WHO and the World Bank in 1987 has been largely stalled in the developing world. There have been some successes, but the pace of reform in the public sector has been outstripped by the widespread growth of private health markets in the developing countries. In the developed and industrialized countries there has been significant attempts at reform in the past decade. In Western Europe the largely public systems have tried and with some success, to instill greater cost control, competition, market driven incentive structures, and greater consumer satisfaction and producer quality into their systems. But in a place like the USA where a major reform effort put before the Congress failed in its entirety to be adopted, the private sector has to a large extent accomplished much of this anticipated reform but without any major governmental or public involvement. In the major public program (Medicare), reform has stalled and there are quite divergent political agendas on how to fix the major reforms of this system.

Placing these developments in the wider context of the reform agenda and in the framework of political and economic reforms of the past decade suggests that there are some significant barriers to implementing the original health sector reform agenda in the developing countries. For the most part, this paper focuses only on the developing countries and the pace of health sector reform there. In particular in places such as Africa, the original reform agenda is barely off the ground and troubles with it abound. In Asia, there have been some notable successes with the original agenda, but a wall of barriers to further reform has been reached. In the Arab states, and especially in the oil rich Gulf States, health sector reform is just beginning and the original reform agenda, if it is appropriate to their reform efforts, is stalled on many of the same structural asymmetries as found in the developing world. But it is clear that the ideas of Alma Ata and of the 1987 reform agenda need to overcome some significant barriers in the years ahead if extent of health sector reform envisioned nearly 20 years ago can become a reality in the developing world. We call these barriers the missing infrastructure of reform and group these elements under three main categories:

---

[40]This Paper was originally written as a Background paper for the International Health Policy Program (IHPP) as the possible basis for an Annual Meeting. This version of the paper was completed 15 December 1996).

(1) **Governance** (2) **Professional Societies and Institutions**, and (3) **Information**. The paper expands on some of these elements and suggests some future directions for health policy research.

OVERVIEW

The reform of health sectors is a continuing drama. Lord Beveridge's inspired reforms of access to health care for all and with quality and dignity is still live. In America, Harry Truman and Lyndon Johnson transformed America's health care system with the passage of Medicare and Medicaid in 1965. In the developing world, Alma Ata in 1978 and the influential World Bank Report of 1987(the Akin-Birdsall-DeFerranti report) and the World Health Organizations Technical Discussions at the 1987 World Health Assembly are also significant landmarks of modern reform efforts. By and large, the reform message in the developing world since at least the last decade has centered on several recurring themes. Ministries of Health should decentralize their activities, countries should shift resources to primary care (the Alma Ata influence) and away from acute care, private sector growth should be encouraged and with better coordination between it and the public sector, new sources of finance, both public and private should be sought (and here insurance, user charges, and other financial innovations were encouraged).

On the whole, the impact of health sector reform on the improvement in health status, on the quality of health care populations receive, and on the greater access to services by the poor has produced a mixed record of success.

Still after at least a decade of reform efforts, countries are still struggling to decentralize their Ministries of Health, widespread adoption of user charges has not significantly expanded resources for care, acute care is still more highly prized and funded than primary care, and private sector growth has probably widened access to care between haves and have nots. It is from this perspective that a new focus on other attributes of health sector reform may be needed in the coming decade. This reform agenda of the past decade, as epitomized by the Alma Ata Declaration and the 1987 World Bank report is certainly correct. But what experience has shown is that this agenda has to dig deeper roots if it is to succeed. The directions suggested in this concept paper are with this outcome in mind. The undercurrent of health policy research for the reform agenda of the past decade has been substantial; but only scholars and researchers have done a fraction of that research from the developing world. (Berman 1995) Those of us in the international research community may well not have helped by pushing this agenda so hard in our own work.

What may distinguish the next thrust of research on the issues outlined here is that the driving support for it originates with the leading policy research scholars in the developing world. (Research underway and supported by the International Health Policy Program (IHPP) in China, India, Thailand, Philippines, Uganda, Kenya, Nigeria, Ghana, and Tanzania is especially important to note).

The Health Reform Agenda

We have mentioned a number of things that would define the content of the agenda for reform above:

- Improved equity in health and health care
- Increased and better management of health resources
- Improved performance of the health system and quality of care
- And, greater satisfaction for consumers and providers of health care.

Obviously, we can add or subtract from this listing. But there is more or less some agreement of the reform agenda over the past decade and it has not deviated very much from this list.

The aspects of the current reform agenda most implemented and to some extent most studied are those regarding health care financing and organization. And here three categories dominate: (1) user charges, (2) health insurance and (3) decentralization. Some sub issues of these three are how Ministries of Health have been reorganized, certain privatization moves such as contracting, and a number of other factors.

One of these other factors is: the frustration level in pushing successfully this reform agenda. In truth this agenda has been stalled and it has run up against what may be called the infrastructure elements for reform. What has happened in many countries is that successful implementation of the reform agenda depends on many things that have to be fixed first and which lie outside the health sector's capacity to fix them. Nonetheless, the sweep of health sector reforms in the past decade has enveloped all types of health care systems and supporting economic structures from very advanced democracies with quite open and growing economies to more authoritarian and/or closed economies with limited growth. All have had some measure of reform in their health sector and the one constant that seems to run through all dimensions of these reform efforts is that the push toward market systems and all it entails seems dominant. Of course, other things are wrapped around this—decentralizing Ministries of Health for example—but usually the intent is to change incentives, to give workers, consumers and producers incentives to economize on resource use, or channel ability to pay for services more equitably. Reforms of financing of care, greater and widespread use of insurance, decentralization of public services is to be found in both the developing and developed worlds. And everywhere the main forces pushing for reform were raising private and public costs of the system, general dissatisfaction with quality of care and access to care. In short, in the past decade, virtually every country has had some impetus toward reform of their health systems and some reasons to pursue reform.

THE WIDER REFORM AGENDA

One must also remember that while the health sector reforms noted above seemed to us in the policy research community as paramount, we must remember the wider framework of reform that has swept the developing and to some extent the industrialized world in the past decade. Economic and political liberalization has dominated the world in the past decade. Reducing the size of government, liberalizing financial and trade structures, private and sovereign debt restructuring, and generating competitiveness in economies frame the larger series of events within which health sector reform was occurring. The parallel economic changes in economic structures, especially in the developing world, were toward reducing the size of government, making it more responsive to peoples needs, also liberalizing financial and trade structures, and with greater attention to macroeconomic policies to contain inflation and exchange rate fluctuations. In the industrialized countries, economic reform has been private sector based and huge job restructuring and corporate downsizing has occurred. In both rich countries and poor, the competitiveness of the world economy has changed so dramatically in the past decade that for any country to lose an ounce of competitiveness can mean economic hardship. The formerly socialist economies are caught in both worlds: they need to liberalize their economies to become world competitive and they also have the overhang of huge debt, inflation, trade deficits, and are badly in need of reform and money for their social welfare services. They resemble in many respects the developing countries of Asia and Africa.

For the most part, these economic restructuring reforms were generated by market rather than governmental initiatives, though some government initiatives were and are present that make such changes happen. Then there have been the parallel reform efforts of political liberalization characterized by a series of reforms that involved greater respect for individual and collective rights, greater freedom of association and expression, constitutional changes toward multi-party states where none existed before, free elections and in many instances greater civilian control over the military. Just as with the agenda of health sector reforms, the record of success on economic and political liberalization reforms have produced mixed results. Some people now live in greater freedom; some countries are now more democratic. But inter-country income inequalities are now greater than a decade ago, and intracountry income inequalities have grown as well. And these results are not limited just to the developing world: the gap between the richest countries has widened, income distributions within rich countries have widened, and the income disparity between rich and poor countries has widened, even as some poor countries have done extremely well in terms of economic growth the past decade.

The connection between the wider political and economic reform agenda and the reforms of the past decade in health care while not seemingly obvious are indeed closely connected. One might describe the health reform agenda as itself emphasizing liberalizing themes: decentralize Ministries, allow private markets to flourish, reduce government regulations and the size and scope of government, find new ways for people who can pay for services to do so, and new ways to insure equity for those who cannot pay. And show concern that the people who use the system are satisfied with their access to it and the quality of care they receive. The growth of inequalities within and between countries makes the task of health sector reform both more needed and more difficult.

THE NEXT GENERATION OF HEALTH REFORM

Much of the health policy research of the last decade, especially that done with IHPP support, has shown several things: the original reform agenda is a good one, but it is much more complicated and intricate than first supposed. Most of us did not anticipate how these wider reforms in politics and economics would spill over into the health sector. Few of us anticipated how rapid would be the transformation of private markets in health in the developing world. To a certain extent, this is where the push of reform has centered and not on the public sector. There are many, many layers to remove before health systems can be decentralized, private systems blended into the public, new sources of finance found that do not propagate already wide income and access disparities, and the like. The rapid growth of the private health sector, in fact, has made all the more urgent the need to define, perhaps redefine, the role of government in health care as a provider of care, a financier of care, and as a regulator of standards and norms of quality and consumer protection and satisfaction.

Behind this first generation of the reform agenda appears another and deeper set of reforms needed if the original agenda is to produce the desired results of better health, efficient delivery systems, equity in access and lower cost, but improved quality of care and consumer satisfaction. We label this next layer of reform as the infrastructure of health sector reform. The first generation defined the overall map for reform efforts; what our research has shown is that the highways and byways for the straightest trajectory from point A to point B on that map is yet to be fully discovered. What we propose here is a continuation of the original research agenda but focused on the inner content, the infrastructure that needs to be built if the ultimate reform agenda is to succeed. Some of this research is already underway in IHPP supported countries. Decentralization, for example, part of the major reform agenda, runs contrary in many countries to the entrenched bureaucracy. If decentralization is a good strategy, and some research suggests it is, then barriers to countries doing this successfully (even defining what successful means) must be found out and overcome. Similarly, the great growth of the private sector in countries has not really relieved the fiscal burden of governments for health care, as one thought would be possible a decade ago. In part this is because governments have not been able to find the right blend between allowing private health markets to grow, maintaining some semblance of equity and equal access, and insuring quality of care (perhaps even consumer satisfaction) through a blend of governmental regulatory powers and the powers to tax and control. Nor has private sector growth lessened the greater role for government as a standard setter, a setter of rules and regulations and as a regulator. Also, from governmental perspectives, the move to decentralize health systems, to allow private health markets to grow, are all part of larger governmental reforms of economic and political liberalization: sometimes the barriers found in the health sector for success in these venues is attributable to the larger governmental reform agenda.

THE CONTENTS OF THE NEXT REFORM AGENDA

There are obviously a number of directions one might go in pursuing the barriers to success in implementing the original agenda of health reform. One line of research is to find the common elements, which permitted some countries to advance further than others. Studies of this kind are under way on such topics as Decentralization, User Charges. Public and Private roles, and several other aspects. One can learn from both the cases of success as well as failure. What some IHPP researchers have been finding in their most recent work is that a number of particular points, what we call the infrastructure of reform, need deeper and sustained analysis. In the spirit of simplicity we group these into three categories:

1. *Governance*

Decentralization as well as a host of health sector reforms comes up against full force governmental rules of personnel and civil service as well as the imbedded incentive structures that inhibit risk taking on the part of the governmental bureaucracy. The World Bank has already recognized the importance of governance issues for economic and social development, in its program lending support for public sector management (PSM). In the context of health sector reform, we see the governance issues of extreme importance in pushing through on the original reform agenda. Decentralization of health services cannot fully succeed until governments fully acknowledge their accountability—much of decentralization has pushed functions to the periphery but not accountability. Similarly, governance issues in health care must have a secure legal framework to underline accountability. Sharpening civil service reforms, reshaping incentive structures through new pay and grading structures, are all elements of reform yet to be fully undertaken in the developing world. The Bank also speaks of transparency and information as being the other prongs of the governance issue. And these too in health care reform have become barriers to effective change. To make public sector managers more accountable they must have incentives for performance and grading performance requires a transparency about what norms and standards are in play. And finally, the great rise of the private sector as part of health reform over the past decade has made one pillar of governance—the legal framework—extremely important. Many countries are now getting around to this in health sector reform through passage of legislation governing health reform, or through executive orders and the like. Accountability and transparency, as the Bank notes, "poor governance is characterized by arbitrary policy making, unaccountable bureaucracies, unenforced or unjust legal systems, the abuse of executive power, a civil society unengaged in public life, and widespread corruption." (From a statement in the World Bank Paper on its World Wide Web Site on Public Sector Management, 1996). What some recent research in IHPP countries shows is that these governance issues are fundamental to any reform effort for it to succeed. In a 1987 paper I (Andreano and Heliminak, "The Role of the Private Sector" also collected in this volume) what we call here infrastructure was called the "real" health system. In a recent ECONOMIST magazine (Nov.30th.1996) there was a large advertisement for Uganda for an Adviser for Human Resource Management for Uganda Civil Service Reform. In the body of the ad they state: "The aim of the Uganda Civil Service Reform (CSR) is to build a civil service which is efficient and effective in providing high quality and appropriate services, supports sustainable national development and facilitates the growth of a viable private sector. The key components of the reform programme are optimising the size and structure of the civil service; developing human and physical resources through training, pay reform and retooling, strengthening control systems; and improving the efficiency and effectiveness of the services delivered by public officials." (Page 99) In the thinking behind the present paper, the concept of Governance and what additional policy research is needed to advance any reform agenda in health care is well embodied in the language of this advertisement.

2. Professional Societies, Associations, and Institutions

A second direction for policy research, now partly underway, is that in many instances well-intentioned reform efforts, perhaps even in the context of countries with good PSM and corresponding governance features, have stalled because of professional opposition or indifference. The role of physicians and their associations and societies, long a subject for policy analysis in the industrial countries, is now a major issue in developing countries. Physicians, perhaps in part because of the growth of legal frameworks (which by the way is extremely important for the private sector) in countries deeply in reform, has energized physicians both publicly employed or in their capacity as providers in the private (especially for profit) health sector. Physicians still have enormous power to control quality, access, and cost decisions in health care systems. How they organize and how they influence policy will be crucial to reform. The opposition of physicians, whether or not they have professional associations, is a major issue for health reform. The former Director-General of WHO, Dr. Halfdan Mahler used to always speak of the Medical Mafia as a barrier to the reforms proposed at Alma Ata. The self-interest of physicians whether they work exclusively for Government, or on their own private account, is no different than the self-interest of other professional groups. But in the case of health care reform, so much of the treatment and finance decisions are the domain of physician decisions, where physicians stand on matters of policy is fundamental to the success of any reform agenda. As such, study of these professional societies, how they function, their relationship to the main reform agenda, how they behave in the private sector, these and related issues, are part of the unknown when it comes to success or failure of reform efforts. The importance of these professional societies, emphasizing here only physicians but there are equivalents for all the medical professions, are an integral part of the infrastructure of reform.

In much the same vein as the above discussion about physicians one must also include the position of importance to health sector reform held by other professional groups. We speak of civil service reform under GOVERNANCE. But in most developed countries and in many developing countries, the people who work in the health sector (often the doctors, but the nurses, the clerks, pharmacists, etc.) have organized, many into trade or labour unions that deal directly with government. These organizations are often an obstacle to reform, for reform threatens their power, status, and perhaps even their incomes. In the last two months, for example, there have been extended strikes in South Korea and in Zimbabwe of hospital workers with the issues being some measure of reform introduced by government. Perhaps the issues are deeper than that, but such organized groups can be a real barrier to reform, especially if the chances involved could affect them adversely. Observation of reform agendas in the developing world show this is a neglected area of research. We need to understand how such groups work, how can their legitimate objections be harmonized and still lead to meaningful reform. Also, these professional and labour groups have much to say about quality, cost, and access in the system no matter what government policy is: as they often control how rules, regulations, and benefits are to be interpreted and implemented, their powers to influence who gets what, when, can be vast. Some country-based research is needed to understand these forces as barriers or aids to health sector reform.

An additional issue with respect to all professional societies of the types described here is how influential they are in setting accreditation and certification rules. These are often the first line of defense against reform efforts. In many instances in the developing world, accreditation standards often impose what could be called internal taxes in the system: to obtain a license, for example, may not only require a fee, but signed acceptance of your qualifications by innumerable governmental agencies. Thus to undo something imposes a real tax in time, effort, and energy on those pushing for change. To simplify rules, say for a generic based pharmacopia, may often require huge transfers of time, energy, and money just to make a change. In most instances, the benefit/cost ratio from elimination of some of the more ornerous accreditation and credentialing rules is usually favorable. We need more country-based research on these issues.

3. Information

It is true that the original reform agenda was based only partly on research and more largely on intuition and theory: we hypothesized that, for example, MOH's would be better able to deliver services—that they would be more efficient—if they and the service delivery system were less centralized. There was really only modest research that led to this reform element; rather it just seemed it should be so based on the underlying perverse incentives, i.e. incentive theory; fixing the incentives should fix the problem. Like other aspects of the original reform agenda, insufficient information on this element showed the problems were much more complex, and the forces working against change, much more intricate. Reformers and policy makers were left with much too little information about which policy choices to make to overcome the barriers. Also, as more information was gathered, it was clear that things outside of the health sector (e.g. civil service rules, etc.) needed to be fixed first. The current drive for data on national health accounts is a vital part of the importance of information to the infrastructure of reform. The NHA can prove to be a useful policy tool for judging interventions past, present, and future.

Other dimensions of information, which are essential to overcome barriers to reform, include data on policy impacts in terms of benefits and costs both before and after interventions. This is especially lacking for public program interventions: we are always surprised after a program has been implemented when we find out it only partially has had an impact on those targeted while large numbers of untargeted people have reaped the benefits. Why is this so? Could such program designs have been conceived better with better information?

In health policies in finance and administration, some of the original reform elements have bogged down because the wider impacts on access and ability to pay caused by inequities in the distribution of incomes were not incorporated into the original program design.

At yet another level, INFORMATION as part of the research agenda of health reform should be thought of in terms of how well informed, how well treated, and how consumers are valued in the reform agenda. Emphasis on consumer satisfaction, which has come to be part of the original reform agenda, requires information on how consumers are treated, how long they have to wait for services, whether or not the services satisfy their needs, as well as a host of other questions. This is a badly researched area and one that seems to be important for the success of the original agenda. Often, we find that consumers are themselves resistant to changes that could clearly be in their best interest; we need to know why this is so, and how it happens. Professional Associations have substantial power to influence consumer perceptions of levels of satisfaction and this is not always done in the public interest.

In short, the lack of information is a crucial reform element of the infrastructure and it is in short supply in the developing world. New policy research strategies are needed to develop the information base needed for successful reform.

GOING FORWORD

Obviously many more details need to be filled in and discussed beyond the comments above. But it is the belief that underlies this paper that the current reform agenda will continue to sputter until some progress is made on the variety of infrastructure issues noted above. Reform of health systems requires both political and economic change and a desire to pursue change; health policy research alone is not the change agent, but perhaps a point on the map to a larger road to reform. To this end, we propose a new push of policy research not just to better define the current agenda of reform, but to discover ways of advancing it into the largely unexplored areas of Governance (and all the issues it contains) and Professional Society and Institutional Constraints and Information. There is research underway in the areas we call infrastructure. In projects supported by the International Health Policy Program significant work on the three areas of Governance, Professional Societies, and Information discussed above is underway in a number of Asian and African Countries. We would like to see the main international bodies that fund and influence health research in the developing world, have a dialogue about the issues raised in this paper, and if the ideas meet the market test, then put more resources into more policy researchers in the developing world. What a cursory review of the literature produced thus far about the success and failure of the original reform agenda shows, is that most of it has been done by scholars from the West. The leading edge of research done by the leading scholars in the developing world has now begun to focus on the ideas of this paper. The international community has to make sure resources are available. Research is not the only tool for change, but if the original and amended reform agenda for health was a good one, and most everyone thinks it is, we will need a research base on the barriers and obstacles to getting that agenda implemented successfully. What this paper suggests is that there is another layer of research needed to push the original agenda to fruition and in some cases just to get it started. The purpose of the paper is to initiate the discussion needed to refine and influence what donors and then researchers are doing.

More Notes on Health Reform
ABSTRACT

This paper is meant to be read in connection with the paper Notes on Health Reform, otherwise called the Concept Paper and printed here above. In this present paper, I survey a whole bunch of areas of the world, add some more detail to the substance of the arguments in the Concept paper, and look at what kind of evidence one would need to conclude anything about the success or failure of health reform. (To readers: I do know there is overlap between the two papers but the repetition is not fatal, I believe. This paper also includes some material also presented in the previous Selection in this volume).

THE CONTEXT OF HEALTH REFORM

We have placed the modern efforts at health reform from the 1978 Alma Ata Declaration, punctuated by the 1987 World Bank Report (Akin, et al) and the Technical Discussions at the 1987 World Health Assembly. There was also a pioneering effort in 1987 in Asia, which examined the progress of reform in some twenty Asian countries. The last piece of the intellectual foundation, of course, is the landmark 1993 World Development Report of the World Bank, Report on Health. The original reform agenda certainly was shaped by these events and publications. But as is always the case, what occurred in international forums or in prestigious publications was a mirror reflection of events that were actually happening in country after country. These events, though primarily in our work stressing the developing countries, really cut across all kinds of health systems and at all levels of economic growth and development. Low-income, middle income, oil rich and high-income industrialized countries have experienced some significant impulses to reform of their health care system. There has been an atmosphere of change that has characterized the entire world the past decade, and not just in health care. But at the risk of oversimplification, let me cast a summation on the factors that seemed to dominate discussion in health care, almost irrespective of the type of system and level of income of the country.

1. There has been a great rise in public and professional expectation of what modern medicine can do or is capable of doing. This has been a source of pride and pressure: pride in that medical miracles no longer seemed uncommon, pressure in that everyone wanted access to the new advances which exerted great upward pressure on expenditures. The advances in

diagnostics, in new therapies, new drugs, and new scientific knowledge have all fueled this rising tide of medical expectations. This has made most health care systems look inadequate in the eyes of consumers: they all want more of these advances when they need them, but resent that the cost and coverage of the new medicine often puts it out of reach of most of the population, except the well-off and rich.

2. The past decade has also seen a major shift in the patterns of disease. New diseases have emerged, especially the auto-immune diseases such as HIV and AIDS, but new bacterial strains with heretofore benign impacts but are now in some cases raging out of control. And the reappearance of old diseases such as malaria. New diseases have placed enormous strains on resource capacity, have challenged the effectiveness and availability of new drugs, and have scared the hell out of a lot of people. Death rates and morbidity levels from the newer diseases have increased, in some countries and cases very dramatically, and with serious economic consequences on the health care systems. Since 1980 there have been three entirely newly identified viral agents: H.I.V.1, 1983 (Acquired immunodeficiency syndrome), Hepatitis C and Hepatitis E, 1989 and 1990, respectively; and Hemorrhagic fever, 1991. Some old viruses now found in new locations: 1992-93 Yellow Fever, Kenya; 1993 Hantavirus, Southwestern U.S. There has also been a newly identified agent for a Rickettsial disease, Ehrlichia chaffeenis, and a newly identified bacterial agent (1992), Vibrio cholarae. A wonderful and useful book, Laurie Garret, *The Coming Plague: Newly Emerging Diseases in a World Out of Balance (1995)*, has details on these and other changes in infectious disease agents, the recrudescence of things such as malaria, and so forth. (Also see, the NEW YORK TIMES Tuesday May 10,1994, page B7).

3. A third force, especially noticeable in the past decade, is the major demographic shifts that have taken place and/or are still underway. In rich countries, countries on the rise economically such as the Asian tigers, the populations have aged dramatically and will continue to do so. In the developing countries, most with high population growth rates, the populations are significantly younger. Both present real strains on the health system as well on other aspects of an economy but importantly the social security and social welfare systems. Populations aging use more resources while the younger populations present real problems in providing a sufficient tax base from which to collect revenues to be used for health care systems. The disease profiles are also quite different between old and young and this presents particularly stressful situations on resource allocation.

Against these wider forces, within the health systems themselves, the past decade has also forced country after country to examine closely what the systems look like in terms of equity and efficiency. The enormous increase in health expenditures has alone sparked the reform agenda in the industrialized world and in the countries on the rise. But rising inequities in access, consumer dissatisfaction, and general inefficiencies because of the nature of health care as a quasi public good, fueled reform efforts. In the developing world, the bias of expenditures on acute care, the ceiling against new resources for health, and the dissatisfaction of consumers were just as fertile a climate for reform as in the rich countries. So when the international community looked at itself, say at Alma Ata, or in terms of the deeply structured analyses produced in the context of the leading organizations such as the World Bank, the World Health Organization and the Asian Development Bank, there were receptive ears for suggestions of what to do about their health care systems in all parts of the globe.

After Alma Ata, what seemed to form as the strategy of health reform in both rich and poor countries, again at the risk of simplification, could be put into a few generalizations.

1. Nearly everybody argued for health care systems to become more competitive and be driven by market incentives. In the developing world this was translated into decentralizing ministries of health, both in their capacity as suppliers of services, but also in other structural dimensions such as consumer satisfaction, access to services, and quality control.

2. Surprisingly, the role of government in health care, while being urged to be reduced as a direct supplier or provider, was asked to expand by assuming a more interventionist regulatory role. In developed countries quality control, provider payments, cost containment policies, new technology and a host of other governmental initiatives were thought to be more central to any reform of health care markets. In the developing world, the growth of private health markets was, in many ways, outstripping governmental points of traditional leverage (e.g. by being the provider of last resort), and cried out for closer government influence on standards, professional certification, quality control, and in some cases consumer protection. In middle income countries government's role was also being redefined, especially in the case of social insurance, to extend coverage more widely, to phase out subsidies to favored (usually better-off groups), expand consumer choices, and to take a greater concern to use its powers to control expenditures and costs in the system.

3. A third, not unrelated aspect, involved innovations in both the finance and delivery of care. In the industrialized countries more ability to pay incentives were used, tighter systems of risk sharing between supplier and recipient of care, and a wider array of financial instruments such as newer types of health insurance, various cost recovery schemes, and the like. These forces were at work in both rich and poor countries.

A REGIONAL SURVEY OF THE CONTEXT OF REFORM: EUROPE

In 1992 OECD summarized the main context of reform among member countries in Europe as (perhaps simplified): gaps in access and income protection when care is prolonged; unacceptably rapid increases in health expenditures and; concerns about the inefficiency and poor qualitative performance of the health systems. (OECD 1992, This report examines seven European Countries: Belgium, France, Germany, Ireland, Netherlands, Spain, and United Kingdom). In Europe one has a cross section of types of systems. The main types of systems range from public contracts (compulsory or voluntary health insurance with direct payments to providers),compulsory health insurance with various payment models, integrated systems where both the provision of care and insurance against health risk is supplied by the same organization (e.g. a "sickness" fund), social health insurance where compulsory health insurance is part of a wider social security system, to voluntary, indemnity based insurance, finance and delivery systems. Virtually all countries have been in one or more aspects of implementing what we have called the traditional reform agenda. A simplified summation would show the reforms concentrated on containing costs (often using what has been called "global budgets"), improving the incentive structure of the payment, delivery, and finance aspects of their systems, and in general instilling various market driven forces with more competition, greater consumer choice, and reduced bureaucratic and government regulatory procedures. Even in the highly consumer accepted and mainly public system in the UK has this been true. In nearly all countries some form of cost sharing has been introduced and in a number of countries eligibility has been extended, in many cases bringing the last remaining groups within the coverage of national schemes. The 1992 OECD report suggests that in the seven countries studied, at least, both inefficiencies in one or more parts of the delivery system still exist and that inequities in access are still larger than socially acceptable. As we note below, it is not clear that system efficiencies have improved or that expenditure growth has been contained.

A Side Excursion

What has been called the public contract model (OECD 1992) was at the heart of the reform agenda in Western Europe over the past decade. It is dominant in Germany and has been followed in most details in the reconversion of health systems in the formerly Socialist countries of Eastern Europe (WHO

1993b;WHO 1991). As defined by OECD (1992 p.9) the model refers to "compulsory or voluntary health insurance, which involves direct payments, under contract, from the insurors or third parties to the providers...In this model providers are often independent and contractual payments are often by capitation or fee for service." This model also makes use of what has often been called by policy analysts as "Global Budgeting." This is where a target expenditure level is set for the whole system, prospectively, and then contracts between insurers and providers are concluded on the basis of these targets. Penalties and rewards for insurers and providers are built into the targets and expenditure caps. Germany is the major user the contract model. The results are mixed; global budgeting works for a bit, but so long as there are no restraints on demand, public policy simply amounts to fixing the targets to accommodate the expenditure growth that fits the allowable amount of political pressure from all the affected groups-insurers, providers, and consumers. Once there is an attempt to squeeze the target caps and contain real expenditure growth in the system, the pressure of labor and trade unions, the professional associations of doctors, etc, and even consumer groups rebel against the changes and political bargaining begins yet again. As will be noted later, if containment of expenditure growth was a goal of health reform, it has failed. If increased efficiencies in the system were a goal, there has been some partial success but not yet enough to show real savings in system costs. If increased access to care and reduced inequities in access were goals, the limits to success of reform outweigh the gains.

Some recent experience in Germany, however, may show how the shape of reform can occur in an advanced economy and one spending a very substantial portion of its GDP on health. In1993 Germany made a major effort to slash 11billion marks (about $7 billion) from its health care spending, a reduction of about 6%. The major cost saving effort was aimed at cutting the budget and expenditures for prescription drugs about 2.4billion marks (about $1.5 billion). The data show that Government policies of scrutinizing physician prescribing practices, denying payment, shifting to more generic drug use, all had some effect in the short-run. But then those affected began their complaints. The corner pharmacies that had their sales decreased, the giant pharmaceutical companies of Germany complained bitterly, and not the least doctors and their patients complained. To their credit, German health policy makers stuck to their guns, but the forces of resistance to change are gearing up and over time these policies, or some other ways of substituting for them, will need to be adopted to quell the criticism. In any case, after a one-year dip in spending, total health spending in Germany, as a % of GDP, has continued to rise anyway. (A nice survey of the events of 1993 is in the *Wall Street Journal*, May 4,1993,p. A12).

The transition in the formerly socialist countries of Eastern and Central Europe and the former Soviet Republics is particularly painful to watch. All of these systems were centrally planned, truly public systems, with free care, financed out of the general budget. There were always private markets for health services but these were not legal. Now with the triumph of democracy and capitalism, these countries have all tried some dimensions of reform of their health systems. The problems are immense and in a few countries there have been some successes, notably Poland, Hungary, the Czech Republic and perhaps others. But in Russia itself the system has not made a successful transition and in some other countries the level, access and quality of health care is very troubling. A recent story in the *New York Times* (Wednesday, Dec. 25, 1996) reports on the situation in Bulgaria with the headline: "Bulgaria Runs Out of Medical Supplies." In the text of the story, a neurosurgeon is quoted as saying that the financial crises was made worse,"...because the Ministry of Health insisted that medical care be provided completely free. We tell the Minister of Health that we have no more money, and she replies that medical care is free." (Page A6)

HEALTH CARE REFORM IN ASIA

Some of the fastest growing economies of the past decade are in Asia. It has as nearly a diverse variety of health delivery and health finance systems as in Europe or Latin America. Private health care markets have a very great presence here and have grown enormously in the past decade. In the landmark 1987 Asian Development Bank study that looked at 15 Asian countries ranging from Fiji, to China, to South Korea, the same system wide problems as exist elsewhere exist in Asia. (A paper of mine from this Conference is included in this volume as Selection 12, "The Role of the Private Sector".) Rising expenditures, inefficiency and inequity and in the poorest countries of the region, widespread consumer dissatisfaction with government services, gross waste, mismanagement, and system inefficiencies. The traditional reform agenda has been widely adopted: purely public systems have tried to reform and decentralize and privatize; more insurance schemes both public and private have been tried, and some structural changes introduced which reduced government control over the sector. In Asia, perhaps more than in any other region, private market growth in health care has outstripped governmental reform initiatives. The problems now are how to reinstill a governmental role as noted in the Concept paper.

In Asia the variety of health care reforms undertaken has been quite rich and has covered nearly all aspects of the original reform agenda. Some countries have engaged in very substantial downsizing of their ministries of health and in privatizing previously public facilities (mainly hospitals). And here several countries come to mind: Malaysia which has both decentralized and privatized, Indonesia which has done the same, and South Korea, China, and Bangkok which all have been innovative in trying new ways to finance care with some interesting health insurance schemes. The Philippines is also another hotbed of reform with decentralization and one of the Region's most comprehensive pieces of Legislation underlining reform efforts. But except perhaps for China, it is fair to say that in virtually all the major countries of Asia (excluding Japan which is lumped with my earlier remarks about industrial countries) the public health sector proportionately is less important than the private sector. Private health markets have grown dramatically in Asia. The point, therefore, is that well-intentioned reform of the public sector, even if it succeeded (which it has not), somewhat trivializes the changes in health care systems in Asia. Not only is the original reform agenda being swamped by the growth of private markets, but this growth needs to redefine Government's role in health care, somewhat away from its role as producer and financier of care and more toward its regulatory, norm and standard setting role, and indeed its legislative role as well. In the private sector in large parts of Asia, many of the innovative forms of insurance and delivery are being tried. Managed care, widely used in America is not uncommon in places like Indonesia, Philippines, and Thailand. The widespread extension of health insurance in South Korea and the health card insurance program in Thailand are also worth noting as innovative reform initiatives of Government. But it is not a stretch to put the cutting edge of reform in the private sector; the responses and impulses of public sector reform seem quite muted in Asia. Is anything working? Perhaps, but not overwhelmingly so. Total expenditures are rising, private market growth may have intensified inequities of access, and again the nature of Government' s role needs to become quite different from that envisioned by the original reform agenda. More on the evidence front later.

An interesting case of how the reform agenda can have been somewhat successful but at the same time have produced empty results is the case of South Korea. This country started on a goal about 20 years ago of covering everyone in an employment based national health insurance program. Services still were delivered, for the most part in the private sector, but an employment based insurance scheme was introduced. Its ultimate goal of covering all parts of the population has now been reached. However, costs in the system have grown so high that over time, the benefits that recipients were covered for were continuously reduced. In South Korea today, the population covered by national insurance is nearly 100% and out-of-pocket costs are so great because the covered benefits have eroded so much. So in a sense, all South Koreans have insurance coverage; but they had best not have the need for and duration of medical and other services not included in the covered benefits.

Another country of real interest is India where many of the reform issues are in the forefront. Decentralization of the public system has gone well apace and the States, which have so much of the public role in health, have also been experimental laboratories. A number of important pieces of legislation have been enacted recently especially in the area of health infrastructure essential to pursuit of the reform agenda. Yet, private markets are still growing, access to care is still uneven, and there are serious questions about quality, cost, and bureaucratic malaise, inertia, and ineffectiveness in the both the private and public health sector.

HEALTH REFORM IN LATIN AMERICA

The reform agenda of the past decade has not escaped Latin America even though health care systems there are dominated by large social security/health insurance systems. It is generally thought that private markets in health care are small in Latin America, but some recent research has shown that the size of the private sector has been underestimated. (Lastiri, 1991). The World Bank estimates that social security systems in Latin America cover about 60% of the continent's population, in some countries more, in some less. These social insurance systems have produced many substantial inequities and inequalities. A nice quotation from Brian Abel-Smith sums up this point: "There are inequalities in the benefits provided by different funds and within funds. There may be inequalities in the benefits provided between the employee and his dependents and between the benefits provided to different hierarchical groups of employees. But the major inequality is between the regularly employed mainly urban worker who has rights to mainly curative health services including high technology services...and the urban poor who are not regularly employed and not only have no rights but also are without much in the way of local services."(Abel-Smith, 1985,p.959)

But like elsewhere, reform efforts have been underway in Latin America for the better part of a decade. Some countries such as Mexico have wrestled with very major reforms, much like those envisioned in the original reform agenda. But here the greatest political barrier to such fundamental change was the social insurance funds themselves who saw their role lessened. But the major pieces of the reform agenda are being tried in Latin America as well, with the special twist of trying also to reform and extend the social insurance systems where high costs, inefficiencies and some consumer dissatisfaction have made reform a hot political issue. Privatizing (e.g. Chile), decentralization (Brazil and Argentina), major extensions of social insurance coverage into rural areas and self-employed groups (Panama and Costa Rica, possibly Mexico), and the use of user charges, market driven incentives, and managed care concepts are all being tried. One interesting experiment worth noting is the PROSALUD program in Bolivia, certainly one of the continents poorest countries. PROSALUD is a private non-profit owned, nearly 91% funded from assessed user charges, has given widespread consumer satisfaction with services and with the providers who work in the system (Ii, 1993). But extension of the model elsewhere has been widely opposed by physicians in private practice. PROSALUD was largely an initiative of Government as a way to challenge public services and to see if payment by poor people for services could be sustained. (Ii, 1993)

HEALTH REFORM IN THE MIDDLE EAST

This is the part of the world where the original reform agenda has penetrated the least. It is also a region of great diversity in wealth, type of system, and access to care. There is also a great diversity and disparity among countries of the region. Egypt, technically in Africa, is a large, populous country, with very severe access and coverage problems in the public sector and a two tier private sector which supports the elite and wealthy not just of Egypt but of other Arab countries who come there for sometimes routine medical care but mostly for exotic or high tech care. In Iraq the health system is devasted by two wars and the five-year trade and oil embargo; health care reform would be an unwelcome problem. Iran and Afghanistan, technically not Middle East, or Arab countries but grouped here for convenience, are at the other end of the spectrum; Iran has a vibrant private health sector living within a largely socialist influenced public sector; Afghanistan is devasted, much like Iraq, and perhaps moreso. In both countries, indeed for all the region, data are hard to come by and not much exists in the conventional data sources about these countries, how they are doing on health status, how much they are spending, and what kinds of reform initiatives may be in the works. In the oil rich Gulf States (Saudi Arabia, United Arab Emirates, Qatar, Oman, Bahrain, Kuwait which form the Gulf Council States) spending on health care is high with both a mixture of the public and private in terms of delivery system. Expenditures have been rising quite dramatically the past decade while the oil revenue necessary to support the quite advanced systems of social support in these countries, has declined precipitously, putting substantial pressure on government. (The past year, 1996, has seen a major gain in oil revenues as the world price of crude oil has risen. It is too soon to say if this represents a new trend). The presence of very large expatriate populations in these countries, most of whom have access to the health system, creates problems of finance, equity, and insurance unique to these countries. But health reform is underway in the Gulf States. Almost all have considered user charges and some are already imposing these for limited activities. Nearly all these countries have underway plans to charge expatriates (and/or their employers) costs more equal to the cost of the care provided, rather than the highly subsidized systems now. And at least one state, UAE, has already implemented a limited insurance payment model for expatriate workers. In the Gulf and other states of the Middle East, there exists the tradition of the classic public health model, government owned, run and provided health system paid for out of general taxation. But alongside this are the other traditions of free markets; open competition, minimum governmental regulation and these are very evident in health care. Private health markets are large in all these countries and in many cases activities there have outstripped the pace, quality, and comprehensiveness of reforms contemplated, or undertaken, by governments in the public sector. There are more aspects of these factors discussed below.

HEALTH REFORM IN AFRICA

Last but not least, of course, no survey would be complete without consideration of Africa. Again, we violate some conventions of geography by having already talked of Egypt earlier. Here we must make the distinction between northern, largely French-speaking Africa and Africa south of the Sahara, conventionally referred to as Sub-Saharan Africa. There is not a lot to write about here. In Sub-Saharan Africa the main story is poverty and health reform takes a back seat to this predominating imperative. Yet reform along the lines of the original reform agenda is underway in many countries: in East Africa with Tanzania and Uganda, and Kenya somewhat in the lead; in West Africa, Ghana is by far ahead of everyone, though Ivory Coast is doing well; Mali, Botswana and Zimbabwe have all undertaken, in a rather serious way, parts of the reform agenda. In so many ways Africa is different and this is certainly true with respect to health reform. There are features unique to Africa such as the huge donor presence in the health sector; the donors can both be a help to health reform or a barrier to it. In many parts of Africa you find the same types of heavy unionization of health workers as found in Western and Southern Europe; these too can be both help and a barrier to reform. (Just recently a several month's long strike of hospital workers in Zimbabwe ended). And in Africa, the widespread prevalence of graft and corruption in the Civil Service system is itself a major barrier to change of any kind. Nonetheless, having all these caveats upfront, one finds many of the same trends with reform in Africa as elsewhere: public systems have tried to decentralize with very limited success, private health sectors have taken off and are very major sectors for provision of care. There is very wide divergence in access to care by income groups, in the quality of care received, and in the performance of systems, public and private. Political instability, slow or even negative economic growth, in some cases wars and militant border clashes, all inhibit an atmosphere in which any priority can be claimed for health sector reform. Yet levels of dissatisfaction with services received, and with access to quality services is the most lacking fundamentally. Africa, south of the Sahara is the most fertile area of the world in need of health reform. But it is here one sees the barriers to reform writ large: incompetent public sector management (there are exceptions, of course), resistance to change by those most affected by the change such as trade unions of health professionals, even the donor community in many instances, and for the most part real disregard for the wishes, aspirations and satisfaction of consumers. Yet in this most unfavorable setting one finds the most interesting research being done on the barriers to health sector reform, especially in Tanzania, Uganda, Ghana, somewhat so in Nigeria and Kenya. So far, at any rate, the failures of reform outweigh the successes.

HEALTH REFORM IN THE UNITED STATES

I have left the United States for last and as a special case because nowhere else are the arguments being advanced in the Concept paper better illustrated than what has happened in the U.S. during the first two years of the Administration of President Clinton. A major effort to reform the U.S. system was put together by Mrs. Clinton and an inhouse team of experts. This effort resulted in an 1000 page piece of legislation introduced into the Congress in the fall of 1992. The main thrust of the Clinton reform was to give, within a reasonable period of time (year 2000 was the final date set at the end of the acrimonious debate) universal access to insurance coverage to the entire population. This was to be provided to those uncovered parts of the population by all employers with a system of government subsidies to ease the phase in to total coverage.

Costs were to be contained by use of managed care incentives—to bias against fee for service medicine—with competition between regional purchasing coalitions, which would purchase care from providers in the region. An elaborate system of market regulation, supposedly to make the markets work and be "competitive" was included as was a fairly elaborate governmental bureaucracy at the Federal and State level to supervise the contract bidding process and to monitor quality control. Major changes were also included on the benefit and provider reimbursement side for the two major public programs: Medicare (for the elderly) and Medicaid (for the poor). The details on the proposed reforms is greater than I am giving here because it is not on the nature of the reforms that is of interest to us but what happened to the reforms. First, one should argue that the Clinton proposed reforms came from the same family as what we refer to as the original reform agenda: expenditures in the U.S. had reached 13% of GDP already, were forecasted to reach 20% in half a decade, and yet there were perhaps 40 million people, somewhere around 20% of the total population, without any health insurance at all, and perhaps another 10million people with very limited insurance coverage, certainly not enough to cover major emergencies. The former were referred to as the Uninsured, the latter to the Underinsured.

All the polls of voter and consumer sentiment taken in the US during 1991 showed that concern for health care was the major, usually the first ranking, issue on the minds of the American population. President Clinton had as clear a mandate for change, as an elected politician will ever get. Every major interest group in the country was on record as favoring change from the American Medical Association (the principal organization for physicians nationwide) to the local, corner pharmacy. At the time Clinton sent his bill to Congress, it had already before it 11 other legislative proposals to reform the US health care system ranging from minor reforms to reforms far more sweeping in scope than those proposed by the President. The climate for change was ripe. What went wrong? There is now a good literature about this but what went wrong is easy to determine: the political savvy of the President and his team was weak, all the interest groups figured out the costs and benefits to them of these changes, and those who could have gained the most from the changes had neither the political clout or the resources to fight off those opposed. A major effort to change and turn public opinion against the Clinton proposals financed by the Health Insurance Association, a major potential loser under the Clinton plan, largely succeeded and the Clinton plan was easily derailed and put in the ash bin of failed reform efforts. What happens in the US always seems to be on a large scale because it is a large country, it is a rich country, and it is a country, which is dominated by private markets, not just in health care but everywhere. Yet, most analysts believe that had President Clinton handled the politics of reform in the proper manner, he could have won a major change in a major sector of the American economy. But the plan was flawed, the way the plan was put together was flawed, and the way the flawed plan was sold was flawed; the result was a flawed effort. One sees many of the same elements at work when reform agenda's are adopted in countries of the developing world: all the affected parties come out of the woodwork and it takes enormous political skill to get things done. The bureaucracy is usually against the change, even the doctors, donors, and other interest groups. But the people who have the most to gain, usually the consumers, either don't have enough political power, or are unorganized to resist these negative forces.

Yet the fact that the American health sector is so dominated by the private sector, the failed Clinton effort may well have had some major effect on changes in the sector originating in the private companies, private health insurors, and private health providers of the country. In the past five years the percentage of the population enrolled in managed care has gone from under 40% to nearly 85% and most estimates say that by the year 2000 nearly the entire insured population will be in managed care. Yet the number of uninsured and underinsured in the US have not lessened. Total expenditures of the system have leveled off somewhat and will not hit the predicted 20% of GDP every expert had predicted. The two major public programs, Medicare and Medicaid, have had some limited reforms imposed, mostly in Medicaid (nearly all Medicaid recipients most now get care from an HMO or other managed care deliverer). Medicare reform is still alive because the predicted expenditure growth will soon exceed the payroll taxes collected to finance the system.

Reform in the U.S. has been substantial, nonetheless, but it is still the health system in the industrialized world where the original reform agenda is still alive. What the Clinton reform episode showed is that the three issues we focus on, Public Sector Management, Professional Associations, and Information came to be the real barriers to reform in the U.S. and were the rocks on which reform failed: nobody believed a Government bureaucracy better at administering a program than the private sector, the physicians and insurance companies used their political clout more skillfully than did the President, and the people, the ones most affected by the reform, had very little say in the outcome.

What is the most interesting aspect of the US situation is that the private sector, already the dominant player in American health care, has become even moreso since the failure of the Clinton health reform. In just the past few years there have been innumerable consolidations of managed care companies, of hospitals and hospital chains, and the once dominant organizational form—non-profit—has been eroding fast. For profit health care firms—Managed Care, Hospital Chains, etc—all publicly owned companies have been buying, in some cases merging, with previously not for profit, HMO's, and university and community hospitals. What the end game of these enormous consolidations will be no one really knows. A common cliché is that all health care is local, meaning that people relate to those who serve them in their community. The consolidations of the recent past defy that cliché and how consumers, and especially physicians, will react to getting care from (and working for) a company whose stock is traded daily on the New York Stock Exchange is yet to be known.

SOME OTHER RELATED ISSUES TO HEALTH SECTOR REFORM

There are two other issues that cut across the brief survey given above and require some special words on their own. One is the special challenge that a large Donor community presents to implementing an agenda of change in the health sector. The other is the rather peculiar tango that exists between the public and private sectors in most countries, especially where private sector growth has overshadowed public sector reforms.

Ralph Andreano

Donors

This is a touchy subject because the donor community has been so important in most respects in bringing needed resources to the health sectors of developing countries. The donor community runs the gamut from the longstanding mission hospitals in many countries to the special aid programs for disease control, drugs, nutrition, water supply, other physical infrastructure and so on. Yet the donor community has become so large in some countries that they are a party to any reform effort and must be consulted and included by Government. There is a fine line between retaining one's sovereignty and dignity and not loosing needed resources to keep a population afloat. NGO's and others in the Donor community have been especially crucial to health care provision in Africa, in some cases with their aid proportionately larger than what the central government itself spends on health care. Yet there are distortions in priorities that countries have willingly permitted just to get the NGO and Donor aid. Like all other institutions, NGO's and other Donors have what we economists call their own objective function: that is they have something very specific they would like to achieve and to which end they commit their resources to in a given country. Sometimes their goals and aspirations coincide with what should be a country's priority, sometimes not. In any case, any attempt at serious reform of the health sector in developing countries, but especially in Africa, cannot occur without inclusion, discussion, and restructuring of the NGO and Donor community roles in health. In the 1993 World Development Report it notes that aid for health care in the developing countries has contributed to spending imbalances and resource distortions. Donors, it notes, tend to prefer spending on hospitals, expensive equipment and other high cost things, much more difficult for governments to maintain because of high recurring costs once the donor has left. In 1988-90, the Report mentions, that Japan spent more than 33% of its bilateral aid on building hospitals, France spent 25% and Italy and Germany each 15%. In the concept paper, I include the NGO's and Donor's in general as part of the Institutional barriers to health sector reform. Very little research is underway on their role in the reform agenda, but this is changing by some original work underway in Uganda and Tanzania.

The Public/Private Dilemma

There is another phenomenon not so easily grouped under the brief survey of reform in the regions and by level of income noted above. I have noted repeatedly that the private sector growth in health care is in some sense a more dominant characteristic in rich and poor countries over the past decade than governmental changes. On the one hand it looks like private sector growth exceeds in importance what shape reform takes in the public sector. On the other,

172

without private sector growth, any reform on the public side is probably very limited. To my observation, reform and the growth of the private sector in health, mostly so in the poorest developing countries but with some exceptions in the rich countries, are intertwined events; one happens with and because of the other. This interconnection is not always good for the people or the country. To simplify the example I have in mind, consider that in the private sector people pay for their care (or an employer does) and in the public sector, society pays either through general taxes or other claims on the central treasury. At the time of use of services, public ones are free, private ones are not. It matters very much, therefore, which public services are free and which are not. What one finds for the most part is that people will stay in the private sector up until the point that they need a highly expensive service (say such as specialized surgery and extensive hospital care) and then they will blend into the public sector, where such services are still offered. There are two kinds of dilemma's here: (1) what rules should govern the services that should remain as public, and hence free, and which should not? And, (2) if the private sector takes a patient through routine care, for payment, and then moves the patient back into the public sector when there is something the private sector has chosen not to provide and which is free, how can it be said that the growth of the private sector is a serious ally of governmental reform? In some of the Gulf States, with very complex and growing private sectors, usually employer financed, what one observes is that as long as Government continues to allocate most of its health investments into specialized and usually high quality physician and hospital care, the private sector will never undertake the investment needed to turn such dimensions of care into profit centers. What this all means, to me at any rate, in the context of an agenda for health sector reform, is that the original reform agenda and nothing much since, has articulated how Government should shape its service delivery system in order to allow private sector growth to do things the Government used to do. The whole point of the original reform agenda, articulated at Alma Ata and reaffirmed in 1987, was to allow the private sector to grow so Governments could spend less on services that people would be willing and able to pay for, and divert those resources into things with very large positive externalities and focus mainly on questions of equity (in access, in costs, in geography, etc.). In so far as one can see on the research done thus far, this main effect of the original reform agenda has not really happened; government's continue to spend most of their resources on acute care, private sectors are allowed to grow quite large (and only in a few countries to let that growth go all the way to private for profit specialized hospitals), but the big, highly specialized, expensive services, are still essentially free (even if there is a user charge attached it is less than the cost of provision of the service). The rational private sector invests in those things it can easily sell at prevailing market prices (say a clinic visit to a private clinic where one pays versus a visit to a free government clinic where one waits and gets indifferent service), and avoids making major capital decisions in diagnostic equipment and institutions for specialized care with the supporting physician and nurse infrastructure. From this perspective, the vibrant growth of the private sector especially in the poorest developing countries is a two-edged sword: on the one hand it is good for consumers who can afford it, it increases consumer choices, and it is good for competition; but, if Government's response is no change in its own delivery and service structure, the private sector is getting a free ride. Government is not able to reallocate public resources to uses with higher social benefits, and the possible benefits to the otherwise poor country are blunted.

WHO NEEDS REFORM ANYWAY?

There are two marvelous and powerful graphs in the WB Development Report on Health (1993). One (Figure 3.0) shows since 1900 the growth in life expectancy and the growth of income with the clear conclusion shown in the chart that as the income of countries grows life expectancy grows and that since 1900 both have increased dramatically. The other chart (Figure 3.1) shows the predicted gains in life expectancy based on the expected ranking of countries according to the level of GDP spent on health. The major conclusion of the graph is that some countries spend much less than others but achieve greater than expected gains in life expectancy (China and Sri Lanka being prime examples), and some countries spend vastly more of their resources and achieve much less than predicted outcomes in life expectancy (the principal case being the US). Both these charts and some additional limited evidence presented below makes one wonder what the fuss is all about when it comes to reform of the finance and delivery systems of health in the rich and the poor countries; where are the great gains in health improvement coming from? From the efficiency and equity (mostly non-existent) of health care systems, or from other things? Well, clearly the delivery systems do produce gains in health; and the better the system in terms of coverage, and in services aimed at disease prevention, and the more access and efficiency of the system all will have some impact on health. Otherwise we would not be so concerned with having efficient and equitable systems and while not having these still insisting on reform to make these systems that way. But the gains in health are only one of the measures of performance one can use to measure the success of a health system and in turn the success of a reform effort. It is unlikely that a health system will be at technical and allocative efficiency and be Pareto optimal; it is theoretically possible, but empirically not observable. Still there are very few voices in the world that would not favor a major overhaul of the health systems of the world both in the rich and poor countries. A measure of success is whether or not people feel they get quality services, that they are available when needed, are delivered for the most part with efficiency and equity, and that people have a right to know what is being done to them, how much it will cost them, and whether or not they are getting the highest standard of care available. To argue for health care reform is to say that most systems do not do, well enough or enough of it, any of these things.

The burden of argument of these two papers on Notes on Reform is that the original reform agenda of Alma Ata and of the extensions and amplifications of 1987 was a good one. If fully implemented, as applicable in countries, would these reforms have produced efficient, more equitable systems, where patients felt they got value for money, got the best treatment at the best level of efficiency and that it was available to all irrespective of income? No one would argue that the original reform agenda was going to produce manna from heaven for the world's health systems. Yet the belief then and now is strong that changes were and are needed and the menu of reform ought to look something like what was outlined at Alma Ata and explicated by the World Bank, WHO, and ADB in 1987. The bottom line is that after the reforms, people would be better off, resources would now be used more efficiently, consumers would be better satisfied, and a key component of economic growth and development—better health as a part of human capital—would now be able to be a key aspect in the economic life of countries. Relative to the expectations, the extent to which this has happened around the world is disappointing. And the argument of these papers is that unanticipated barriers to pursuing the health reform agenda, what we have called the traditional agenda, have developed and without overturning these barriers, further gains in reform will be stifled.

There is another level to our arguments that needs some discussion. If one looks at the major thrust of the original reform agenda, there is being preached a certain universality which looks much like what in other circles has come to be called "globalization." Indeed the pursuit of economic efficiency has become a universal goal, since as a recent Newsweek story put it:"those who run countries fear that they will be punished if they do not provide the capital markets with tribute. This economic imperative has squashed political discourse into narrower channels than once seemed possible—to call yourself a socialist is to call yourself a dinosaur." (*Newsweek*, Dec.30, 1996-Jan.6, 1997, story by Michael Elliot, pp. 39-42. The quotation is from page 41.) Two new recent publications, one an article in Foreign Affairs by Ethan Kapstein and the other a book by Samuel Huntington (Huntington's book is *The Clash of Civilizations*) challenge these concepts of globalization and in ways that seem relevant to some of the arguments in our two papers. Kapstein is quoted in the Newsweek article as saying: "The global economy is leaving millions of disaffected workers in its train. Inequality, unemployment and endemic poverty have become its handmaiden." And Huntington in the same article is quoted as saying:"what

Westerners see as benign global integration, such as the proliferation of worldwide media, non-Westerners see as nefarious Western imperialism. To the extent that non-Westerners see the world as one, they see it as a threat."

Perhaps some of this anti-Western thinking is at work in the health reform agenda and how it has been translated in countries both rich and poor. In the struggle between economic systems of the past 50 years, it appears that capitalism wins. Therefore, the health reform agenda, indeed the economic reform agenda, is to make competition work, make markets free, allow entrepreneurs to invest and retain their profits, etc. etc. In essence that is the crux of the reform agenda in health: push incentives, give those with a stake in the system a chance to earn something from it, let consumers be satisfied, let them have choices, let private markets and competition reign. Well, this hasn't exactly worked as planned as we have noted throughout our papers: something is missing. We placed the missing elements on what we called the infrastructure of reform, but the backlash against the globalization of ideas may also suggest that our Alma Ata and 1987 reform agenda does not describe what the world was waiting for. This is just a point of view. My own belief is that while the critics of globalization such as Kapstein and Huntington have a solid point of view—at times their insights are tellingly on the mark—we still believe the original reform agenda in health is a good one.

The arguments of these papers need to be brought back to full circle. While we assert the vailidity of the reform agenda and its essential needs in nearly all countries, it is still true that we cannot fully quantify at least just what difference this will make in health.

EVIDENCE?

Just what evidence would be needed to judge whether or not health sector reform has succeeded or not is certainly not obvious. At the time of the World Bank 1993 Development Report on Health, it was clear that efforts since Alma Ata and since the reaffirmation and extension of the reform agenda by the World Bank, WHO, and Asian Development Bank, in various reports in 1987, had not produced much change worldwide. Of course, some countries had succeeded in some aspects of reform and these are duly noted in the 1993 Bank Report. Yet, virtually the same reform agenda is reoffered to the world, suggesting that the pace and volume of reform was still yet to be achieved. If you look just at health improvement, evidence such as life expectancy, infant mortality, and some other measures such as premature mortality, health improvements have continued to grow in both the developing and developed worlds. So in some sense, the pace and intensity of reform of health sectors has not deterred some major improvements in health. There is still very wide divergence in life expectancy within poor countries, and between rich and poor countries. Yet life expectancy has grown quite substantially in the developing world. In 1993, using the World Bank's Social Indicators of Development Data Set, average life expectancy for the entire world is 66 years at birth for males. In the high-income economies alone, it was 77 years for males at birth. For all low-income countries except China and India, average LE was 56 years, and in India 61yrs, and China 69 years. The low-income country figures are dominated by Sub-Saharan Africa where in 1993 average life expectancy was 52 years. The picture on infant mortality rates is brighter. In low-income countries between 1978 and 1994 average rates per 1000 live births fell from 135 to 89. Even in Sub-Saharan Africa the rates fell from 132 to 93. In the Middle East and North Africa from 136 to 52. These declines are roughly comparable to the world average decline for the same period of from 81 to 48 and for the rich country decline from 19 to 7. Yet having noted this, one can also be sure that the gap between the richest countries within the poor developing country group do better than the poorest in that group; and between all poor countries and rich, the gap is huge. Will reform of the health system eliminate these gaps? Perhaps, it certainly can't hurt (unless some things go wrong quite unexpectedly), but health improvements of dramatic magnitudes will require more than just health reform; the best predictor of success for health improvement on these statistics is growth of income. If the poor economies do better, up to a point, these crude indicators of health will improve.

Other possible measures of the success or failure of reform efforts might be data on access to health care. Regrettably this data is almost non-existent on a global scale. Both the OECD data set (Health Data 1996) and the World Bank two data sets, World Development Indicators, and Social Indicators of Development have few country entries for this and there is little data over time to measure such changes. If you look at expenditure data, in the rich countries, the median annual growth rate of total expenditures on health (all measured in purchasing power parity dollars) for the period 1985-1994 are still at stratospheric levels: Germany, 7.92%, France, 6.80%, United Kingdom, 9.17%, the USA, 9.25%. Only Japan's growth rate seems anywhere close to the general annual growth of GDP over the same period, at 4.91%. Per capital expenditures in PPP $ in 1980 in Germany were $802 and in 1994 were $1,869, in France by the same measure and for the same years, $711 to $1,866, Japan $522 to $1,473, and of course, the winner and still champ, USA from $1051 to $3,516. But even a centrally budgeted system such as UK rose for the same period and on the same dollar terms, from $453 to $1,211. (All these numbers are from the OECD data set, Health Data 1996). So one does not exactly find major slowdowns in the rate of spending on health care in the rich countries, and that certainly was an aim of all reform efforts. Of course, one could argue that without reform, the expenditure levels would have been higher yet, and there is some merit to this

Ralph Andreano

view. But not enough to proclaim reform efforts, at least on the cost containment front, of having been a ringing success. For the developing countries, the World Bank data are ambiguous. On the one hand, it is pretty clear that in most developing countries total expenditures have risen in the past decade simply because of the explosive growth of the private sector. But health expenditures as a percentage of central government expenditures have not risen except in a few countries. At present, spending on health care mops up about 8% of total world product with 87% of that amount (and 42%alone in the U.S.) in the rich countries. Developing countries average about 4% of their GDP spent on health (but this includes public and private expenditures) with the respective per capita averages being $41compared to $1,900 in the rich countries.

Cost containment is not an objective of reform in the developing world; rather, what is more important is redressing the misallocation of public resources from such high cost treatments (such as expensive surgeries and hospital care) to cost-effective uses of resources such as primary care. Yet in the Barnum and Kutzin study, it shows that even at this mid-point in the decade somewhere from 40% to 80% of their entire health budgets are still spent on these high cost items. So redressing the misallocations of resources in the developing world has barely begun. What is more disturbing, however, is that on the supply side, the doctors, nurses, and capital invested in developing countries is still heavily biased on acute care. This is no less true and, of course, more so in the rich countries. However, in the rich countries one is now observing a shift at least away from hospital care to outpatient care, which is somewhat cheaper. In the U.S., for example, for the period 1985 to 1994. the median annual percentage growth rate for inpatient care (8.39%) is well less than the growth rate for outpatient or ambulatory care over the same period (10.27%) (Data from OECD Health Data 1996). Major resource shifts are underway in the rich countries, especially in the largely dominated private sector in the USA. And in these resource shifts one can see the promise of Alma Ata and the hope that similar resource shifts can be done on a massive scale in the developing world. A variety of research in the US has shown how cost-effective it is for patients to be seen first by a primary care physician. A number of regression models have shown that first contact with a primary care physician, on average, reduces expenditures (for both inpatient and ambulatory services) for 24 of the most common acute (not chronic) conditions. (Reported in APHRSD, Agency for Public Health Reasearch and Development Vol. 197, Oct.1996, and page 5). Research on the cost of lives saved and on the QUALYS, (Quality Adjusted Life – Years Saved) and DALYS, (Disability Adjusted Life – Years Saved) gained from various cost-effective interventions reaffirms the wisdom of the Alma Ata reform agenda to push primary care in all its dimensions. The median cost, for example, of a year of life saved for childhood immunizations has been estimated at "less than zero" and for prenatal care the same. Obviously, the actual cost is not zero, but compared to other uses

178

of the same amount of resources, to save a year of life, these interventions are practically "free".

SUMMING UP

I am not sure how to sum up all the arguments of this supplementary paper and the earlier one. But I think it is simple, even if a somewhat watered-down version, to note that the original reform agenda of Alma Ata and of 1987 is still a good one. Few countries, rich or poor, have really accomplished much in the way of major structural reform. And I say this while still noting that some countries both rich and poor have accomplished lots of great things: my assessment is overall. Yet the ideas are still good ideas and worth pursuing. What I am asserting and with a limited amount of evidence, to be sure, is that there are certain barriers to implementing that agenda that rear their ugly head when things start to push ahead especially when there are inklings of some success with reform. I have cast these barriers as a missing infrastructure needed to implement the original reform agenda, and I have noted that the three classes I single out (Public Sector Management, Professional Associations and Institutions, and Information) all emerge in the reform efforts, at least as I have observed them, in rich and poor countries. Yet health gains continue even while poverty and inequality grow: poverty and inequality are not just developing country problems as these exist in large degree in rich countries with just a few exceptions. (Of course the scale of poverty and inequality is massively different between rich and poor countries). I have argued that policy research on these three elements is needed and really is already underway in a number of countries. But the larger argument is not that new research alone will show us the way to overcome these barriers, although one hopes this will happen; but, rather, that these three elements represent barriers in and of themselves and they stand in the way of any worldwide and major success with reform efforts of the public systems in the developing world. What I find the most intriguing point is that private sector growth has outstripped the pace of change and reform in the developing world, and the three elements I have singled out are now more important than ever. Not just to get to the original reform agenda, but also because of the growth of private medical markets, the urgency and need for governments to redefine their roles in health must become part of the agenda of reform. I hope all of this makes some sense.

Ralph Andreano

BIBLIOGRAPHIC NOTE

As with the Concept paper, I have barely cited all the papers and sources that have in one way or the other been noted or cited in the two papers. This is at best a partial bibliography.

Abel-Smith, Brian (1985), "Global Perspective on Health Services Financing," *Social Science and Medicine,* Vol. 21, No. 9, pp.957-963.

Asian Development Bank (1987), *Health Care Financing (Regional Seminar on Health Care Financing, July 27-August 3, Manila)* Published by EDI, ADB, Manila, 1987. See especially the papers by Charles Griffin on user charges, John Akin on Health Insurance, and Ralph Andreano and Thomas Helminiak on the Role of the Private Sector.

Gertler, Paul and Jacques Van der Gaag (1990), The Willingness to Pay for Medical Care: Evidence from Two Developing Countries. (World Bank, Washington).

Korte, R (1996), *Planning for Health Systems Reforms* (I pulled this off the Internet on the Afro-nets page. I do not know where it was given or if it was published elsewhere. But I found it useful).

Lastiri, Santiago (1991), Financing of the Mexican Health Care System: The Role of the Private Sector in the Financing and Delivery of Services, (Ph.D. Thesis, University of Wisconsin, Madison, Wisconsin, USA).

Ii, Masako (1993), *Willingness to Pay for Medical Care: Evidence from Urban Areas in Bolivia.* (Ph.D. Thesis, University of Wisconsin, Madison, Wisconsin, USA).

OECD (1992), The Reform of Health Care: A Comparative Study of Seven OECD Countries. Health Policy Studies, No. 2 (Paris, France).

—————(1990), *Health Care Systems in Transition: The Search For Efficiency,* Social Policy Studies, and No. 2. (Paris, France).

World Bank (1993), *World Development Report on Health* (Oxford University Press, Washington and Oxford).

—————(1987), Financing Health Services in Developing Countries: An Agenda For Reform. A World Bank Policy Study (Washington, DC).

World Health Organization (1993a), *Evaluation of Recent Changes in the Financing of Health Services* (Report of a WHO Study Group, Geneva, Switzerland).

—————(1993b), *Antidotum.* The First Meeting of the Expert Network on the Health and Health Care Financing Strategies. Warsaw/Ryma, May 31-June1 (Warsaw).

—————(1991), *Organization and Financing of Health Care Reform in Countries of Central and Eastern Europe.* Report of a WHO Task Force on Health Development. (Geneva, Switzerland).

————(1991a), The Public/Private Mix in National Health Systems and The Role of the Ministries of Health (Special Meeting, held in Mexico City, Mexico) (Geneva, Switzerland).

Ralph Andreano

Notes on Economic Aspects of Governance[41]

OVERVIEW

In the two earlier papers (Notes on Health Reform and More Notes on Health Reform) I speculated on the barriers that seem to exist in developing countries that inhibit change in the public health sector. Some key elements identified were: governance, or as we called it in the above papers, public sector management; professional associations (such as medical associations, trade unions, etc.), and information gaps on a wide variety of reform issues such as programs and policies evaluation. It is clear that these barriers exist not just in the health sector but also throughout the social sectors in developing countries. In this memo we refine some of these concepts. Governance has become the new cliché inside the UN system so we take a peek at what it may mean there. Governance has come to mean all three of the elements noted above and that is what is dealt with in this note.

SOME DEFINITIONS

The reality in most developing countries is that public services are mostly in disrepair, in bad standing with the public, and losing out to private markets and institutions, which are growing rapidly everywhere. Most countries, beyond health care, are moving toward, or are already deeply committed to, market driven growth. This has led to movements for privatization of governmental institutions and the like. The role of government is being lessened, allegedly. The new orthodoxy is market driven, individual centered, and incentive laden approaches supposedly lead to faster and more sustained development. The actual evidence is mixed. But experiences now suggest that the role of government in the developing world is still relevant, still potentially large, and still needed. Its functions and scope of influence is being rethought and redefined and this is desirable. If one thinks first of health care, market driven growth and the subsequent decline of so-called "free" services have probably increased inequities with regard to access and quality of services. Extending beyond health care to the social sector generally, the same generalizations persist: inequities in

---

[41]This note was written for the World Health Organization in 1997 after some UN and WHO administrators had read the earlier two papers; Notes on Health Sector Reform and More Notes on Health Sector Reform. I was asked to develop the Governance issues a bit further and suggest some possible programs for WHO to work on. I have left out here that part of the paper dealing with the specific programmatic suggestions to WHO. (Authors note, Feb. 10, 2001).

access, income, wealth, and opportunity are widening as private/market driven initiatives have taken hold. This is not all bad and one is not asserting that the clock should be turned back. Our perception of the problems of government and the way they govern in the developing world, in principle, should not be different from perceptions of the changing role of government in the industrialized countries. There are certain standards and norms of what constitute "good government". And these are at the heart of what we now call governance.

Many attempts to outline the characteristics of "sound governance" have been made (UNDP, Report on the Workshop on Governance for Sustainable Human Development, 24-26April, 1996 New York, p. 8/9) and the temptation is to include everything one can think of. There is considerable confusion, I think, in the UN system papers on the subject. There is a wide spectrum of government types from democratic to authoritarian but the quality of the governance may not necessarily depend on the type of government provided certain principles exist. These are:

(1) Government and its services are centered on the people they are supposed to serve. (2) The perception of the people is that those who run government and provide services are accountable for their actions. And, (3) the behavior of government officials is what is euphemistically called "transparent." Each of these requires some explanation. The reason private markets have grown (not the only reason) is that if a provider does not put the person it aims to serve first, i.e. is not consumer friendly, the consumer will seek providers that do offer this. Some recent exit interviews with consumers who use private medical clinics, often just across the street from "free" public ones, reveal that among the top reasons for choosing to use these facilities is that the staff are accommodating, accessible, friendly, and seem to care about "your" needs. (Other important reasons were drug availability, hours of operation, and location). On point (2), in democratic societies there is some balance of power with different levels of government having some checks and balances on each other. And there are other disinterested groups such as the media, which hold government as a whole, and agencies and individuals to account when wrongs, in general, or on particular sets of consumers, are committed. Some body, or institution, has to hold government accountable for its actions and in non-democratic, or near democratic governments, these elements of governance are often missing. On point (3), one of the most damaging things to the public's perception of government being at best ineffective, at worst, corrupt, is the widespread favoring of special interest groups, open bribery and under the table payments to jump a queue or secure a governmental advantage. This is the meaning of transparency; when a law says such and such should be followed, or rules are prescribed, if the public's perception is that they are not, it is an open invitation to disapprove of the

governance citizens get and to sow interest and ambition in finding ways of seeking your own advantages and to advance your own special interests.

This infrastructure of governance, therefore, encompasses the basic institutions of government: its legal structures, rules, regulations, standards, and norms; its fiscal, budgetary, and personnel structures including the power to tax and collect revenues legally; and finally, an internal structure or system with elements of checks and balances between different levels of government and different agencies. If there is a strong judicial system and tradition, the principle of transparency and even accountability is believed to be much stronger. A separation of powers and roles between different levels of government, an executive, a legislative body, and a judiciary are common features of democratic governments; but elements or near substitutes of these can be found if there is a real desire for and expression of "good government", regardless of the constitutional foundation of a country.

OPERATIONALIZING THE CONCEPTS OF GOVERNANCE

If we reduce for sake of discussion the basic principles of good governance to three concepts it may simplify how one thinks about initiating changes in countries. First, learning from the lessons of private sector growth, governance where the targets are people, consumers, clients, or whatever one calls it, form the central focus of government actions, is the first major concept. Second, accountability at all levels and an endogenous process of checks and balances is another major component of good governance. And, third, all governmental actions of its institutions and its providers should be above board and transparent; an internal system of checks and balances should minimize if not eliminate the under the table payments, graft and other forms of monetary and non-monetary corruption. These concepts are deceptively simple and if it were easy to achieve and implement them, what country wouldn't want to do so? The reality is that only a few states can claim their governance meets these three tests and where there is widespread support and approval of government performance. Most of the world falls into the much larger group where governments are mistrusted, where government workers are surly and discourteous toward people (consumers, clients), and where unvarnished self-interest governs both individual and group behavior. If we are now targeting governance as a barrier to effective change in health and in development in general, how can these trends be reversed? Not easily! The documents emerging from various parts of the UN System, especially the United Nations Development Program (UNDP) but also the World Health Organization (WHO), are suggesting a comprehensive set of principles to meet the tests of good governance, but their prescription for implementation is that "everyone should work together" to make it all possible. The reality is that in most countries, self-interest of individuals, groups, communities, governments, officials of government—whatever—present disharmonious situations, not harmonious ones. For the three principles we single out above (all envisioned in an endogenous system of checks and balances) they may indeed conflict with each other. Why would governments want to be responsibly disposed toward their populations in services delivered by viewing them as clients or consumers such as is done by the private sector? The only reason one can think of is if they had some incentive or set of incentives to do so: if government officials' careers depended on consumer satisfaction, if government revenues depended on the use and reception of government services by the population, then perhaps governance would be people focused. Similarly, even if governments did target client satisfaction, if they are unaccountable for their actions, and if there is no internal system of rewards and punishments, what incentives exist to continue such practices? The answer is: none! Self-interest drives groups and individuals to seek advantages of a personal or institutional kind from government and this leads to monetary and non-monetary forms of bribery and corruption. A system, client focused, could not survive very long if at the same time there were no internal corrective processes to divert perceptions of self-interest into constructive alternatives. If we knew the answers to all these questions and we knew how to suggest ways for countries to implement the principles of good governance, we would have done so already! That is why one needs further study of these issues to see how governance and the institutions and incentives required can be found and activated in developing countries. In health care, in principle, the elements of good governance would be no different than in other social sectors. So the comments in this memo are not always just geared toward the health sector. But for WHO it is the relevant place to start and it must study the cases of where good governance persists, find out, if it can, why it persists, what internal institutions make it work, and the extent to which these findings are exportable to other cultures and states. A modest approach for WHO would be to flesh out the concepts and analytical principles of governance somewhat along the lines suggested above. As the leading UN agency responsible for world health, it is incumbent for WHO to find a way to relate its mission to good governance in developing countries.

Governance and WHO: A look at the UN "Governance"

A point of major significance which is not discussed in this memo, but is elsewhere, is that the same investigation of principles of governance summarily noted above are equally relevant to study within the context of WHO, or for that matter, the entire UN System. The UN does not meet most tests of good governance: it focuses on governments, not people, its actions and programmes

Ralph Andreano

and personnel are often not appointed by merit or performance evaluated, and accountability and transparency within the UN system is clouded by the dynamics of international politics. The UN and WHO are organized as if they have an internal system of checks and balances, but they do not. I see a moral dilemma: how can WHO or the UN system as a whole advise countries to improve their governance, suggest ways of their doing so, if their own house does not meet the simple tests of good governance? A good question, I think and one, which needs some discussion.

SELECTION 10

HEALTH ECONOMICS AND HEALTH POLICY IN GLOBAL PERSPECTIVE[42]

INTRODUCTION

The countries in the Eastern Mediterranean Region of the World Health Organization (EMR) represent as diversified and complex a grouping of countries as one could imagine. The range of problems and choices facing countries in this diverse region, however, are common to those found elsewhere. And many of the policy initiatives and policy issues in this region are being tried or addressed by other developing countries. In this paper, I will try to give a framework to shape our thinking both for this Inter-country Meeting (IC) and for future initiatives for Member countries of EMR to consider in the years ahead. The outline of the paper is as follows: 1) a brief global overview of world economic conditions and health care, 2) the situation in EMR, 3) some underlying policy issues, 4) global policy development, 5) the potential for health economics.

I. GLOBAL OVERVIEW: DEVELOPMENTS IN WORLD ECONOMIC CONDITION AND HEALTH CARE THE PAST SEVERAL YEARS

The past three years have intensified the negative economic trends affecting economic welfare and health in the developing countries and especially in the least developed countries. The worsening of the debt crisis and the rising proportion of export revenues needed to service international debt in the developing countries (especially of Africa and Latin America) have had substantial impact on resources available for health and health status. The continual decline of commodity and raw material prices and the increased demands of structural adjustment programs (SAP), and the number of countries now under SAP's in the past three years may have also worsened the economic capacity of developing countries ability to maintain existing levels of health. In oil producing countries, the decline in world oil prices has also had an impact on health budgets as well as other social policy objectives.

---

[42]Paper prepared for the 1st IC Workshop on Health Economics, WHO, EMR held in Riyadh, Saudia Arabia, February 20-24, 1989.

The immediate and longer-term prospects for the developing countries have also not been enhanced by other recent developments on the world economic scene. The international liquidity crisis stimulated by the worldwide crash of world securities markets on October 19, 1988 has made structural adjustment programs (SAP's) more difficult to implement and worsened the ability of developing countries to move out of their resource scarcities for health through economic growth. Except for a few countries of the developing world, long-term growth prospects are very bleak and this does not portend well for human resources development. A buoyant economic growth in the industrialized countries could help the developing countries to achieve success with their SAP's and to reduce the international transfer of resources from poor to rich countries indigenous to today's debt problem. But modest economic growth in the industrialized countries, growing protectionism, widening trade deficits, rising nominal and real interest rates all work against the economic possibilities for countries in the developing world.

In the developed countries including a number of oil export based economies, the past three years has also seen a continuation of recent trends: rising total expenditures for health care and as a percent of GDP or GNP; slippage in problem areas of access and health status for very poor, high risk populations, especially in urban areas; and concerns for quality of care, among other developments. In the rich countries the emphasis on containment of costs, with the need to improve health system efficiency, and with a continuing concern for equity deterioration has dominated public policy debates and legislation. In the developed countries with predominantly publicly funded and operated services, concerns about resource constraints, system efficiencies, and access and equity gaps have also been more evident than in recent years.

In the socialist countries where economic growth has also been modest over the past several years (excepting China) there has been a remarkable movement to improve productive efficiency and to expand the scope for consumer choices. Market liberalization policies in these economies in general have also had some spillover effects into the health system and have resulted in continuing concerns for new sources of financing, cost containment, quality of care, and maintaining equity.

Around the world, in all economies, private sector (profit and not-for-profit) expenditures on health care have been growing in the past several years. This growth is in part due to severe resource constraints faced by public systems but also because of the desire of consumers for alternatives to obtaining health services. The growth of the private sector health care system, especially in the developing countries, has presented both problems and opportunities; problems in the sense that all health care costs have been pushed upwards and some inequities intensified; opportunities in the sense that countries can reconsider the amount of public resources they need to commit to health care to cover entire populations.

In summary, in all countries, the past several years have seen attempts to find new sources for financing services, including Primary Health Care (PHC), and to restructure health service delivery systems so as to reach some socially acceptable equilibrium between costs, quality, and equity. The health sector is confronted with serious conflicts, contradictions, and pressures within this global economic environment and its implications for health systems. Health budgets in developing countries are being cut or not allowed to grow in real terms; recurrent costs continue to mount; and the demand for services rises faster than the supply of those services. This is especially so in countries where the services are largely publicly provided and funded by public revenues. WHO and member states agreed in the World Health Assembly (WHA) in 1987, that the challenges to the health sector are to use existing resources as efficiently as possible without compromising acceptable standards of equity and quality and to find new resources to meet enlarged and growing population demands. Developing countries are not likely to acquire more or new resources for the health sector from outside; except for famines and disease-specific crises that challenge the world's conscience, developing countries will have to depend on themselves to generate the resources needed to meet HFA goals and objectives.

II. CONDITIONS IN THE EASTERN MEDITERRANEAN REGION (EMR)

The EMR has experienced most of the macroeconomic impacts of the world economic situation—in some cases with greater intensity than elsewhere and in others to a lesser degree. But all Member States of the EMR face economic issues that have the impact of constraining the growth of resources and economic support for Health For All (HFA) strategies. Quantitative data are sparse for EMR but judging from what data does exist, it is fair to conclude that the same problems found elsewhere in the world are found here—some more pronounced, some less—but all with the special problems unique to this region. These problems are: managing resources efficiently, growing inequities in access and finance, private sector expenditure growth, rising consumer expectations, and declines in real resources, available or likely to be available, for the economic support of HFA. In some countries user charges are being proposed. In others vast schemes of health insurance are contemplated. In the wealthier countries of the region cost escalation, especially hospital cost, is a problem and governments are unsure of how to cope with this. In a few countries governments are being urged to "cooperate" with the private sector; in others, decentralization of services management, greater community participation, and more intersectoral coordination are being urged as ways to deal with the declining resource base for health.

All countries of the region stress the great deficiencies in information on demographic data, demand for services, health utilization patterns, costs, and effectiveness of services, and data on financing of the health system. In some countries of the Region, extensive bilateral aid to the health sector may be distorting incentives and the capacities to deal, over the long term, with rationalizing and improving the internal efficiency of the health sector.

On the whole, per capita expenditures on health care (with a few exceptions) in the region are low. The Regional average of Gross Domestic Product (GDP) spent on health is below the desired level of "at least 5 percent", though of course there is great diversity in the Region. (The 5% threshold was proposed by WHO as a standard to achieve for a country 's health expenditures as a fraction of its GDP.)

Against this background, it is clear that the Region faces grave and growing concerns in providing economic support to meet the commitments of HFA. Few countries of the Region have the resources and tools to deal effectively with declining real resource support for health; and economic conditions suggest these problems will persist for some time to come.

III. SOME UNDERLYING POLICY ISSUES

A variety of policy advice is being offered to developing countries on what to do to facilitate a transition to these new economic conditions. The World Bank in a recent report has pinpointed three major problems facing countries and has proposed four policy reforms to deal with these problems. The problems are: allocation: insufficient spending on cost effective health activities, internal inefficiency of public programs, and inequity in the distribution of benefits from health services. The four policy reforms proposed are:

1. Charge users of government health facilities.
2. Provide insurance or other risk coverage.
3. Use non-government resources effectively.
4. Decentralize government health services.[43]

---

[43]See World Bank, *Financing Health Services in Developing Countries* (Washington, DC, 1987).

In another paper these issues are further explored within the context of HFA and PHC.[44] I do not have sufficient space in this paper to recount all the details of either study. Instead, let me focus on the main challenge:

- How can governments muster, for the year 2000, the resources necessary for health care maintenance and growth in their countries?

Resources for Health by the Year 2000

It is fairly obvious to most observers that the resources for health in most developing countries in the coming decade will be in short supply. External resources for health will not be forthcoming in significant amounts. So if countries are to maintain existing health levels and do so for increasing populations, the resources necessary for maintenance will have to be generated internally. Incremental improvements in health levels beyond pure maintenance will add further strains upon resource availability. So the existing and future pressures on developing world health ministries will be unbearable and politically explosive. Actual and existing health levels may deteriorate. This is the context that leads to the broad policy prescriptions for reform of health systems such as those proposed by the World Bank and other international lending agencies and other economists as well.

The issue is: Where will resources for health come from in the decade ahead? Developing countries, generally cannot hope to generate such resources from high rates of economic growth. Only a few will be able to do so; the rest of the developing world will be struggling in the decade ahead with economic adjustment policies rather than growth policies. From my perspective the policy agenda needed to successfully address the issue of resource availability are simple, but devastingly complex politically. The agenda involves three major policy choices:

1. How should governments in the developing world spend their limited resources?
2. What can governments do to generate more resources for how they decide to spend for health?
3. How should governments manage effectively the available resources for whatever policies and objectives they decide to spend?

A brief discussion of each of these questions. *First*, how should governments spend their resources? The issue here is that not everything can be done. You cannot hope to achieve "true equity" (whatever it is!) and be efficient at the same

---

[44]See Andreano and Helminiak (1987).

time. (See Annex I) You cannot provide equal amounts of hospital services as you do PHC services in rural areas. In economics parlance, the question as I've posed it is this: What is "appropriate" in health care for governments to do and what is "appropriate" to be left to private markets to solve? In health care in the developing world, governments, again with few exceptions, have for a variety of reasons (historical, cultural, and/or political) elected to provide most, if not all, health services. And they have usually done so from general tax revenues. In a world where resources are now limited and demands on the resources approach infinity, is it appropriate for governments to continue providing services that private markets could provide better (i.e. more efficiently)? Government services in the developing countries, provided "free", and for reasons based on equity, are neither actually free (consider travel and/or waiting times, for example) nor equitable (i.e. hospital care, urban-based is favored over PHC, rural-based). Governments could limit themselves to what we economists call "public goods" and let private markets allocate resources through changes in prices and incomes. The theory of public goods applied to health care suggests that governments should provide basic sanitation services, mass campaigns (such as immunizations, nutrition, etc.), individual immunizations (because of the high externalities), health education, and perhaps basic and applied health and biomedical research. In these instances of public or quasi-public goods, governments could not count on private markets to supply the socially desirable amounts of consumption, i.e. private markets would "fail".

In the developing countries, however, governments provide or attempt to provide public as well as private goods in health care. Public sector activity seems based less on reasons of market failure than on concerns for equity. If equity is not being satisfactorily achieved, however, it is perhaps time for governments to decide to husband their resources so as to pinpoint more carefully their equity objectives—i.e. by providing public goods to those most in "need" and/or unable to purchase from private markets. Resources "saved" (withdrawn) by governments competing (and generally doing so poorly) with the private sector, should be reapplied to more specific targets such as public goods, equity, and underprovided goods from private markets. This would be a way to generate huge amounts of resources in the developing countries. The resources could be used to achieve a different level of equity. The private sector (profit and non-profit) can produce these services much more efficiently than can the public sector. So the answer to the first question is this: Governments should consider not providing health care services that duplicate those better provided through private markets and apply the resources "saved" by pinpointing their application to well-defined equity objectives, pure public goods, and controls and regulation (cost and quality) over the private sector. In an ideal world these things might be done easily; however, in the real world governments cannot privatize or close down traditionally provided health services without incredible political risks.[45]

The *second* question may be more grounded in the real world. If governments can't (or are unwilling) to restructure their systems, how can they still generate more resources? The answer here is also simple: Charge those who can pay something for the services and, most importantly, manage the services more efficiently, i.e. manage them as if they were in the private market. Imposing user charges or cost recovery is controversial politically, but if circumstances are right it can be done. The reality is this: real resources available for health may decline and if so, existing health levels will as well. Can governments continue to maintain full services, strain their budgets to meet operating and recurrent costs, and adversely select the population between private and public facilities? Private sector health care is growing in the developing countries and there is precious little governments can (or should) do to prevent this. The sensible policy is to make public facilities, if they are going to be maintained, as competitive from a price and quality standpoint—as the private sector.

The *third* question addresses the status quo: If governments can't or are unable to change the distribution of production, and can't or won't use incentives for cost recovery, how can they manage their systems better to squeeze out additional resources? There is much that can be suggested on this question but space limitations limit me to discuss just one aspect: How can managerial performance be improved in the public system? The answer is: Improve the reward/incentive structure for managers at all levels. We must look at a health care system in terms of what is motivating its managers: the potential for generating new resources through improved managerial efficiency is enormous. Personnel rules, reward structures for performance, and the panoply of disincentives public employees face all have to be changed if managerial performance is to be improved. The point is this: If governments can't or won't change the financial or the production basis of their health care system, they can gain extraordinary amounts of resources by just managing "what they got" better.

IV. GLOBAL POLICY DEVELOPMENTS IN HEALTH CARE

Let me now summarize some of the changes in health care policy under way and which lie behind the discussion in Section III. Countries in the developing world have been pursuing five lines of policy intervention. Sometimes these have

---

[45]An excellent analysis of the public *vs.* private issues in health care is in A. J. Culyer and Bengt Jonsson (eds.), Public and Private Health Services (1986), Basil Blackwell, Oxford).

been done together, in combination, or in some countries only a few interventions have been tried. These five policy directions are:

- <u>Micro management</u> of the public health delivery system (i.e. trying to induce greater worker productivity, improve responsiveness to patient demands, etc.); often this policy approach has involved changes in work rules and career incentives as well as restructuring and decentralizing management, planning, and responsibilities of public health delivery systems. Restructuring is greatly restricted because of the rising and heavy burden of recurrent costs, most of which are for personnel.

- <u>New sources of finance</u>. In this area some countries have shown greater willingness and have had some success with community sources of finance for health care. In a great many countries user charges are being assessed in an attempt to generate more revenues. Several countries have combined both approaches and with some modest successes.

- Initiation and expansion of the <u>coverage of health insurance</u> schemes, private and public. A large number of countries are experimenting with health insurance schemes as a way to generate resources, and redirect the demand for services toward the most cost-effective level of delivery. A number of the middle to high-income developing countries have also either underway or in experimental stages, prepaid/capitation and/or managed care systems in their public and private health care systems.

- The growing level of expenditures in the private health sector has been seen in many developing countries as an additional way to expand total resources for health care and to find points of substitution and complementarity with the private health care sector.

- Finally, many countries in the developing world have been forced by the current stringency of resources for health to reexamine their <u>policies and programs toward the most vulnerable, highest risk, and poorest people</u> in their populations. Many countries have come to realize that the limited available resources have to be allocated both more efficiently and more equitably.

It is too soon to know whether or not these policies can succeed in generating more resources, in managing public resources more efficiently, and to protect the most vulnerable and poor. The limited amount of research thus far on these policies produces a mixed record. Some of the policies may themselves contribute to further inequity in a country, however well intentioned the policy. Concern, for example, about user fees is growing and a number of studies have pointed out (perhaps from bitter experience) the do's and don'ts of this initiative.[46] The point is, however, that these five areas for policy intervention represent the range of choices countries face. To examine what will work best in one country setting and how any individual country can overcome its resource constraints requires sound empirical analysis and some basic concepts in economics. Countries should not undertake major changes in policy without a first pass analysis of the expected benefits and costs and the distribution of both on key population groups. To do this type of policy analysis, countries need to apply basic concepts of economics.

V. THE POTENTIAL FOR HEALTH ECONOMICS

Health economics is a way of analyzing the efficient allocation of resources, of evaluating choices and options, of judging the performance, operation, and capacities of the health sector. Health economics is a part of general economics and as such is a way of analyzing what is produced, how much is produced, who gets what is produced and how all these are done with resource efficiency and equity. It can be especially useful in assisting the analysis of the range of problems and policy issues we have discussed thus far: namely, how to manage resources efficiently and how to expand or mobilize the base of resources needed for health care. Both are central issues that the analytical and practical content of health economics are equipped to examine.

Member states are turning to WHO for technical assistance, training, and above all guidance in ways to respond and meet these challenges to economic support for HFA strategies. Countries must have the capacity to deal with the economic analysis of their particular situation. Cost-effective strategies which do not compromise quality but reach the poorest populations are needed. Ways of coping with distorted resource allocations that produce both inefficiencies and inequities are desperately needed. Alternatives to taxation as the main basis for generating new resources for the health sector need to be explored. Analysis on these and other policies central to the basic issues of how the health sector is to be financed and whether or not it is equitable require hard economic analysis of choices and options governments may have and the risk or benefits of doing one thing as opposed to another.

Health planning must also be based on a foundation of health economics principles. In the health sector efficient choices must be made because resources are limited. Alternatives always exist and governments must know the benefits and cost of alternatives if they are to make efficient and equitable choices. Health manpower planning, for example, entails major economic consequences

---

[46]See Paul Gertler, et al, "Are User Fees Regressive?" Journal of Econometrics, Vol. 36, 1987, pp. 67-88.

depending on the options that are pursued. Planning how to generate the financial support needed for the health sector and what is the most equitable or efficient way(s) to do so require hard economic analysis. Planning support within Member States must embody basic principles of health economics on resource allocations, the incentives—good and bad—that policies adopted generate, and on the economic capacities of a country to generate the resources needed for their health sector.

As has been noted, a major key is efficient management of the health sector and here economic principles require broad and intensive application. The bias toward curative care as opposed to PHC is a policy, resource, and management issue. Rising hospital costs and ways of containing these so as to still keep quality levels high but to reduce the inequities produced by rising costs—these too will require strong application of health economics in terms of efficient resource allocation choices. The role of government in containing costs needs to be explored. How can resources in the private sector be tapped? Linking up planning activities with management goals and objectives, say, especially on such issues as efficient planning and use of resources, also contain the applications of economics.

The countries of EMR are varied and diverse; there are some few wealthy countries but the Region also has some of the poorest countries of the world as well. Economic resources, planning and management capacities vary from passable to poor. Basic data available on the health sector—expenditures, utilization, demand, etc.—are available for only a few countries. As already noted the underlying economic infrastructure of support for the health sector varies from poor to non-existent in the Region. People and institutions inside or outside of government to apply economic principles to the health sector are scarce or non-existent. Implementing new health care policies is done without much data to know whether such policies would be effective or counter-productive and with virtually no basic data to evaluate which outcome has been achieved. With the exception of a few of the richer countries of the Region the use and applications of economic principles in health is in a totally underdeveloped state. Member States, however, have expressed great concern over this situation and recognize their deficiencies and gaps. There is a willingness and acceptance of the role of health economics in the Region because the problems are so great and the tools and people needed to resolve the problems are so poor. The range of policy issues and changes being contemplated by some countries of the Region covers all the main currents being discussed worldwide. The desire to incorporate economic thinking into health policies and to generate the required base of information is a felt need between both the rich and poor countries of the Region.

Three major problem areas may be noted: (1) the lack of basic information needed for planning, management, analysis, and evaluation; (2) the urgency of analysis needed for major policy changes that are contemplated as governments try to cope with the problem of declining health resources and rising consumer expectations in health, and (3) the need to build in the Region a critical mass of professionals in health and health related *institutions* who know how to use basic economic principles in any work related to health policy formulation, implementation, and education.

Introduction to the IC Workshop

What I have tried to cover in this paper is the range of problems and policy issues in health care that most directly affect countries in the developing world. This IC workshop is the first major organized effort for EMR to build the economic foundation for the analysis of policy issues and concerns facing member states. The country reports that will be presented are the first attempts to systematize the inclusion of economic analysis in the health sector. In the next few days we hope the interaction with colleagues from other countries and with WHO experts will build the level of enthusiasm that can be successfully transmitted to your governments.

BIBLIOGRAPHY

Akin, John, (1987), "Health Insurance in Developing Countries: Prospects For Risk-Sharing," (paper delivered at ADB Health Finance Seminar, Manila, 1987)

Andreano, R. and Tom Helminiak, (1987), "The Role of the Private Sector in Health Care in the Developing Countries," (paper delivered at ADB Conference on Health Care Finance, Manila, 27 July-3 August 1987)

————, (1988), "The Challenges to HFA and PHC: An Economists Perspective," (paper delivered at Joint WHO/ICN Meeting, Geneva, 1-3 August 1988)

Andreano, R., "The World Economic Crisis and Its Impact on Health and Health Services," (paper prepared for the EB, WHO, October, 1988).

Bell, David E. and Michael R. Reich, (1988), (eds.), *Health, Nutrition, and Economic Crises: Approaches to Policy in the Third World*, (Auburn House, Auburn, MA, USA 1988)

Cho, Yoon Je, (1988), "Some Policy Lessons from the Opening of the Korean Insurance Market," *The World Bank Economic Review*, Vol. 2, No. 2, (May 1988), pp. 241-254.

Cornia, G. A., R. Jolly and F. Stewart, (1987), (eds.), *Adjustment with a Human Face: Protecting the Vulnerable and Promoting Growth*, (Oxford University Press, 1987)

Fuchs, Victor, (1988), "The 'Competition Revolution' in Health Care," *Health Affairs* (Summer 1988), pp. 5-24.

Gertler, Paul, Luis Locay, and Warren Sanderson, (1987), "Are User Fees Regressive?" *Journal of Econometrics*, Vol. 36 (1987), pp. 67-88.

Griffin, Charles, (1987), "User Charges for Health Care in Principle and Practice," (paper delivered at ADB Health Finance Seminar, Manila, 1987)

Grilli, Enzo R. and Maw Cheng Yang, (1988), "Primary Commodity Prices, Manufactured Goods Prices, and the Terms of Trade of Developing Countries: What the Long-Run Shows," *The World Bank Economic Review*, Vol. 2, No. 1, (January 1988), pp. 1-48.

Heller, Peter S., et al., (1988), The Implications of Fund-Supported Adjustment Programs For Poverty: Experiences in Selected Countries (IMF, Washington D.C., 1988)

Lal, Deepak, (1987), "The Political Economy of Economic Liberalization," *The World Bank Economic Review*, Vol. 1, No. 2, (Jan. 1987), pp. 273-300.

Lewis, Maureen A. "The Private Sector and Health Care Delivery in Developing Countries: Definition, Experience, Potential (Project REACH, Washington D.C., April 1988)

Musgrove, Philip, (1987), "The Economic Crisis and its Impact on Health and Health Care in Latin America and the Caribbean," *International Journal of Health Services*, Vol. 17, No. 3, 1987, pp. 411-441.

OECD, (1985), *Measuring Health Care, 1960-1983: Expenditures, Costs, and Performances*, (Paris, 1985).

OECD, (1987), *Financing and Delivery Health Care: A Comparative Analysis of OECD Countries* (Paris, 1987).

Psacharopoulos, George, (1988), "Education and Development: A Review," *The World Bank Research Observer*, Vol. 3, No. 1, (January 1988), pp. 99-116.

Schieber, George J. and Jean-Pierre Poullier, "Trends in International Health Care Spending," *Health Affairs*, (Fall 1987), pp. 105-112.

Shepard, Donald, Guy Carrin, and Prosper Nyandagazi, "Self-Financing of Health Care at Government Health Centers in Rwanda," (paper prepared for Project REACH, January 23, 1987)

Sisk, Jane E, "The Costs of Aids," *Health Affairs*, Summer 1987), pp. 5-21.

Smith, Brian Abel and Ajay Dua, (1987), Community Financing of Health Care," (paper delivered at ADB Health Finance Seminar, Manila, 1987).

UN, Economics and Social Council (1988a), "Main Research Findings of the System in Major Global Economic and Social Trends, Policies and Emerging Issues," (Second Regular Session of 1988)

————, (1988b), "Net Transfers of Resources from Developing to Developed Countries," (Second Regular Session of 1988).

————, (1988c), "Overall Socio-Economic Perspective of the World Economy to the Year 2000," (Second Regular Session of 1988)

————, (1988d), "Summary of the Economic and Social Survey of Asia and the Pacific, 1987" (Second Regular Session of 1988).

————, (1988e), "Summary of the Survey of Economic and Social Developments in the Region of the Economic and Social Commission for Western Asia, 1987" (Second Regular Session of 1988).

————, (1988f), "Summary of the Survey of Economic and Social Conditions in Africa, 1986-87," (Second Regular Session of 1988).

————, (1988g), "Summary of the Economic Survey of Latin America and the Caribbean, 1987," (Second Regular Session of 1988).

United Nations Economic and Social Council, (1988), Committee For Development Planning, Report on the 24th Session (New York, 12-15 April 1988), Supplement No. 6, Official Records 1988.

United Nations System, (1988), Administrative Committee on Coordination, "Report on Substantive Questions," (Geneva 6-8 April 1988), especially IIC.

The World Bank, (1984), *World Development Report 1984*, (Washington, DC 1984).

The World Bank, (1987), *Financing Health Services in Developing Countries: An Agenda for Reform*, (Washington, DC 1987).

The World Bank, (1988), *World Development Report 1988*, (Washington, DC 1988).

World Health Organization (1987a), "Economic Support for National Health for All Strategies: Background Document," (Fortieth World Health Assembly, Geneva, May 1987).

————, (1987b), "Final Report of the Interregional Workshop on Economics of Health Manpower Development in Support of Primary Health Care," (Manila, 22-26, June 1987).

————, (1987c), "Evaluation of the Strategy for Health for All by the Year 2000. Seventh Report on the World Health Situation. I, Global Review, Geneva 1987).

ATTACHMENT I

Equity in Health: The Concept of Trade-offs

The concept of "trade-offs"—the necessity of giving up something in order to obtain (more of) something else is fundamental to economics. For national economies, this concept is often illustrated by a "production possibility frontier." Figure 1 depicts a simplified version of a production possibility (PP) frontier for an economy.

With the available two dimensions of the surface of the figure, just two separate goods (or separate bundles of goods) can be shown. The figure indicates that if all of the economy's resources are devoted to the good(s) measured on the vertical axis, amount A of that good cold be produced and 0 amount of the horizontal axis good). Intermediate positions on the curve AB describe the rate at which either of the two goods must be sacrificed (traded-off) to obtain a given increment in the other. Thus, e.g., if the economy's resources were distributed to produce amount A_1 of the one good and B_1 of the other (point X on the PP frontier), it could increase the production of the second from B_1 to B_2 if it is willing to reduce the production of the former from A_1 to A_2 (at point Y on the PP frontier).

But this assumes that the economy's resources are already operating with maximum achievable efficiency. If, as in Figure 2, instead of operating on the maximum efficiency PP frontier (i.e., on curve AB) the economy is at point Z (on a less efficient PP curve), it could, by improving the production efficiency of the system, achieve more of both goods. This is not easy to do, however.

Within the health sector, it is believed that there is a trade-off between the total amount of health services that can be produced (termed "efficiency") and the degree of equity of health services distribution, we necessarily must sacrifice some total output of health services—as in moving from X to Y in Figure 1. So, if the health sector is unable (or unwilling) to improve the overall efficiency of the system, it must decide how much additional equity it is willing to produce—at the expense of some, corresponding amount of total health services.

Figure 1: Production Possibility Curves: Maximum System Efficiency

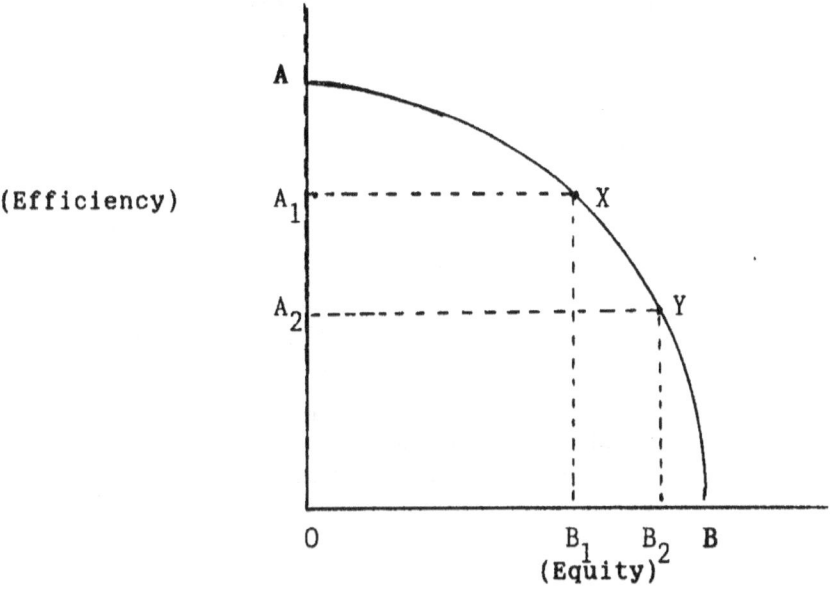

Figure 2: Production Possibility Curves: Less than Maximum System Efficiency

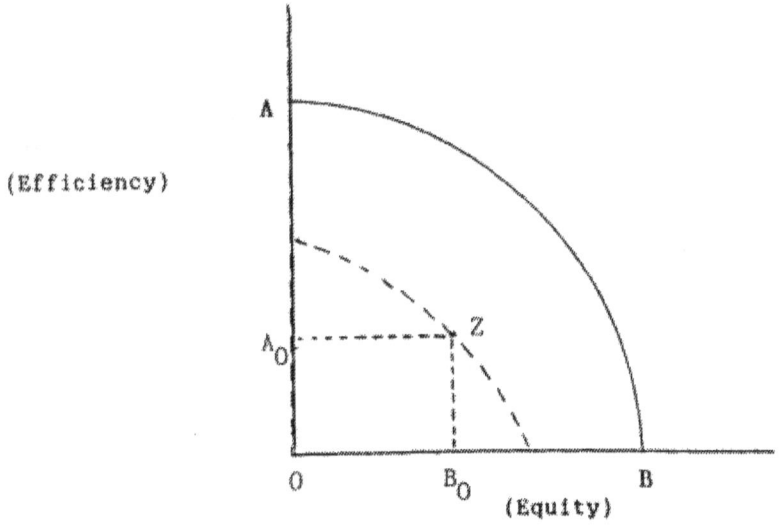

SELECTION 11

ARE WE SPENDING TOO MUCH ON HEALTH CARE? AN INTERNATIONAL SURVEY[47]

INTRODUCTION

The title of this paper was assigned to me and is not necessarily the choice of title I would make to examine the issues that are likely to be involved. At the outset, the question title of the paper begs yet another question: is there some "optimal," or, "correct" amount a country should spend on health care? In theory, perhaps there is an optimal or "correct" level: in practice it is very hard to ascertain just what that level may be for any single or group of countries. More than a decade ago, I had the same question put to me with regard to America. Nearly all serious policy analysts believe America spends "too much" on health care. But how much is too much and how would one know when the "correct" amount has been achieved.[48] There are two ways to illustrate the complexity of the problem: (1) country data relating expenditures to key measures of health status and (2), theoretically, in terms of some social preference function and a production possibility function (PPF). In terms of the latter, as shown below, a given country trades-off expenditures on health for expenditures on all other goods; the PPF traces all efficient combinations of these tradeoffs. A social preference function tangent to the PPF describes an optimal point (c) for a given country. Some countries lie within the PPF and could thus spend more on health and other goods because it would be efficient to do so (Point A). Other countries might prefer a social preference function beyond the PPF (Point B) but the economy would have to grow significantly before Point B could be attained. The difference between both social preferences functions might be, say a gain in LE, and this is not clearly asymmetric to the expenditure level. Points inside PPF, such as A, could be say an IMR: here countries would clearly benefit, and it would be an efficient use of resources, to reduce IMR.

---

[47]Paper prepared for WHO EMRO Inter-Country Meeting, Muscat, OMAN, October 25-29, 1991.
[48]See Andreano (1980), "Does America Spend Too Much on Health Care," *Bulletin of the New York Academy of Medicine*, Vol. 38, No. 1, pp. 19-25.

Chart I

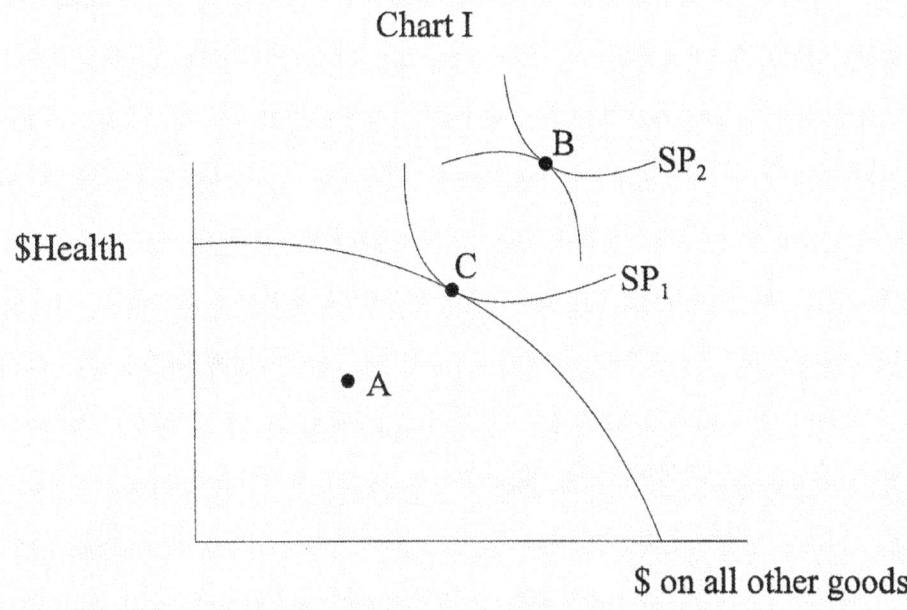

$Health

B

SP_2

C

SP_1

• A

$ on all other goods

Theory aside, an optimal level of expenditures on health for a society to achieve, is a very imprecise concept. Nonetheless, as developed further in the paper, most developing countries are within their PPF, Point A, and could benefit from spending more on health. But it requires further analysis of the system of delivery of services and the financing system before one can conclude such additional spending in health could be accomplished efficiently.

The difficulty of discovering an optimum expenditure level may be further illustrated by two pieces of data. One, Figure 1, relates GDP per capita and public expenditure as health for some selected countries for 1985. A regression line is then calculated. As one can see there is no clear linear relationship between the two except at low levels of GDP and low levels of public health expenditure. The countries inside the square of Figure I are most probably countries in Point A of the earlier PPF diagram. Nonetheless, there are yet, as shown in the figure, countries with high GDP per head with very low levels of public health expenditures. In truth, the most precise comparison should be total health expenditures, public and private, regressed against GDP because, especially in some very poor countries, private expenditures on health exceed those originating from the public sector. This point is well illustrated in Chart II, which shows the private share of total health expenditures against GDP per capita.

Figure I

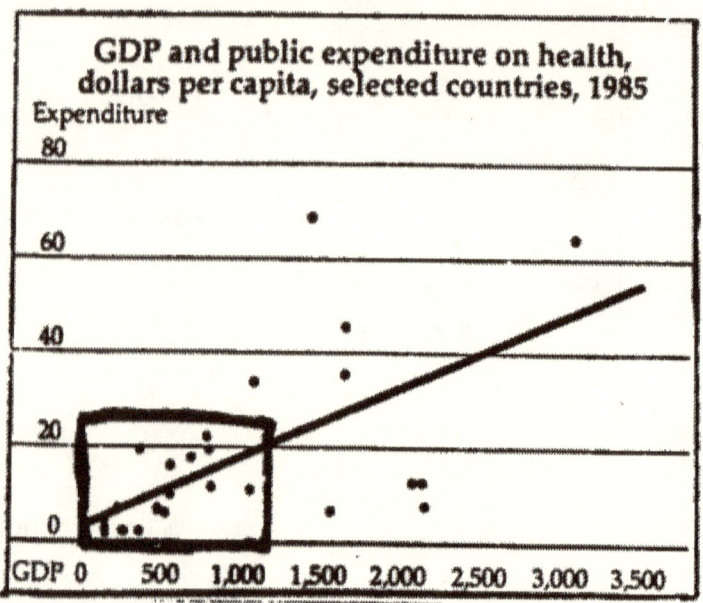

GDP and public expenditure on health, dollars per capita, selected countries, 1985

Yet another measure can reveal the inherent difficulty in answering the question "Are we spending too much on health care?" That is some sort of performance measure: i.e. looking at resources invested against some key measures of health performance. This is done, for illustrative purposes, in Table I for 5 rich countries comparing per capita health expenditures against certain inputs (MD's per 100,000 population) and outputs: Life Expectancy (LE), Infant Mortality Rate (IMR), Heart Disease deaths. As can be seen from Table I, countries that spend the most do not always produce the highest health outcomes.

In any case, what one wants to convey in this overly long introduction is a sense that viewed from a number of different prospectives, theoretical, analytical, and quantitative, it is difficult, if not impossible, to capture what an optimum level of health expenditures might be for any given country.

Chart II

PRIVATE SHARE OF TOTAL HEALTH EXPENDITURE COMPARED TO GNP PER CAPITA
(Countries below $2,000 GNP per capita)

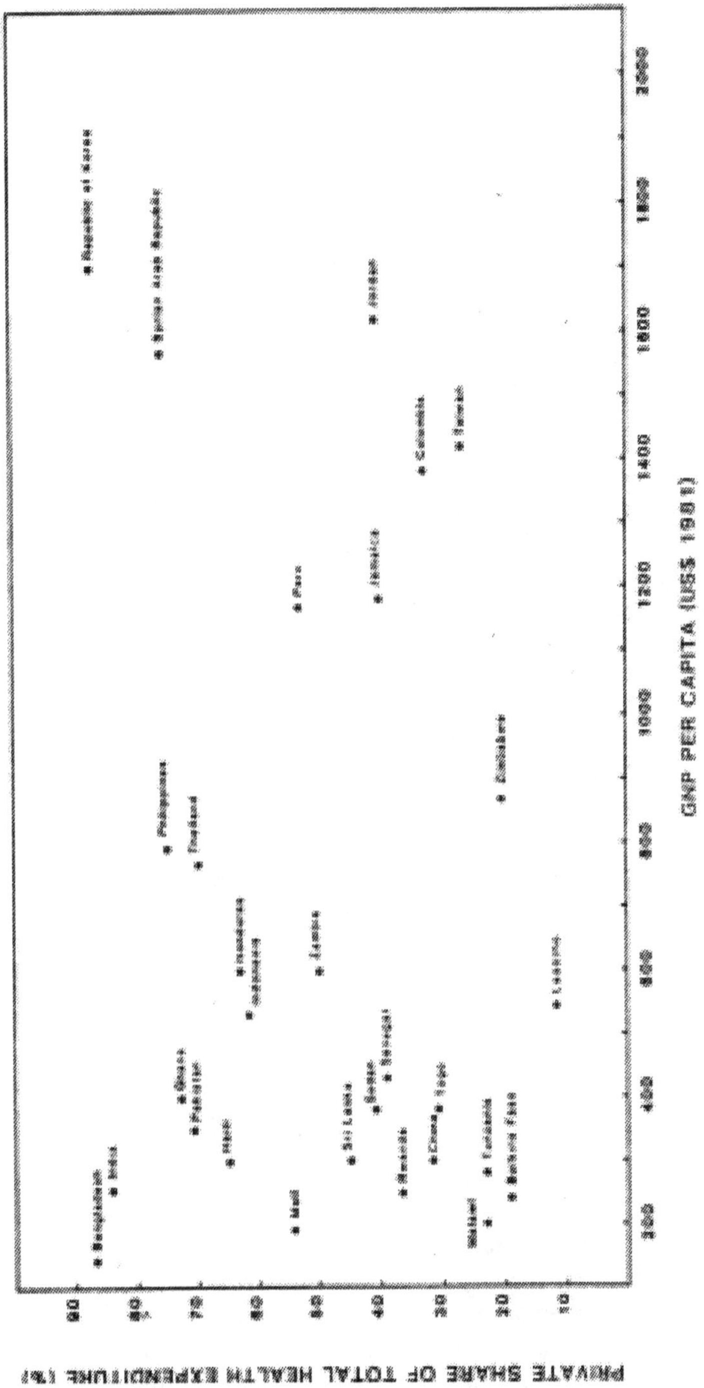

GNP PER CAPITA (US$ 1981)

PRIVATE SHARE OF TOTAL HEALTH EXPENDITURE (%)

Source: R. Andreano and T. Helminiak (1989), "The Role of the Private Sector," in *Health Care Finance*, (Asian Development Bank, Manila).

		Table I			
Expenditures and Performance, 5 Rich Countries (1984)					
Country	1984 $P.capita	No. Of MD's per 100,00 Pop.	LE at Birth	IMR	Deaths from Heart Disease per 100,000 Pop.
USA	$1,500	192	75	12	435
W. Germany	900	222	73	13	584
France	800	172	76	10	380
Japan	500	128*	77*	7*	266*
U.K	400*	154	74	12	579

Source: All data from World Bank Development Report (1988, 1990) and <u>Economist</u>, April 28, 1984, p. 18.
* = "Best" performance.

With these introductory notions out of the way, the remainder of the paper addresses two major questions: (1) do countries, especially developing countries, spend what they spend on health care wisely, efficiently, and equitably? And (2) what could countries do to increase both the amount of resources allocated to health care and to do so both efficiently and equitably. (Appendix Table A contains some basic data, which should be referred to for all parts of this paper.)

Resources Devoted to Health

Before addressing these two questions we first develop what data we have to show patterns of spending across countries. It is not truly possible to quantify all the resources devoted to health; at best one can trace what governments spend on health delivery services and the real revenues expended on related health actions such as immunizations, drugs, water supplies, etc. To get a true measure of real resources devoted to health one would need a separate line item in the national income accounts. Some attempts have been made in this direction, but except for the industrialized countries it is not even possible to approximate this calculation. We have only fragmentary evidence of what individuals and households (perhaps even communities) may spend on health care services and related health activities. With all the flaws, omissions, and ambiguities the three most commonly used measures of real resources devoted to health are: (1) proportion of GNP or GDP spent, total (i.e. both public and private) and per capita, (2) individual and/or household expenditures on medical care, and (3) government expenditures on health care, total, per capita, or as a percent of total government expenditures. While data of this kind are readily available for most industrialized countries, it is less available as one goes down the scale and level of development. Most of the data generated in measures (1) - (3) are self-reported by governments and to a much lesser extent based on survey data. Further, to make comparisons in expenditure levels over time and across countries are difficult because of differences in exchange rates and domestic rates of inflation. What one wants in such comparisons are real rates adjusted for domestic and international differences in prices and exchange rates. (See Appendix B).

Against all the above qualifications, we know precious little about how real resources devoted to health care have changed in the past decade. Comprehensive and comparable information on trends in expenditure levels is available for only a few countries. Only 13 developing countries have been reporting to the UN system on current health expenditure in both the public and private sector since 1977. In 10 of these, health expenditures were a higher proportion of GDP in the early 1980's compared to the mid 1970's. Some developing countries report on health expenditure in the public sector only: in a majority of those reporting (15 countries) it has risen as a percent of GDP. But as GDP itself has fallen in real terms in some countries this does not mean, per se, higher expenditure levels on health. Reports to the IMF show that more developing countries reported reductions in proportions of government budgets devoted to health care than reported increases. For the poorest, least developed countries, the data reported are much more sparse and hard to compare: in only 4 of the 36 least developed countries in 1987 were such data available. In some of these countries, health care spending has most probably been falling because income per head has declined. This is undoubtedly most true for African countries, a few in South East Asia, and in Central and South America. (See data in Appendix Table A.)

In the following three tables some additional data on each of these three categories is assembled. Spending on Medical Care as percent of total household consumption, from limited household expenditure survey in a few countries, shows that even in the poorest countries 3-4 percent is spent out of pocket on medical services. This is usually for drugs. Table II shows, by WHO Region, the wide variations between countries. In rich countries such as the U.S., the medical expenditures are usually for premium payments for health insurance. Proportions of the GNP spent on health by WHO Regions are also shown in Table 111.

Again great variations exist between rich and poor countries. Table IV shows the percentage of total central government expenditures on health for the years 1972 and 1987. In very few countries in the developing world have these proportions increased.

Table II

Medical Care as % of Total Household Consumption
(Range of Years 1980-85)
Selected Countries, WHO Regions

Africa		EMRO	
Ethiopia	3%	Egypt	14%
Zaire	3%	Iran	6%
Malawi	2%	Morocco	7%
Nigeria	3%	Pakistan	3%
Botswana	4%	Jordan	5%
Americas		**South-East Asia**	
U.S.	14%	India	3%
Venezuela	8%	Sri Lanka	2%
Brazil	6%	Bangladesh	2%
Canada	5%	Thailand	5%
Jamaica	3%	Indonesia	2%
Europe		**WPR**	
Spain	7%	Australia	10%
Switzerland	15%	Japan	10%
U.K.	8%	Philippines	2%
Portugal	6%	Republic of Korea	5%
Sweden	11%	China	1%

Source: Compiled from World Bank, <u>World Development Report</u> (1989), and pp. 182-183.

Table III

Proportion of GNP Spent on Health
By WHO Region and Level of Development
(1987)

WHO Region	Weighted Average of % Spent on Health of GNP
Africa	3.0%
Americas	6.8
South-East Asia	2.8
Europe	5.5
EMRO	4.6
WP	5.3
Average (all Regions)	4.6%
Development Level	
Least Developed	2.2%
Other Developing	3.6%
Industrialized	6.8%

Source: *Global Strategy Health For All*, Detailed Analysis of Global Indicators, Monitoring 1989, p. 9.

Table IV

Percentage of Total Central Government Expenditure
On Health, 1972-1987

World Bank Category	% Of total	
	1972	1987
Low income (excl. China and India)	5.4%	3.4%
Middle Income	6.3	5.1
High Income	11.1	12.1
WHO Regions (Selected Countries)		
Africa		
Zambia	7.4%	4.7%
Kenya	7.9	6.6
China	6.3	8.3
Americas		
U.S.	8.6	12.2
Paraguay	3.5	3.1
Chile	8.2	6.0
Euro		
Sweden	3.6	1.2
Italy	13.5	9.6
U.K.	12.2	13.1
South-East Asia		
India	1.5	1.9
Sri Lanka	6.4	5.4
Indonesia	1.4	1.5
Western Pacific Region		
Australia	7.0	9.5
Philippines	3.2	5.5
New Zealand	14.8	12.4

Source: Compiled from World Bank, *World Development Report* (1989), and pp. 184-185.

From the limited data available, however, certain not unreasonable conclusions can be offered.

1. There are very wide disparities in levels of spending between countries according to their level of development as measured by real income per head.
2. These disparities have widened during the past decade: Industrialized countries now spend proportionately more per head than a decade earlier; poorer countries less, and the gap has widened.
3. In the poorest and many near poor developing countries spending by governments in real terms has remained stable or declined; it has seldom increased.
4. The burden of paying privately, and out of pocket, for health care services and products, has risen in most countries, but especially in low and middle-income countries.
5. The future levels of real resources required to maintain the gains in health status of the last decade, or to improve them still further, have increased dramatically. This is because health services are faced with increasing demands due to population growth, ageing populations, the spread of new medical technologies and the general higher aspirations and expectations people have for improved health. Slow or declining economic growth, reductions in real income per head, reductions in public spending, and the impact of structural adjustment packages, all place enormous pressure on the health sector in the least developed and developing countries.

Do Countries Spend Resources Wisely?

This question, like all others on this topic, is exceedingly complex and there is no single, uniform, answer, which can apply to all countries and at all, times. Some countries even among the poorest do very well; some, if not most, less so. Some rich countries do very badly on both efficiency and equity grounds; others do surprisingly well. Two tables in the recent UNDP, *Human Development Red* (1990) illustrate the problem. In one chart (A) social sectors—health and education—receive less priority than do military and national security expenditures. In another set of countries chart (B), the situation is just the reverse. Similarly in countries with low under 5 children's mortality, the percentage of GDP spent on health is about (on average) twice as high as in countries with very high under 5 mortality (based on data in World Bank, *World Development Report 1990*, p. 46).

The problem of making wise choices in the use of health resources cuts across levels of development. In rich countries, as the chart below (c) shows, three equally effective, but disparately costly, heart drugs are available. In the U.S., the most expensive of the 3 drugs (TPA) is the drug of choice. Perhaps, the most glaring example of questionable choice is the proportion of public expenditures on health, which go to hospital care, especially in poor countries. (See Appendix Table A, last column). So without exception in rich countries and poor, one can find glaring examples where both public money and private money being spent involves questionable choices. And further, the equity consequences of inappropriate choices can be very severe: in the U.S. some 40 million people have no health insurance; in many poor countries in some cases up to 50 percent of populations have no access to any services—primary or acute. Inequities and inefficiencies are about the two most common characteristics one can find for health care delivery and finance systems. And this is not a problem just for poor countries and it is a characteristic whether a health care system is predominantly public (i.e. "free"), or private (i.e. most people pay).

If one accepts this assessment, however harsh it may be, it seems logical to ask why is this so? Why do countries and individuals often, if not usually, make "bad" choices in health care? Part of an explanation lies in the nature of health care as a commodity itself: many view it as a "right" so there is logically no level or amount of consumption that is sufficient. There is always something more that could be done. Demand is insatiable even though resources are inevitably limited and cannot satisfy all demands.

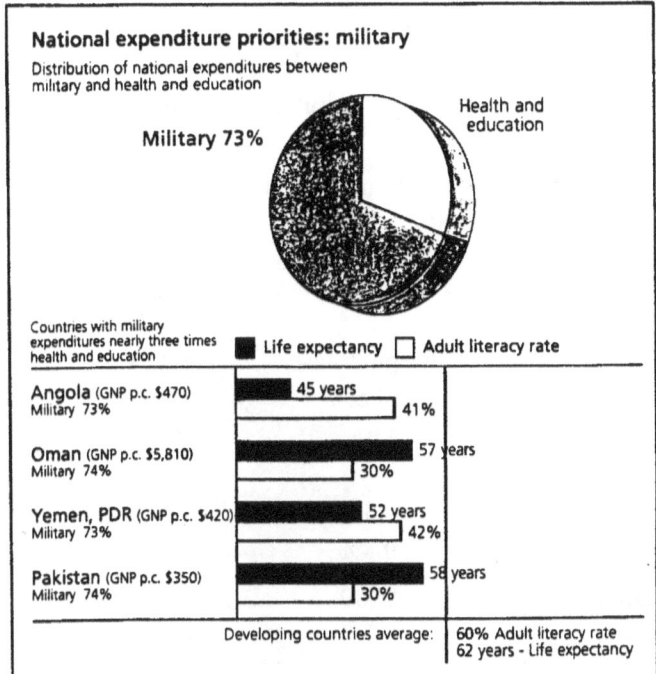

National expenditure priorities: military

Distribution of national expenditures between military and health and education

Military 73%

Health and education

Countries with military expenditures nearly three times health and education

■ Life expectancy □ Adult literacy rate

Angola (GNP p.c. $470)
Military 73%
45 years
41%

Oman (GNP p.c. $5,810)
Military 74%
57 years
30%

Yemen, PDR (GNP p.c. $420)
Military 73%
52 years
42%

Pakistan (GNP p.c. $350)
Military 74%
58 years
30%

Developing countries average: | 60% Adult literacy rate
62 years - Life expectancy

Chart A

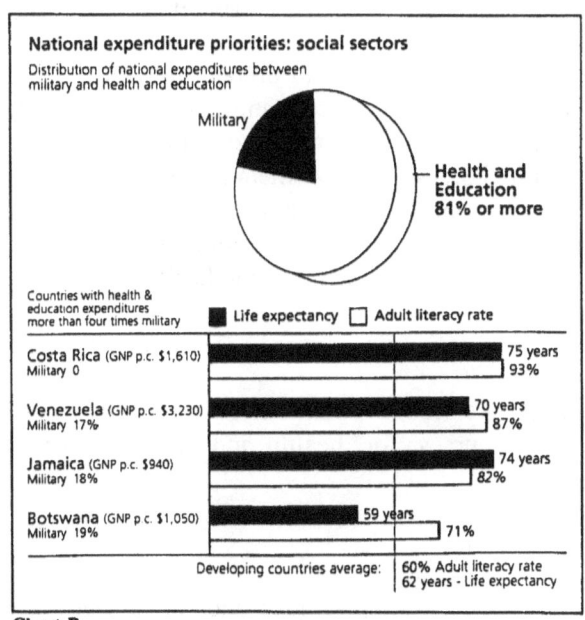

National expenditure priorities: social sectors

Distribution of national expenditures between military and health and education

Military

Health and Education 81% or more

Countries with health & education expenditures more than four times military

■ Life expectancy □ Adult literacy rate

Costa Rica (GNP p.c. $1,610)
Military 0
75 years
93%

Venezuela (GNP p.c. $3,230)
Military 17%
70 years
87%

Jamaica (GNP p.c. $940)
Military 18%
74 years
82%

Botswana (GNP p.c. $1,050)
Military 19%
59 years
71%

Developing countries average: | 60% Adult literacy rate
62 years - Life expectancy

Chart B

213

Chart C

Equally Effective, but One's Cheaper

Figures for drugs used to break up blood clots, from a study completed January 31, which included 46,092 patients at 936 hospitals in 16 countries, including the United States. The three drugs were given to equal numbers of patients. The death and stroke figures were taken 35 days after the patients received the drugs.

	Streptokinase	T.P.A.	Eminase
Deaths	10.5%	10.3%	10.6%
All strokes	1.1%	1.5%	1.5%
Strokes, probably from cerebral hemorrhage	0.3%	0.7%	0.6%
Other strokes	0.8%	0.8%	0.9%
Price per treatment	$200	$2,000-2,700	$1,700

Source: *New York Times* (undated).

In poor countries, the tragedy of unwise choices, private or public, is more severe. A rich country can make mistakes even in its extravagances; a poor country does not have that luxury. What seems an appropriate and pragmatic line of reasoning is for both public bodies and private individuals to re-examine the rationale for making choices regarding consumption and use of health resources. Governments appear to spend resources on many inappropriate things; individuals make health choices—or have them made for them by government— which does not afford them the chance to live pain free lives. Economic deprivation, of course, of individuals and governments lies at the root of many, if not all, the inappropriate choices that get made in health care resource usage.[49]

What Can Countries Do? Policy Responses in Developing Countries

Five policy approaches seem to characterize country responses in trying to generate more real resources for health and manage available resources efficiently.

---

[49]In another paper I examine the conceptual foundation of individual and governmental behavior on health care choices. "A New Paradigm for Health" (This paper is included in the present volume).

1. "Micro-management" of the public health delivery system (i.e., specific measures to induce greater productivity among health workers, improve responsiveness to patients' demands, etc.); often this has involved changes in work rules and career incentives as well as the restructuring and decentralization of management, planning, and responsibilities in public health delivery systems.

2. New sources of finance: some countries have shown greater willingness to experiment in this area than in others, and they have had some success with community sources of finance for health care. In a great many countries, user charges are being assessed as a source of revenue. Several countries have combined both approaches, with modest success.

3. Initiation and expansion of the coverage of health insurance schemes, private and public: a large number of countries are experimenting with health insurance schemes as a way to generate resources and redirect the demand for services towards the most cost-effective level of delivery. A number of the middle-to-high-income developing countries are either introducing or experimenting with pre-paid/capitation and/or "managed" schemes in their public and private health care systems.

4. To increase expenditure in the private health sector has been seen in many developing countries as an additional way to expand total resources for health care and substitute and/or complement the resources expended by the public health care sector.

5. Finally, many countries in the developing world have been forced to re-examine their polices and programmes in the interest of the most vulnerable (high-risk) and poorest among their populations. Many countries have come to realize that the limited available resources have to be allocated both more efficiently and more equitably. Often this means reallocating away from acute care to primary care.

It is too soon to know whether these policies can succeed in generating more resources, in managing public resources more efficiently, and in protecting the most vulnerable and the poor. The potential to do so is there but the limited amount of research done so far on such policies has produced mixed results. Some of the policies, however well-intentioned, may actually be contributing to further inequity.[50] Concern, for example, about user fees is growing, and a number of studies have pointed out the "dos" and "don'ts" (perhaps based on bitter experience) of this initiative.

All five policies, however, are conditioned by external events often not under control of any single country. For example:

---

[50]See Paul Gertler, et. al. (1987), "Are User Fees Regressive?" *Journal of Econometrics*, Vol. 36, pp. 67-88.

- there is still a huge gap in the spending levels for health between rich and poor countries; some countries spend as little as $2 per head, some over $1000. Difference in economic growth rates between rich and poor countries will only increase this gap further.
- Medical care technology is changing and its capital and operating costs continue to escalate. This is a major problem in both developing and developed countries and represents, given the high level of expectations for health care services in developing countries, a problem. These forces already exacerbate the problem for developing countries in covering recurrent costs.
- New diseases—such as AIDS, Lyme disease,—and the recrudescence of old ones, such as malaria, present new demands for resources devoted to health protection and services. These developments have the potential to devastate levels of health spending in developing countries and containment of the diseases is beyond the limits of resources countries can generate internally.
- Worsened economic conditions, especially in the least developed countries, jeopardizes past health improvements if real resources grow, at rates less than population growth rates.
- The demographic effects on demands for health care resources from both growing populations and aging populations are now and will continue to remain large.

As we have noted already, there is no precise relationship between the amount of resources a country spends on health care and health levels—because of other factors intervening with both positive and negative health effects—it is clear that to maintain past gains in health status, especially in the developing countries, is going to require resource level expenditures of a much higher magnitude than presently exists. WHO has set a minimum standard of 5 percent of GNP on health. But of 129 countries (out of 166 member states) reporting expenditures, 60 percent of member states have spending levels below 5 percent GNP; those countries spending above 5 percent (57 member states) are the industrialized countries of Europe and the Americans, the oil exporting countries of the Gulf states, and the Nic's and several of the near and emerging Nic's. For the majority (at least 65 percent of the world's population) of the world, spending levels are within the range of 1-3 percent of GNP. With such low levels of resources available for health, developing countries must manage what they have efficiently and re-examine what areas of health are appropriate for government resources. Private sector development can augment government resources if governments choose to apply their resources to those things that count; protecting equity, providing health care where private markets would fail and other health programs with positive social externalities and benefits.

Surveys in the Latin American and Caribbean region have conservatively estimated the average wastage of health resources to be 40 percent of total expenditures—at least US $10,000 million each year. In one major industrialized economy half of recent cost increases have been attributed to basic mismanagement in the health system. It has been found that savings of half of current expenditures on pharmaceuticals could have been made through better management in one of Is the world's poorest countries. The health plan of one African country identifies potential savings of over a quarter of the recurrent budget of its central hospital by simple management improvements. Inefficiencies on a similar scale are also reported in industrialized countries. (These comments have been collected from internal unpublished sources within WHO Geneva). Inefficient decisions for resource allocation and wasteful management practices damage the prospects of health for all in two ways. In the short term they reduce the amount and quality of health care that can be made available at a cost countries can afford. As a result people suffer unnecessarily. In the longer term they undermine the health sector's case for additional resources, thus contributing to the cycle of inefficiency, underfinancing and avoidable illness. Achieving better value for money in health requires managers with skills in practical economics, and the incentives and information to act in cost conscious ways.

CONCLUDING NOTES

The title of the paper asked: "Are We Spending Too Much on Health Care?" The analysis and discussion in the paper suggests: we can never really know the answer but experience suggests that for some countries, perhaps most in the developing world, more resources for health could—I emphasize could—be effectively used to improve health status. But the great burden is for countries to make better and wiser choices in using limited resources experience to date shows they have. For human development and health levels to increase over the next decade in the developing world will require favorable world economic conditions and major reform in management, delivery, and financing efficiency.

Appendix Table A

Selected Health Indicators, Most Recent Estimates

Country	Per Capita GNP	Life Expectancy at Birth	Infant Mortality (per 1,000 Live Births)	Health Inputs/1,000 Population Physicians	Nursing Persons	Hospital Beds	Health Spending as a % of GNP	Hospitals as a % of Public Health Expenditure
Low Income Countries								
Mozambique	101	48	139	0.03	0.17	1.09	4.4%	36.0%
Ethiopia	122	47	135	0.01	0.19	0.30	3.6	48.6
Tanzania	157	53	104	0.04	0.40	NA		
Malawi	162	47	149	0.09	0.32	1.54		80.8
Guinea-Bissau	165	40	145	0.14	0.89	1.86		
Somalia	166	47	130	0.06	0.65	1.43		70.0
Bangladesh	168	51	118	0.15	0.11	0.28	1.7	51.7
Nepal	174	51	126	0.03	0.21	0.17	1.4	24.5
Chad	179	46	130	0.03	0.29	1.31		
Bhutan	193	48	127	0.04	0.33	0.71	2.0	
Gambia	215	44	143	0.09	0.46	1.67		45.4
Lao, PDR	215	49	108	0.73	1.88	0.93		
Mali	225	47	168	0.04	0.74	0.71	0.8	
Sierra Leone	234	42	152	0.07	0.92	1.21	3.0	
Burundi	236	49	73	0.05	0.33	1.11		66.4
Myanmar	244	60	68	0.27	1.11	0.85	3.2	
Madagascar	251	50	119	0.10	0.58	2.50		
Zaire	257	52	96	NA	0.57	3.33		
Uganda	277	48	101	0.05	0.49	1.52	2.1	43.4
Nigeria	281	51	103	0.13	0.98	0.73		
Niger	294	45	133	0.03	2.23	0.50		
Zambia	294	53	78	0.14	1.35	3.54		
Burkina Faso	300	47	137	0.02	0.59	0.57		
Rwanda	322	49	120	0.03	0.27	1.49	3.5	
China	330	70	31	1.00	0.72	2.00	4.0	66.0
India	338	58	97	0.40	0.59	0.77	4.3	
Guyana	350	63	44	0.16	1.13	3.33		
Pakistan	352	55	107	0.34	0.20	0.59	3.5	
Kenya	366	59	70	0.10	1.05	1.67	2.3	72.9
Togo	368	53	92	0.11	0.81	1.43		
Benin	369	51	115	0.06	0.57	1.13		
Central Afr Rep	376	50	102	0.04	0.46	1.58		
Haiti	379	55	116	0.14	0.44	0.72		
Guinea	401	43	143	0.02	0.16	1.53		
Ghana	404	54	88	0.07	1.56	1.25	.1.2	
Maldives	407	60	87	0.07	1.63	NA		
Sao Tome/Principe	409	65	49	0.50	3.49	26.49		
Lesotho	411	56	98	0.05	0.26	1.67	2.0	74.0
Sri Lanka	423	71	21	0.18	0.78	2.94	2.3	70.0
Sudan	424	50	106	0.10	0.80	0.90		
Comoros	443	56	80	0.08	0.44	2.10		
Mauritania	448	46	125	0.08	0.83	0.77		
Indonesia	468	61	68	0.11	0.79	0.55	2.2	37.3

Appendix Table A (continued)

Selected Health Indicators, Most Recent Estimates

Country	Per Capita GNP	Life Expectancy at Birth	Infant Mortality (per 1,000 Live Births)	Health Inputs/1,000 Population Physicians	Nursing Persons	Hospital Beds	Health Spending as a % of GNP	Hospitals as a % of Public Health Expenditure
Low Income Countries with Missing GNP Data								
Afghanistan	NA	38	172	0.16	0.11	0.27		
Kampuchea	NA	46	130	NA	0.73	1.08		
Liberia	NA	50	130	0.11	0.74	1.67		
Viet Nam	NA	66	44	1.00	1.60	3.64		
Middle Income Countries								
Yemen, PDR	526	51	118	0.23	0.95	1.56		
Solomon Islands	546	64	43	0.13	1.69	5.72		
Bolivia	570	53	108	0.65	0.40	2.00	2.3%	
Zimbabwe	605	63	49	0.15	1.00	1.43	4.2	56.0%
Equatorial Guinea	606	46	127	NA	0.80	NA		
Yemen, Arab Rep	615	47	128	0.16	0.37	0.45	6.0	
Philippines	629	64	44	0.15	0.36	1.67	2.4	71.0
Nicaragua	631	64	60	0.67	1.87	2.50		
Western Samoa	641	66	50	0.27	2.43	4.36		
Senegal	648	48	78	0.07	0.48	1.25	0.8	50.0
Kiribati	649	55	62	0.51	4.38	4.78		
Egypt	661	63	83	1.27	1.25	2.04		
Cape Verde	679	65	66	0.19	1.36	2.14		
Dominican Republic	721	66	63	0.57	0.83	2.50		
Swaziland	813	56	118	0.05	0.95	3.37	5.5	52.0
Papua New Guinea	828	54	61	0.16	1.12	4.74	3.8	45.0
Morocco	831	61	71	0.21	0.95	1.24	1.2	
Tonga	832	66	26	0.61	1.79	3.64		
Vanuatu	837	64	56	0.19	2.14	6.08		
Honduras	864	64	68	0.66	1.49	1.25		
Cote D'Ivoire	878	53	95	NA	0.49	1.16	1.1	45.5
Congo	891	53	117	0.12	1.74	4.59		
Guatemala	896	62	57	0.46	1.17	1.67		
Botswana	937	67	41	0.14	1.42	2.37		48.8
El Salvador	961	63	57	0.35	1.07	2.00		61.6
Paraguay	971	67	41	0.69	1.00	1.67		
Cameroon	997	56	92	NA	0.51	2.50		
Thailand	1,034	65	30	0.16	1.40	1.54	3.8	53.0
Jamaica	1,070	73	11	0.48	2.03	3.30	4.6	72.3
Ecuador	1,106	66	62	1.21	1.62	2.50	3.4	
Peru	1,117	62	86	0.96	0.99	1.69		
Jordan	1,123	66	43	0.88	0.77	0.91	6.8	75.4
Colombia	1,178	68	39	0.84	1.60	1.72	4.9	67.0
St. Vin/Grens.	1,201	70	25	0.23	1.48	4.99		
Tunisia	1,228	66	48	0.46	2.73	2.13		
Turkey	1,282	64	75	0.72	0.97	2.13	3.5	62.7
Belize	1,462	67	50	0.45	2.02	3.31		

Ralph Andreano

Appendix Table A (continued)

Selected Health Indicators, Most Recent Estimates

Country	Per Capita GNP	Life Expectancy at Birth	Infant Mortality (per 1,000 Live Births)	Physicians	Nursing Persons	Hospital Beds	Health Spending as a % of GNP	Hospitals as a % of Public Health Expenditure
Middle Income Countries (continued)								
Chile	1,506	72	20	0.81	2.70	3.41		
Fiji	1,518	71	21	0.56	2.11	2.44	3.8	
St. Lucia	1,669	71	21	0.26	1.90	5.07		
Dominica	1,680	74	18	0.32	1.88	4.44		
Syria	1,680	65	46	0.76	1.12	1.13		
Costa Rica	1,684	75	18	1.04	2.22	3.41		
Grenada	1,707	69	34	0.47	NA	5.95		
Mexico	1,753	69	46	0.81	1.14	1.25	3.4	57.6
Mauritius	1,803	67	22	0.53	1.72	3.33		
Poland	1,848	72	16	2.05	5.35	7.64		
Malaysia	1,934	70	23	0.52	0.99	2.50	3.5	65.1
Panama	2,124	72	22	1.00	2.57	3.33	5.6	
Brazil	2,157	65	61	0.93	0.83	5.00	5.6	68.1
South Africa	2,290	61	70	NA	2.43	NA		
Algeria	2,356	64	72	0.43	3.33	2.50	5.4	
Uruguay	2,436	72	23	1.99	5.29	3.32		
Hungary	2,456	70	16	3.26	5.76	9.17		
Yugoslavia	2,510	72	25	1.82	3.92	5.98		
Argentina	2,573	71	31	2.68	1.02	5.59	7.1%	
Suriname	2,605	67	42	0.79	3.62	8.90		
St. Kitts/Nevis	2,860	69	40	0.45	7.95	8.65		
Gabon	2,968	53	101	0.36	3.67	1.25		
Venezuela	3,130	70	35	1.43	2.71	0.37		
Trinidad/Tobago	3,474	71	16	1.04	3.87	4.98		
Korea	3,598	70	24	0.86	1.70	1.67	4.3	33.5%
Seychelles	3,644	70	18	0.45	5.03	4.92		
Portugal	3,645	74	14	2.42	1.59	5.00		
Antigua/Barbuda	3,884	73	22	NA	3.07	6.53		
Greece	4,774	77	12	2.85	2.20	6.16	5.3	
Oman	5,000	55	100	0.92	2.57	1.80		
Malta	5,194	73	10	1.14	8.78	10.00		
Libya	5,419	61	80	1.44	2.85	4.83		
Puerto Rico	5,630	75	15	NA	NA	NA		
Barbados	5,920	75	12	0.89	4.49	8.53		

Appendix Table A (continued)

Selected Health Indicators, Most Recent Estimates

Country	Per Capita GNP	Life Expectancy at Birth	Infant Mortality (per 1,000 Live Births)	Health Inputs/1,000 Population			Health Spending as a % of GNP	Hospitals as a % of Public Health Expenditure
				Physicians	Nursing Persons	Hospital Beds		
Countries Believed to be Middle Income, but with Missing GNP Data								
Angola	NA	45	135	0.06	0.99	2.72		
Djibouti	NA	47	122	0.24	1.99	3.64		
French Guiana	NA	73	NA	1.40	16.65	12.15		
Gibraltar	NA	NA	5	NA	NA	NA		
Guadeloupe	NA	74	15	1.38	1.90	11.41		
Iraq	NA	64	68	0.55	0.58	1.85		
Lebanon	NA	67	40	150	1.59	4.34		
Macao	NA	71	12	1.80	2.31	5.49		
Martinique	NA	75	13	1.43	NA	10.06		
Montserrat	NA	69	32	0.42	NA	NA		
Namibia	NA	57	104	NA	NA	NA		
Pacific Isls T.T.	NA	72	20	NA	NA	NA		
Reunion	NA	71	14	NA	3.62	8.66		
Romania	NA	70	24	1.76	3.60	8.77		
High Income Countries								
Cyprus	6,260	76	12	1.34	3.67	5.56		
Bahrain	6,341	68	26	1.24	2.75	3.19		
Iran	6,358	63	64	0.36	0.92	1.56		
Saudi Arabia	6,476	64	69	1.45	3.12	1.47		
Ireland	7,741	74	7	1.48	7.22	9.71	7.4	
Spain	7,780	77	9	3.16	3.86	5.20	6.0	
Israel	8,944	76	11	2.90	9.37	5.00		
Singapore	9,058	74	7	0.76	2.96	4.05		
Hong Kong	9,252	77	7	0.93	4.15	4.89		
Qatar	9,931	70	31	2.06	5.31	3.03		
New Zealand	9,991	75	11	1.74	12.37	10.13	6.9	
Bahamas	10,688	68	26	0.94	4.85	4.40		
Australia	12,331	76	9	2.29	8.73	12.00	7.1	
United Kingdom	12,797	75	9	1.64	8.33	9.32	6.1	
Italy	13,311	77	10	4.28	NA	10.59	6.9	
Belgium	14,472	75	9	3.02	9.26	9.38	7.2	

Source: Howard Barnum and Joseph Kutzin, Public Hospitalization in Developing Countries (manuscript, World Bank, May 1991), pp. 2-41/43.

Appendix B
Some Notes Concerning Making International Comparisons of Spending Levels on Health Care

Data on expenditures for health care services and provisions are available for only a limited number of countries and for only a limited number of years. Comparability in coverage of classes of expenditures, including expenditures that occur outside the public sector, and differences in national income accounting conventions also complicate inter country and time trend comparisons. Similarly, differences in internal and international prices, especially in currency exchange rates, makes conversions into a common value (such as US$) subject to aggregation of measurement error and under or over inclusion of relevant categories of expenditures. The problems presented by these factors in making informed judgments on trends in spending levels and expected levels and potential requirements for the future, are fraught with danger. Resources expended on health care services and actions within a country must be expressed in real terms if any meaningful trend or sectoral comparisons are to be made. The same holds true for comparisons across countries; differences in what a currency within a country can actually buy (the "market basket") get suppressed or overestimated when that currency is expressed in a common unit such as US$. These errors of commission can often lead to incomplete or incorrect conclusions; and, hence, policy actions based on such comparisons may be insufficient or in some cases, wrong.

An example of these issues is in comparing the percentage of central government expenditures as a percentage of total public expenditures over a period of time. Aside from other factors at work—such as reductions in total public expenditures, sectoral reallocations, and the like—a comparison of changes between countries in relative values (percentages) based on calculations made in nominal (i.e. not real expenditures can be confusing. World bank data (*Financing of Health Services*, p. 15) show that Central government expenditures as a percent of total public expenditures to have fallen from about 5 percent to 4 percent for low income countries: over the same period the fall was from slightly above 6 percent to just about 4 percent, or roughly a 33 percent decline. Industrialized countries rose from around 10 percent to just under 12 percent, or an increase of approximately 20 percent. Question: how much of this relative decline in poor and middle countries is due to: (a) increased spending in the private, non-governmental sector, (b) falling values of the domestic currency, (c) rising values of the US$? Does the nominal decline approximate a decline in the real amount of resources governments are allocating to health services or is it a statistical illusion? The truth is we cannot satisfactorily answer any of these questions; the best we can do is make some informed guesses as to what has occurred. What is needed in this, as in other cross national measures of spending are a common way to convert current spending levels at whatever source into a common measure of resource efforts expended.

One method by which this conversion can be made is to correct all national expenditures (whether of central government, private spending, or as a percent of GNP or GDP) into purchasing power parity (PPP). The accompanying chart compiled by OECD for its member countries shows such a conversion: both the GDP's and the health expenditures have been converted into PPP's. If nominal values are used the relative level of spending effort changes. For example, 1982 US GDP per capita is $13,160 the same as in the chart but per capita health spending not converted to PPP is $1,403. Sweden, which by PPP ranks very close to the U.S. in per capita health spending in nominal rates, shows a level of $1,173 or some $230 per head less. Italy's GDP per head converted to PPP is nearly $9,000 but its nominal GDP per head was actually $6,840. PPP converted health spending for Italy is $650 but in nominal terms was actually $445 for 1982.

The point of this note is that one must be very cautious in making judgments on comparisons of National spending levels.

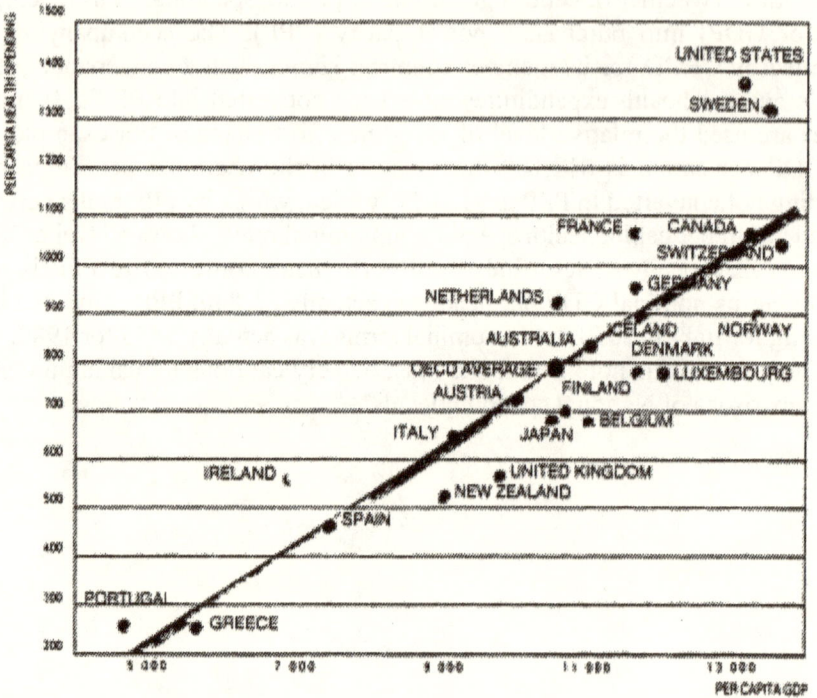

PER CAPITA HEALTH SPENDING AND PER CAPITA GDP, 1982
23 COUNTRIES

$ AT PPPs

Note:

Health spending and GDP converted into dollars from local currencies using GDP purchasing power parities.

Source:

Financing and Delivering Health Care. Paris, OECD, 1987.

SELECTION 12

THE ROLE OF THE PRIVATE SECTOR IN HEALTH CARE IN THE DEVELOPING COUNTRIES[51]

This paper was given at a Regional Seminar on Health Care Financing held at the Asian Development Bank in Manila, from 27-July to 3-August, 1987. The background papers of this Seminar, of which the present paper was one, were published jointly by the Asian Development Bank, The Economic Development Institute of the World Bank, and the East-West Center in 1987. The present paper was in pages 239-299. (My long-time colleague, Dr. Thomas Helminiak is also a co-author for much of this paper and his contributions are gratefully acknowledged.

INTRODUCTION

The recent attention focused on health service financing and delivery systems in the form of publications[52] and conferences has made public a range of issues that up to now have been discussed privately among economists, policy analysts, and decision makers in the Third World. Many health economists who have advised governments and ministers of health have, for years, been urging that attention be paid to some simple theorems of economics to analyze, restructure and reposition the health sector. The 1987 World Bank report has captured many of these arguments of the last decade and put them forward in a package of policy reforms that should command the attention of ministers of health and other ministries in the Third World. Not all of the policy package will be accepted without debate and not all of the analogies will apply uniformly across all Third World countries. But the report establishes the tone and analytical basis for the debate that is now taking place throughout the developing world. Our paper is directed to one aspect—perhaps the most urgent one—of this debate, that is, the role of the private sector. In the context of this paper the private sector means all the nongovernmental sources of care, both not-for-profit and for-profit.[53]

---

[51]This paper was given at a Regional Seminar on Health Care Financing held at the Asian Development Bank in Manila, from 27-July to 3-August, 1987.

[52]See, especially, *Financing Health Services in Developing Countries: An Agenda for Reform,* The World Bank, and Public *and Private Health Services,* Culyer and Jonsson (eds.), 1986.

[53]The private sector typically consists of the following: (a) salaried government physicians with part-time practices (there are cases where private practice is also

Ralph Andreano

The main point of this paper is that the private sector in developing countries can be a vast potential resource to expand services, to reallocate publicly provided funds and services, and to improve the internal efficiency of the country's health sector. The parallel point of the paper is that to utilize the private sector in meeting health care needs is not without difficulty and pitfalls. Consequently government policies toward the private health sector in most developing countries will have to change in many important, but difficult, ways.

The outline of the paper is as follows. The first part deals with some simple theorizing notions regarding private and public health care sectors and the distribution of effort between the two. The middle part of the paper deals with some proposed policy interventions for governments relating to private sector growth. In particular, policies to stimulate insurance markets are examined. These interventions are aimed at market efficiency objectives. The last part of the paper focuses on equity intervention. That is, efficiency objectives achieved through the private sector may conflict with equity objectives of governments. What can be done?

There are four appendices to this paper and a word or two about each seems appropriate. Appendix 1 draws upon the theory of market failure to analyze what ought to be provided in private markets and what ought to be the rationale for government intervention in private markets. This material expands on the analytical framework used in the World Bank (1987) report and in de Ferranti (1984) to help sort out candidates for user fees, to determine the public goods that could be privately provided, and to determine the public goods that the public sector is best capable of supplying. Appendix 2 provides an analytical framework with which to evaluate the financing system-related research going on around the world. The main text of this paper is an expansion of the private sector part of the framework represented in Appendix 2. This framework shows that health care financing and delivery are parts of a complex, interdependent system; policies directed toward one part of the system have effects (costs and benefits) on other parts of the system. Analysis and policy advice now being given to the developing countries must be viewed in this larger context. What theory tells us is optimal does not mean that countries can actually do it. Appendix 3 also expands on another aspect of this general framework, the "real system". Public sector performance in the developing countries must improve; the discussion on the "real system" is intended to help analyze ways of

---

permitted by other nonmedically trained personnel such as nurses and aides; (b) physicians in full-time, private fee-for-service practice; (c) pharmacists, many of whom diagnose, prescribe and treat; (d) missions, charities, churches and other not-for-profit nongovernmental organizations; (e) medical services run for employees by private or quasi-government enterprises, often including dependents of employees; (f) indigenous or traditional practitioners; and (g) private, for-profit hospitals and clinics.

improving that performance. The last appendix is meant to fill the gap between what theory says is a good thing for countries to do and their ability to do it. This material is a general primer on managing change. And in the context of this paper, countries deciding on what policies and posture they wish to take toward private health care will be addressing change of a major kind. The basic material of Appendix 4 is to help the thinking of decision makers and analysts in the developing countries. The basic principles involved in managing major policy changes are discussed.

"OPTIMAL" PRIVATE/PUBLIC SECTOR PROPORTIONS

One can characterize differences in the private and public roles in health care markets in two ways: (1) how and where services are produced and administered; and (2) how services are financed. A major role for the private sector in either of these dimensions does not preclude the possibility of a strong public role in the other. When one sees such disparity around the world in private/public sector roles both in service delivery and financing, it seems unlikely that there is a universally defined optimal distribution.

A fourfold dimension of hypothetical roles is illustrated in Figure 1.

Figure 1

Hypothetical Roles of Financing and Services Delivery

		Public	Private
Delivery of Services	Private	(1)	(2)
	Public	(3)	(4)

(1) A system can be publicly financed but have privately delivered services.
(2) A system can be both privately financed and privately operated.
(3) A system can be both publicly financed and publicly operated.
(4) A system can be privately financed but publicly delivered.

Obviously, within this matrix, many possible combinations and hybrids are possible. Most countries have hybrid combinations of public and private involvement in both financing and service delivery.

The public role is not limited to either direct financing or direct service delivery. Governments influence the production of services through legal

227

frameworks that establish how health care markets will operate. Governments also have the power to impose specific regulatory requirements on what, how and for whom health care services are privately produced. Government financing interventions can also take a variety of forms: (1) direct budgetary support to the private sector; (2) subsidies (or taxes) on either the supply or demand side of private sector markets; and (3) direct subsidies to the production of health manpower, notably physicians.

The wide variety of private/public sector proportions is illustrated in Figure *2*, which shows, relative to gross national product per capita, the private share of total health expenditures for countries with GNP per capita of US$2,000 or less. As the chart indicates, some very poor countries (Bangladesh, Haiti) still have large private sectors. And some relatively well-off countries (Colombia, People's Republic of China) have lower private sector shares. In Africa, as Table 1 shows, the pattern is much the same with a relatively well-off country like Zimbabwe (21% private) and a very poor one (Burkina Faso) with nearly the same private/public sector proportions. This wide variance is much the same for Asian countries (as shown in Table 1) as well as for industrialized countries.[54]

---

[54]The basic published data on private sector shares in various countries is relatively sparse. The main and most recently collected is D. de Ferranti (1984). The way private sector shares are usually calculated is as a percentage of total spending in a country. This method can, however, mask some important differences in the actual size of a private sector in any given country. What would be helpful is if private sector shares were calculated on the basis of final consumption spending. For a limited number of countries, such data based on final consumption spending are available in the United Nation's report (1986). An example of the differences between both methods can be found in the United States. As a percentage of total expenditures, the private sector share in the United States is usually listed as 57 per cent. However, because public insurance pays for services in private facilities, one might argue that the private sector share in the United States should be larger. Indeed, as measured by final consumption that is indeed true (i.e., 88°/ in 1983: see United Nations 1986). The point is that a consistent data set on private sector shares in the developing countries does not really exist. The de Ferranti (1984) data, the World Bank (1987) report, and scattered, anecdotal evidence is all that is available. It would be useful if countries were given a consistent way to measure private shares and if the international agencies compiled data using a consistent definition.

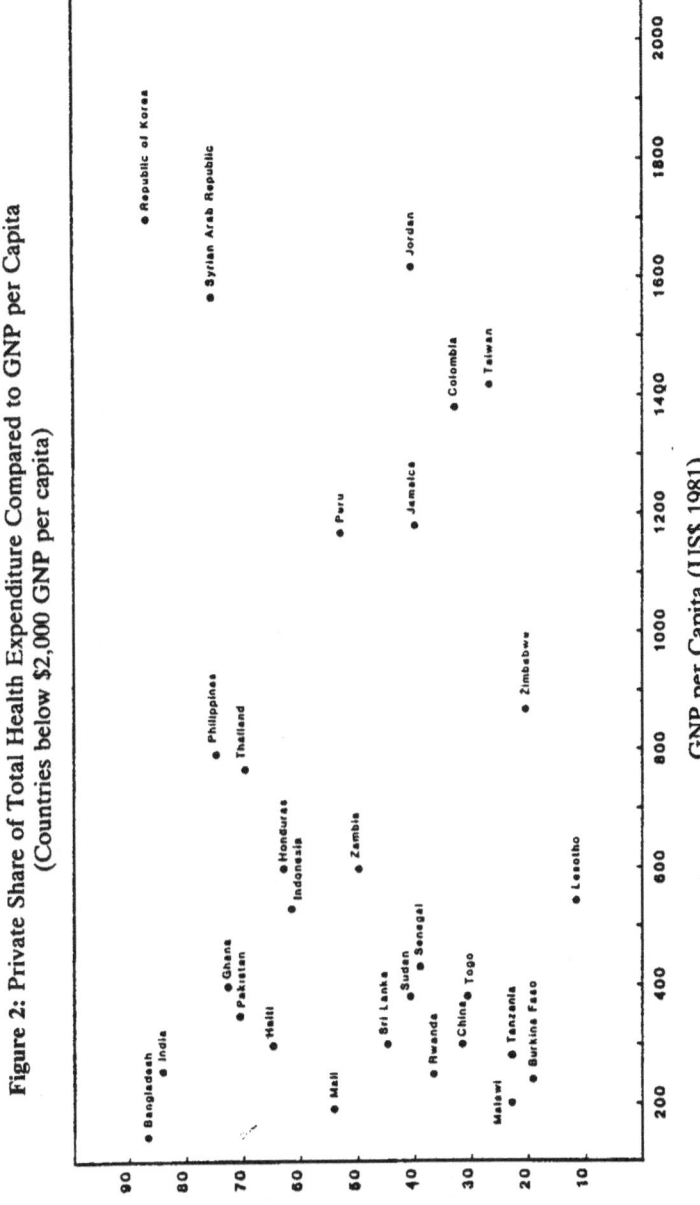

Figure 2: Private Share of Total Health Expenditure Compared to GNP per Capita
(Countries below $2,000 GNP per capita)

Sources: Private share percentages from D. de Ferranti, "Strategies for Paying for Health Services in Developing Countries," *World Health Statistics Quarterly*, Vol. 37, No. 4, 1984; Table 3, p. 448.

GNP per capita from *World Development Report 1983*, Table 1, pp. 148–149.

Table 1

Private Sector Share of Total Health Expenditures: Selected Countries

Country	Private % of Total
Bangladesh (1976)	87
China (1981)	32
India (1970)	84
Indonesia (1982/83)	62
Korea (1975)	87
Pakistan (1982)	71
Australia (1975)	36
Philippines (1970)	75
Sri Lanka (1982)	45
Thailand (1979)	70
UK (1974/75)	7
US (1974/75)	57

Source: de Ferranti, D.M., "Strategies for Paying for Health Services in Developing Countries," World Health Statistics Quarterly, Vol. 37, No. 4, 1984, Table 3, p. 448

INTERVENTIONS AND OPTIONS: SOME SIMPLE THEORY

It is clear that there is a gap between what economic theory forecasts should be done and what governments actually are in a position to do. A redistribution of effort and resources between public and private sectors looks appealing. But how can it be done? The principle derived from theory is relatively simple: Efficiency is achieved through private markets (under perfect competition) but government must intervene to achieve equity objectives (or appropriately compensate for market imperfections). We can distinguish at least two types of equity (financial and distributional) and three types of efficiency (production, financing and utilization).[55] There are trade-offs within and between each of these two groupings. However, for simplicity of conceptualization, we can reduce the optimization problem to one of trade-offs between net equity and net efficiency.

This is depicted graphically in terms of a production possibility curve, such as the AB curve in Figure 3. Each country, with a given health care financing and

---

[55]These equity and efficiency criteria are more fully discussed in Appendix 2.

delivery system in place, will have a production possibility (PP) frontier (curve) that reflects possible trade-offs (dictated by the nature of the system) between (net) efficiency (total effective health care services) and (net) equity. Such trade-offs would occur for modest policy changes, within the existing system format, that sought to increase either efficiency or equity.

For any production possibility frontier, such as that shown in Figure 3 above, there might exist various social welfare functions, reflecting acceptable trade-offs between net efficiency and net equity. In the graph, the social welfare function represented by the indifference curves C_1, C_2, C_3 indicates a greater relative concern for equity, in contrast to the function indicated by indifference curves D_1, D_2, D_3, which give greater relative emphasis to efficiency objectives. As depicted in the figure, for the financing/delivery system offering this production possibility frontier, social welfare function C would result in a welfare maximizing situation at point X, whereas if the country possessed social welfare function D, optimization would result at point Y.

A number of different problem categories exist in regard to a country operating a financing/delivery. system at a non-optimal social welfare point. For the country at point X, in Figure 4, the production possibility frontier has not been attained, perhaps due to poor management, bureaucracy or inappropriately constraining rules and regulations. In the situation represented by point Y, the system is operating efficiently in that the production possibility frontier has been attained; however, sector administrators suffer from a myopia, whereby they fail to understand or recognize that by trading off some equity, enough efficiency could be gained to improve social welfare. At point Z, social welfare is maximized, in that system production efficiency has been achieved and optimal efficiency and equity trade-offs have been made.

Figure 3: Production Possibility Frontier with Different Efficiency-Equity
Preference Function

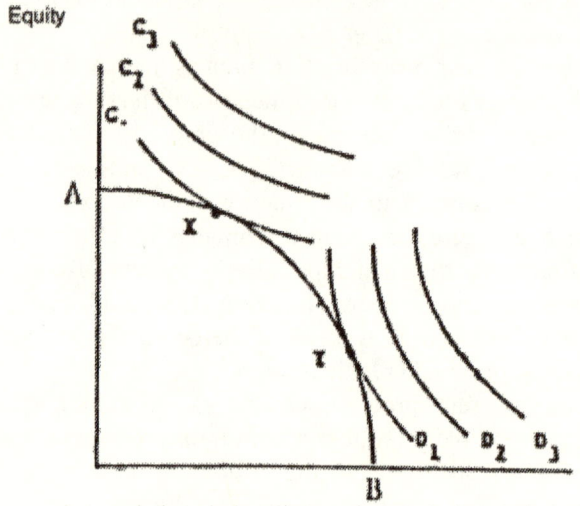

Figure 4: Situations of Suboptimal Production and Production Trade-off
Myopia

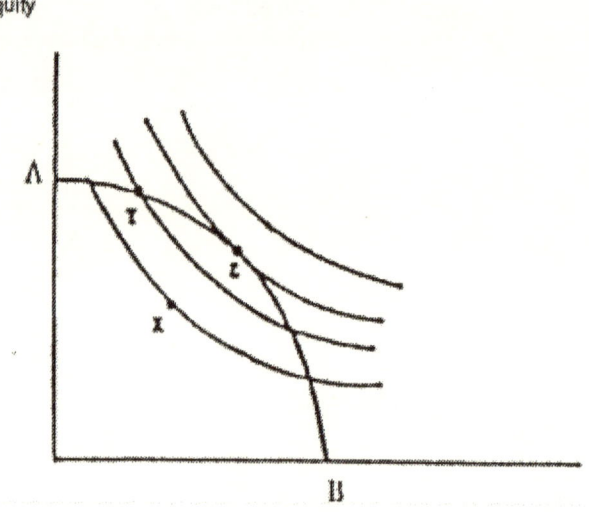

Figure 5 represents another type of production possibility myopia. Each financing/delivery system may be viewed as defining a PP frontier. PP frontier AB above might represent a publicly dominated system. The country operating within this system would optimize, in terms of efficiency-equity trade-off, at point X (tangency with social indifference curve W_1). On the other hand, an alternative system, represented by PP frontier CD (possibly privately dominated), might allow a higher social welfare attainment at point Y (tangency with W_2). Finally, some hybrid system, represented by AD, might allow a still higher social welfare attainment at point Z (tangency with W_3).

The point is that the appropriate production possibility frontier is not that which is defined by any single financing/delivery format, but rather the envelope frontier comprising the outer limits of all feasible financing/delivery systems for the country. Commonly, however, sector administrators will have highly limited, if any, appreciation of the existence and definition of the envelope frontier. Thus, a country with a predominantly public system, such as that of AB in Figure 5, might only perceive the efficiency-equity trade-off possibilities for the existing system, ignoring the possibility that a system format shift (such as to CD, or better, to AD) could offer significant efficiency improvement with °a modest and acceptable equity trade-off.

Figure 5: Envelope Production Possibility Frontier

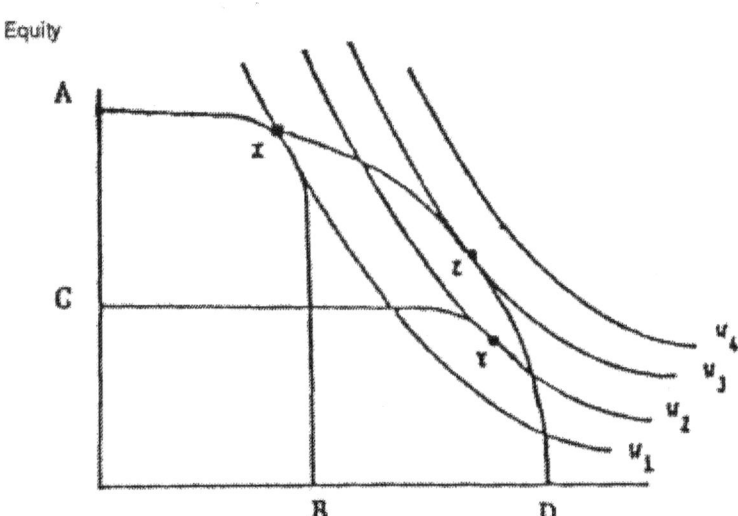

An added complexity to the simple conceptual analysis presented above is that, due to various market imperfections, social efficiency may diverge from private efficiency in the production of at least some health services. Such market imperfections, which include public good status, externalities, natural monopoly, and imperfect information,[56] may call for some form of public intervention with respect to those health care services where significant loss of social efficiency results. More precisely, for the services characterized by such market failure, the cost of specific potential public interventions, including possible offsetting reductions in other private/social efficiency aspects of the private market solutions, must be compared with the presumed (gross) benefit of the reduction of the market imperfection. In many instances, it is quite possible that the net social efficiency benefit of such interventions will actually be negative.

Obviously, a critical aspect of opting for public intervention to counter some element of market failure is to select the appropriate public intervention for the task, that is, the option that offers the maximum net social efficiency improvement. With a range of interventions—extending from combined public administration/delivery and financing, through public full or partial financing only, to various forms of public regulation affecting administration or financing—a starting rule-of-thumb might be to consider the least-intrusive intervention that might remedy the market failure.

In terms of the preceding production possibility frontier conceptual analysis, the circumstance of social efficiency market imperfections variously affecting different health care services suggests a disaggregation of the analysis in the form of separate PP frontiers for individual services or service groupings. That is, the relative shapes and loci of the PP frontiers—describing alternative financing/delivery formats (including varying levels and types of public intervention)—will probably be considerably differentiated according to whether curative, preventive, or community health services are being produced. For example, according to theory, tangency solutions are expected for public-financed formats in the case of preventive services and for formats with greater emphasis on private financing in the case of curative services.

The World Bank has emphasized this differentiation of health services categories with regard to their relative suitability for private versus public financing (de Ferranti 1984). This research has employed economic theory, with attention to the implications of market imperfections, and some highly limited empirical evidence. The policy proposals that have emerged from this research are (implicitly) based on plausible hypotheses regarding the relative shapes and loci of the production possibility frontiers for the advocated formats, with reference to generalized social preference functions. Further theoretical, as well as empirical research, are nevertheless sorely needed with regard to the ideal

---

[56]More detailed discussions on this are provided in Appendix 1.

blends of private and public financing and the particular system formats, which will optimize health sector social efficiency, equity and aggregate resource funding. At the same time, research is also needed in regard to specific methodologies (what in Appendix 2 has been termed "tools and strategies") which, within given financing/delivery formats, capture and maximize individual and group incentives to: (1) optimize equity and efficiency objectives of the system (i.e., to operate on, rather than within the PP frontier); and/or (2) overcome political and inertia constraints to the establishment and success of the system. The remainder of this paper emphasizes this area of research in the context of the private sector option.

Countries are presently struggling to meet the World Health Organization's (WHO) established goal of Health for All by the Year 2000. If this goal is to amount to anything more than rhetoric, countries formulating strategies to pursue the goal need to identify the real economic problem (assuming one does exist) as to why those countries do not have Health for All in the year 1987. It is largely a matter of allocative inefficiency, which can be remedied by allocating existing sector resources to a more efficient delivery mode (such as primary health care) instead of to inefficient delivery modes (such as hospitals). Or, in a similar vein, is there a problem of one of the other forms of allocative efficiency (described in Appendix 2) or of financial or funding efficiency? If the problem is one of efficiency, does it represent inefficiency within the existing financing/delivery system (operation at some point inside the production possibility frontier of the system—point X in Figure 4)? Or does it represent a failure to take advantage of desirable production possibility trade-offs in favor of increased efficiency either due to intra-system production possibility myopia (point Y in Figure 4) or due to inter-system production frontier envelope myopia (point X in Figure 5)?

Alternatively, a Health for All problem interpretation based on inadequate equity under the existing system seems dependent on either (1) the intra-system myopia view, which says that socially acceptable trade-offs of less efficiency for more equity are available under the existing system or (2) the inter-system (production possibility frontier envelope) myopia view, which says that an alternative financing/delivery system that offers lower sacrifices of efficiency for more equity is both feasible and desirable. (These two interpretations would be represented by reversals of the latter two examples described above, involving Figures 4 and 5, depicted most simply by imaging the vertical axis as measuring efficiency and the horizontal as measuring equity, with the shape of the curves unchanged.)

Another alternative interpretation of the Health for All problem is that there is an intersectoral allocative inefficiency resulting in the underfunding of the health sector. (That is, an outward shift of the health sector's production possibility frontier is socially desirable.) This suggests that societies would be willing, in order to obtain more health care services, to give up some resource

235

allocation to other sectors (e.g., education, housing, military defense, or consumer goods). If this is so, then what is the basis for the underfunding constraint and how should it be dealt with? Intersectoral allocative inefficiency is certainly difficult to measure, especially given the market imperfections characterizing the health sector; nevertheless, many might consider the tendencies for unconstrained private health systems to rapidly expand as support for the underfunding argument.

In attempting to pursue the Health for All objective, it is critically important that countries first determine the real economic problem that lies behind the objective so that appropriate strategies can be developed.

When one compares these observations with what is happening to health systems in the developing world, policy arguments of the type advanced by WHO, the World Bank (1987) and others begin to make some sense. Total government resources for health care in the developing countries are not likely to grow very much in real terms and in many cases may actually decline. The choices facing the developing countries are to reallocate public sector resources, to allow the private sector to grow, to adapt policies to make the public sector more efficient and competitive, and to strive to recognize and implement those feasible trade-offs between output, equity and efficiency that are socially desirable. Evaluating and selecting from these choices is easier said than done!

HOW DO WE PROCEED?

Theory advises us that public interventions, either in administration/delivery or the financing of health services, should be undertaken only: (1) where market imperfections would yield inefficient outcomes with the private sector operating freely and where the cost of the public intervention is less than the benefit of the amelioration of the market imperfection; and (2) where the equity result of the private sector approach is undesirable and can be improved by public intervention at socially acceptable cost, including that of efficiency trade-offs.

With respect to both of these theoretical principles, the obviously large challenge to sector administrators is, again, to select the optimal public intervention from the range of options (including that of no intervention at all), such that: (1) net social efficiency is maximized; (2) minimal necessary sacrifices are made to achieve desired quality improvements; and (3) that the efficiency trade-offs that are minimally necessary are really socially acceptable.

This limited statement of the problem reflects an optimal stationary state in terms of total resources allocated to the health sector. In fact, in the real world of developing countries today, the level of public intervention in the health sector determines not only the public/private split for a given resource allocation level; the level (and form) of public intervention also influences the quantity of resource allocation to the sector. This public influence on the level of health sector resource allocation reflects not just the amount of private sector financing, which may be strongly constrained, accepted with a laissez-faire view, or actually encouraged by government action.

Given the various elements of health sector market failure, as well as the various public interventions (which while attempting to correct some market imperfections probably create others), it is doubtful whether the levels of resource allocation to the health sectors of developing countries approximate levels that would be determined by intersector allocative efficiency. The presumption of most health sector administrators in these countries is that their health sectors are under funded. Although we must carefully scrutinize the extent to which underfunding—in terms of intersector allocative efficiency is real,[57] unconstrained or encouraged private sector expansion has been observed to offer an avenue for increased aggregate funding of health for many countries, in addition to providing an opportunity for substituting private for public resources.

The link between theory and specific operational advice is only partially developed, and solid empirical studies to support and fine-tune the theories are mostly absent. Still, there is a large body of belief among analysts such as us, that social optimization in the health services of developing countries could be advanced by increased reliance on the private sector. Before governments can begin to sort out and evaluate the types of trade-offs (benefits and costs) described in the preceding theories for any expanded private sector role, a greater understanding will be needed of the various possible formats and associated implications offered by the private sector option.

WHY USE THE PRIVATE SECTOR?

The private sector includes a wide range of activities and entities, not all of which have profit maximization as their organizing principle. Our excursion into a bit of economic theory highlighted the main dichotomy of efficiency and equity between public and private provision of health goods and services. We now pose a series of questions that are hardly abstract and hardly theoretical: Why should a country want to use the private sector? International agencies such as the World Bank, the Asian Development Bank and WHO are urging countries to explore the option of "using", "cooperating with", or "taking advantage of" the private

---

[57]Intersectoral resource allocation should, in principle, be governed by marginal productivities for resources allocated to the respective sectors. To the extent that health sector needs are poorly met due to low efficiency in the employment of existing resources, the case for added resources to the sector will be improved insofar as the efficiency of existing resources is first raised.

health sector. What do these different exhortations mean? How can countries "use", "take advantage of", or "cooperate with" the private sector? What do these words mean? What policies do they imply? There is a considerable amount of rhetoric on this subject, some theory to support the potentiality of a private sector, and some successes in countries where private sector growth has been extensive. But, in truth, is there an agenda for action available to countries? The answer seems to be that there is none. The one fact that seems irrefutable is that a private health care sector exists in almost every country, rich and poor, socialist or capitalist. And the existence of that sector indicates a number of things about a country's health care system, for example, unhappiness with the current public system, growing personal income inequality, and nonmarket prices allocating public resources. So, if countries are intent on "using" the private sector they must be very clear about the objectives and benefits of doing so. We think that the current climate of opinion has been short of assistance of this type and long on advice to countries to plunge into activities with unknown costs and benefits.

What are some of the objectives countries might have if the private health care sector is to be "used", "taken advantage of", or "cooperated with"? Some possible objectives are as follows:

(1) To substitute private resources for currently used public resources in health care provision where consumers can get the same services and pay for them while reallocating public resources to areas of greater priority (preventive care, free public health, rural areas, etc.).
(2) To use the competitive influence of the private sector to reform the efficiency of the public services and thus increase consumer satisfaction with the system, and, through efficiencies, reallocate resources back into the public system to achieve still better (i.e., more equitable and efficient) delivery, financing and production systems.
(3) To use the private sector, by permitting its growth, as a way to expand total resources in the country devoted to health care by permitting the "efficient" sector to grow relative to the "inefficient" sector.

In the parlance of economics, using the private sector can mean that the two sectors (public and private) have services and products that are substitutes for each other and complements to each other. Alternatively, by permitting private sector growth a country may be consciously trying to increase the total fund of resources to health care, and hence influencing the ultimate output, namely health status.

Our theory has shown that—on the probably correct consumption that production efficiency is greater in private than in public provision of services— governments will face an equity trade-off depending on which set of objectives (and policies) they seek to follow with respect to the private sector. If pure substitution of resources between the two sectors is the objective, then certain explicit policies follow. Governments should permit private sector growth in acute care services, withdrawing public resources from these services for use in the provision of pure or quasi-public goods such as mass campaigns, public health and sanitation, nutrition and family planning. Government's role also would be to maintain, even in acute services, the desired equity level it deems appropriate. (Equity here meaning access and financial.) The benefits of the "using" objective are gains in sector efficiency, a savings of previously used public resources, and extensions of the public system into more intractable parts of the health sector such as rural health. The costs are that some equity levels may be compromised—especially issues of access, quality control, and, potentially, cost escalation (another equity variant) in the private system.

But if substitution is the objective, then the policies to achieve this are fairly obvious:

(1) Close down or privatize acute care services—mainly hospitals.

(2) Keep a tertiary care hospital in the public sector for access, quality control, and cost control objectives.

(3) Withdraw partially or completely, all public subsidies for medical education. (For equity, loans can be substituted for direct subsidies and loans can be tied to government service.)

(4) Reorganize the public system so as to bias it toward provision of services not amenable to private sector provision, that is, pure public health and equity concerns.

(5) Liberalize rules and regulations (if any) inhibiting private sector growth and follow policies such that all who can afford to pay for services are permitted opportunities to obtain such services in private markets. This could mean encouraging private sector growth through insurance and risk-sharing, taxation policies, and other price and market incentives.

There are, of course, generic things that can be done if the objective in using the private sector is to substitute privately paid services for those paid for through public revenues. None of the above five policy directions are easy and there is no general rule or blueprint that all countries can follow; in each country the circumstances will be different and each country has to pursue its own policy course. It is clear, however, that none of these things will be easy to do; it is just as difficult to close a public hospital as a private one. A loss of education subsidies will be painful and not easily accepted. Restructuring the public delivery system means reassigning and retraining personnel; the personnel in the public system would surely resist these changes and civil service rules may even prevent them. And, similarly, to liberalize a regulatory climate will redistribute political power and influence; and those who lose out in such changes can be expected to fight them fiercely (see Appendix 4). So the message is if a country's objective in "using" the private sector is resource substitution, policies implied by this objective are likely to be controversial and not easy to implement. This does not mean the objective should not be pursued; it merely suggests that countries should be cautious. The private sector is not a palliative for the entire health sector funding problems a government may be facing.

The policy menu above is much the same if pursuing "uses" of the private sector involves some variation of pure substitution or complements. Depending on how far governments wish to go in seeking private sector substitution, some of the above policies can be partially implemented, or delayed, or even abandoned—whatever is appropriate to the facts of that particular country. What does seem certain, however, is that even if governments have no explicit objectives toward the private sector, these markets are likely to grow anyway. Government policies can foster that growth, but it is unlikely that the private sector can be completely eliminated. The message we want to deliver is simply this: Countries are being urged to "use" the private sector; we are saying that countries should know why they are doing this before they plunge into objectives of government. The more the production and delivery of health goods and service that can be obtained by risk-sharing and incentive-based behavior by consumers and providers, the better off the health care system will be in terms of efficiency. And empirical evidence shows that people are willing to pay for most important services (especially hospital care and drugs).

Governments can use principles of market behavior, including risksharing and incentives, to reform public systems toward efficiency and still maintain high consumer satisfaction levels for the services. But all the discontinuities of the real system (see Appendix 3) suggest that reform of the public system will not be any easier than pursuing an objective of letting the private sector grow autonomously or in a controlled way. There is no a priori reason why governments could not move their systems closer to efficiency objectives, but in practice, imposing user charges, decentralizing the delivery system, or making managers responsible for performance and policies of these types may be just as difficult to achieve as those discussed above when letting the private sector substitute for some of the major public services. Governments should reform their systems because it is unlikely that any health care system in the developing countries can be wholly public or wholly private. The nature of health care demands and priorities in the developing countries will require both public and private markets.[58] Although the

---

[58]This prescription is not exclusive to developing countries. Even in the United Kingdom where, despite austere Thatcher budgets, expenditure for the National Health Service has risen by a third in real terms in eight years, there are calls for greater private sector participation. A recent article in The Economist (1987) remarks, "The most promising solution...is competition between health authorities and hospitals, between

evidence suggests that public markets cannot produce (or finance) goods and services as efficiently as private markets that does not mean that government output should be accepted as inexorably inefficient in production of financing. To "use", "take advantage of", or "cooperate with" the private health care sector does not mean governments have to abandon the requirement to use their resources efficiently.

EXPANDING THE PRIVATE SECTOR

If countries are intent on letting their private health sector expand, for whatever combination of objectives they may have in mind for doing so, what can be done? There are two areas of overlapping importance here: (1) stimulation of the incremental demand for services delivered in the private sector; and (2) increases in the incremental supply of private sector facilities and services. Obviously, demand and supply side policies are interrelated. There is also another issue (derived from the above) that affects the composition of output—the types (services) of private sector demand that should be expanded and supplied. Using this as a way to organize the policy options of countries pursuing an expanded private sector, what can be suggested?

Demand Side

To expand the private sector would mean increasing the demand for services. Some private sector growth will be autonomous because of income growth, perception of public services, time costs, and the like. In this instance we are not talking about autonomous growth in demand for private sector care, but growth fostered through governmental policies and initiatives. These policies and initiatives are:

(1) tax policies: encourage market insurance, discourage self insurance; tax breaks to consumers for insurance;

---

doctors...More competition would do much to improve the NHS' efficiency...should start looking at ways of encouraging the voluntary and private sectors to take more of the strain." Interestingly, a report by the Health Education Council in the United Kingdom indicates that National Health Service performance even in the equity area has been less than hoped. The report reveals that inequalities in health have not only persisted into the 1980s, but the gap between social classes has widened. (See "Editorial: The Health Divide—The Policy Gap," Health Economics Bulletin, Health Economics Research Unit, University of Aberdeen, June 1987, p. 1.)

(2) pricing policies: increase prices in the public sector above the private sector;

(3) regulatory incentives: for example, let public sector donors have a private practice, encourage physician output; and

(4) subsidy policies: target subsidies to consumers for private sector use.

Supply Side

On the supply side, a number of policies seem useful as ways of increasing or expanding the private sector. (Again, we are speaking of expansion of supply above what would otherwise take place.) These policies are:

(1) tax advantages for certain types of financing and delivery systems (e.g., insurance, capitation);

(2) education subsidies to stimulate output of medical professions personnel, without being extensively tied to government service;

(3) seed capital for new ventures such as health maintenance organizations (HMOs) and large group medical practices; and

(4) restraint of regulatory policies so as to permit easier entry into the private sector for delivery institutions.

Composition of Output

In expanding the private sector, countries may also wish to capture some of the efficiencies obtainable in private markets for the provision of quasi or pure public goods health outputs. For example, if the private sector expansion is primarily in acute care, a country may wish to offer incentives to the private sector to provide services such as immunization, family planning, nutrition, counseling and other forms of preventive care. Similarly, if the private sector will underprovide services in rural areas or in other poor areas, incentives (such as subsidies or tax breaks) could be used to stimulate private sector expansion in the traditionally publicly provided areas and services. The notion here is that by expanding the private sector a country should be sure it is not building in disincentives to seek care from the lowest cost provider. For example, outpatient types of services should not be done on an inpatient basis. Governments can use their power to set incentives and create disincentives (through taxes, loans, subsidies and overt regulation) to insure that the composition of output in the private sector is consistent with equity objectives, without sacrificing the efficiency gains that are expected to come when most health services are delivered through private markets. Policies to increase demand or supply will interact with each other; and it is a government's responsibility to see that the composition of output and the delivery mechanisms in the private sector are not thwarted because of perverse incentives. To expand the private sector using some or all of these policies requires that a country have a clear idea of what is intended, why it is being done, and what outcome is desired.

One final note on the importance of the composition of output: An expanding private sector may raise certain equity issues such as access and quality. One way countries can deal with a part of these equity problems is to retain control and pricing over tertiary care facilities, certification of certain medical specialists, and control over acquisition of new capital and equipment in private sector facilities. This does not insure that an expanded private sector will not generate other inequities, but at least maintaining control of tertiary care services will permit countries to keep important components of medical output under social control. The same principle could be applied to other aspects of the system as well, such as outpatient care and rural clinics.

DEVELOPING PRIVATE INSURANCE MARKETS

The development of insurance (or coverage) arrangements is currently being advocated by some of the international donor agencies as an attractive strategy for the expansion of private sector financing. The case for insurance arrangements has been advanced, based on:

(1) the financial equity offered, due to (a) the fact that health care expenses are shared by the well and the sick, rather than just the sick. alone under full user charge formats, and (b) the greater feasibility of graduated payments according to income than with user charges; and

(2) a perception of consumer demand (i.e., willingness-to-pay) for such arrangements.

Thus health insurance formats, in general, offer appeal in terms of financial equity and aggregate funding enhancement. The impact on distributional equity, however, is a matter of some debate, depending on the breadth of coverage of the individual arrangement and other factors. Funding efficiency will vary among arrangements, depending, for example, on the association with some existing employment financial activity and geographic concentration of enrollees. Finally, production and allocative efficiency are often perceived as being adversely influenced, at least in third-party arrangements where appropriate price incentives are muted.

The different specific rationales for the utilization of insurance arrangements should be noted:

1. *Private risk aversion.* The private demand for health insurance—relating to the uncertain need for costly health services—is, in theory, based on the presumed declining marginal utility of wealth and the consequent superior utility of a small certain loss (insurance premium) relative to the expected value of an uncertain loss (possible uninsured medical expense). With a continuously declining marginal utility of wealth, health insurance will always be attractive (a rational purchase) if sold at an actuarially fair premium (i.e., there are no administrative or other transaction costs). The monetary equivalence of the utility difference between the expected value of the uncertain medical care expense loss and the "actuarially fair" premium, which will vary with the probability of the medical expense, defines the potential allowance for transactions costs for both insurance sellers and buyers. For transactions cost premium supplements below this allowance, health insurance will still be attractive to a rational buyer, based on a private calculus of costs and benefits, but above that allowance insurance will not be attractive.

2. *Social equity enhancement.* Insurance arrangements can also be used to meet social preferences for financial and distributional equity in health care services. This objective can be pursued by charging premiums that are related to the income level of the enrollee, while providing health care benefits that are either equal (regardless of premium payment) or differentiated by less than an actuarial translation of the levied premiums. To the extent that the redistribution strength of the arrangement results, for some income classes, in a premium exceeding the private risk aversion benefit (as defined above, taking transactions costs into account), the insurance arrangement would need to be made compulsory or suffer the loss of the redistribution base.[59]

3. *Budgeting tool for health care expenses.* In the case of relatively routine health care expenses, it is likely that transactions costs exceed any risk aversion benefit. Consequently, a "rational" insurance purchaser would not buy health insurance for such routine expenses. However, in explaining an apparent preference of many for such routine expense coverage, it has been suggested that insurance mechanisms, with regular monthly premiums, are valued for their enforced budgeting for routine health care expenses. Still, it is quite possible that the real cost of the

---

[59]Compulsory social health insurance premiums amount to an earmarked tax. The benefit of the protection of this revenue from alternative program competition for general tax revenues must be assessed against the cost of a separate tax collection mechanism and associated bureaucracy. W. Wlodarczyk (1987) argues that for health insurance to be economically and socially effective, there must be differentiation of both services and premiums, with the level of services related to the level of premium.

budgeting benefit might not be carefully evaluated by purchasers of the benefit.[60]

4. *Production and allocative efficiency enhancement tool.* Generally, health care insurance has (as suggested earlier) been considered antithetical to production and allocative efficiency in health care, due to its effect of separating consumers from price incentives. However, it is possible for insurance arrangements to be constructed to encourage competition among suppliers of health care services and to establish incentives for production and allocative efficiency.

John S. Akin's paper (also in this volume) appears to emphasize the second rationale above, that is, the potential of health insurance as a social equity tool. Mr. Akin also notes the possible need for government intervention in health insurance markets to compensate for the various aspects of market failure in these insurance markets. However, in our view, the government role should be to shape the structure and specific formats of health insurance markets such that those markets offer internal incentives for production and allocation efficiency in the health sector in general.

The market for private and group health insurance in the developing countries is typically small and confined. Reinsurance markets are also generally limited (Wasow and Hill 1986). Capitation schemes, such as HMOs, require application of some basic insurance principles, if not a well-developed health insurance market.

What can government policy do to develop and widen health insurance markets in their countries? In most developing countries, various forms of self-insurance already exist through large enterprises (usually industrial firms) that provide health care services to their employees. These are frequently provided with company-owned facilities and employed personnel, but it is also common for a company to contract for services with the private sector and, in some instances, with the public sector for provision of services to its employees. In most countries, public or government employees also have some health insurance coverage financed by government; most frequently, services must be obtained in public facilities, although on occasion government contracts with some private providers for servicing publicly insured government employees and dependents. And, of course, there are many countries with health benefits as part of employment-financed social insurance schemes. Usually, in social insurance

---

[60]In the United States, tax treatment of employer-paid insurance premiums can reduce real premium costs enough to make insurance a rational purchase (from a private, though not a social perspective) even when transaction costs exceed the risk aversion benefit.

schemes, services are received in government-owned facilities, but there are some exceptions.

The point in recounting these general conditions is that in most developing countries there is some base upon which to build if government wishes to develop or expand individual and group health insurance markets. In the developing countries, these markets are not likely to develop spontaneously, although as wealth increases in a country it does lead to a substantial increase in the demand for insurance. But a basis upon which group insurance markets can be expanded does exist in virtually all developing countries. What policies can government pursue to use this base? Let us list seven policies that could be considered. Some countries are beginning to try or are already pursuing such policies.

SEVEN POLICIES TO EXPAND HEALTH INSURANCE MARKETS

(1) Couple existing government employee insurance plans with private sector plans.
(2) Couple existing private sector employment-based self-insurance plans to private insurance markets.
(3) Expand existing government insurance plans to include nongovernment employees.
(4) Encourage use of capitation and managed care.
(5) Convert existing government insurance schemes into capitation schemes.
(6) Convert existing government acute care institutions into parastatal enterprises.
(7) Nationalize or limit insurance enterprise competition.

We want to give a few points under each of these potential policy interventions. Many of these seven policies are interactive and though listed separately, following one policy may mean following others as well. The point of all the policies is that government is taking a proactive role to stimulate private sector growth through use of insurance and by exerting the power and leverage of government. Government tax policy and the form, kind and level of subsidies government chooses can also do much to change relative prices and to induce desirable changes in behavior. With insurance markets, governments can benefit from the net efficiencies of the private side and utilize or reallocate any public resources substituted for in order to achieve equity objectives and to produce pure or quasi-public goods that the private sector cannot or will not produce.

1. Couple Existing Government Employee Insurance Plans with the Private Sector

In most countries, government employees have some insured health benefits. This represents buying power. Governments could do several things:

(a) Put the insured government employee benefit package up for competitive bid to any private organization. Government specifies the terms of the bid, that is, how and where the benefits are to be received (private or public provider facilities) whether the bid should be capitated or not and which organizations are qualified to bid (insurance companies, clinic groups, etc.).

(b) Governments can put the package up for bid by adding certain incentives and disincentives to government employees and to potential bidders. For example, governments can offer to pay 100 per cent of the employees' benefit policy if in a capitated scheme, but only 90 per cent if the employee opts not to switch. Successful bidders could purchase (at competitive rates) reinsurance for capitated contracts from the government.

(c) Governments could directly subsidize the formation of HMOs or other private insurance companies through direct loans and subsidies.

In the United States many state governments have followed policies similar to these and it has had the effect of restructuring competition in both the insurance and provider markets. In the 1970s, for example, loans and grants were made in the United States to stimulate the development of HMOs. In our own state, Wisconsin, the state government put on the market about $200 million of state health insurance employee benefits in order to stimulate the start-up of HMOs and other prepaid or capitation insurance plans (Luehrs and Hanson 1984). If governments choose to follow this line of approach they should be very clear about their objectives and do considerable front-end research before acting.

2. Couple Existing Private Sector Employment-based Self Insurance Plans to the Insurance Market

Again, nearly all developing countries have some large companies that self-insure their employee health benefits. Self-insurance plans can be taxed so as to force companies to seek alternatives to self-financing. The Government of Indonesia has done this and has forced many large employers to either join other existing government insurance plans or to expand and broaden inclusion of other recipients into the company plans. Again, the taxing power of government can be

247

used to adjust the relative prices between self-insured plans and the rest of the market.

In the United States, self-insured plans escape most of regulatory requirements faced by other insurance companies; such plans are supposedly governed by another federal law (Employee Retirement Income Security Act of 1974). Taxing self-insurance plans in the United States to increase insurance competition is being discussed. In the developing countries, if there is a desire to encourage private insurance plans to promote capitation and prepaid plans—all finance and delivery types thought to be more efficient than either public sector free care or fee for service private care—then the government has the power and policy tools to encourage private plans.

3. Expand Existing Government Plans to Include Nongovernment Employees

This policy is a variant of (2). Here the government, through subsidy or incentives, can extend its plan to private sector employers. It can also expand its plan to have services delivered privately. And government can set the relative prices it wishes to prevail so as to govern market behavior. The health card scheme in Thailand and the Dana Upaya Kesehatan Masyarakat—fund for the health of people plan in Indonesia are examples of this strategy being pursued in the developing countries.

4. Encourage Use of Capitation

It is in the best interest of government to have its own insurance plans and to stimulate prepaid or capitated plans in the private sector. These are the plan types that will best promote the most net efficiency on the finance and service delivery side. Again, government can use its power to tax and to subsidize and its buying power to promote these types of insurance plans. As we shall note later, this is being done now in some developing countries.

5. Convert Existing Government Schemes into Capitation Schemes

Obviously, this is an extension of (4) but it is a more aggressive use of government's leverage to affect change in health care markets. Governments can offer its employees a choice of plans and a choice of service delivery and it can govern how behavior will be changed what government does about coinsurance rates, deductibles and the proportion of a plan paid by government (i.e., if employees opt out of capitation they bear higher out-of-pocket costs).

6. Convert Existing Government Acute Care Institutions into Parastatal Enterprises

This strategy is supply side; it is an indirect way to stimulate competition between private and state institutions (i.e., to advance net efficiency) but is also a way to foster insurance development. A parastatal institution, for example, could be made available for inclusion in other private sector insurance plans, especially for tertiary care. This would be a way to avoid some of the build-up of high technology and capital equipment costs in private institutions that might otherwise occur. Services in parastatal institutions could be offered at some discount to private plans as an inducement for use. There are many variations possible here and these will vary from country to country. But two points are valid regarding this strategy: (1) development of parastatal institutions would improve public sector efficiency and stimulate competition with private institutions; and (2) efficient and high quality parastatal institutions could be a powerful inducement to private insured plans to keep their capitation rates low, knowing that tertiary care does not fully have to be actuarially recovered in the capitation rate. Many developing countries are pursuing this strategy and one, Kenya, is about to undertake a substantial experiment.[61]

7. Nationalize or Limit Insurance Enterprise Competition

This is another supply side policy governments can (and have) followed to get an insurance and reinsurance industry started in their countries. I think this is a major escalation in government policy over those discussed above. But it can work and has worked (for example, in Korea) as a way to get a private market for insurance started in a country where otherwise private market forces would not be able to develop an insurance market. The idea of this strategy is to limit firm competition so as to permit the establishment of sufficiently large market shares so that all firms can be profitable. In such cases, however, government has to use its regulatory powers to be sure premium rates and equity concerns are kept within the boundaries of what government wishes to achieve (see, for example, Wasow 1986).

These seven possible policies do not exhaust all the possibilities, of course. But the point of this exercise is that between leaving the private sector alone and privatizing everything, there is a range of insurance type interventions governments can consider, if they do, indeed, wish to restructure their health care markets and make them more private (i.e., more competitive). All of the seven policies above are ways of saying that if public resources for health are fixed or not growing, some major gains in efficiency on the financing and delivery sides

---

[61]Informal report to the authors from USAID. Washington, DC.

will expand services with existing resources. These policies still require governments to balance their drive for efficiency with their concerns for equity. What these seven policies also assert is that health insurance markets can be stimulated and developed through government initiative; the alternative is to wait for these markets to develop spontaneously and, unless they do (which is doubtful), government will have lost an opportunity to foster a more efficient financing and production (delivery) system. Private sector competition and public sector response have the best chance, in the long run, to offer developing countries a chance to restructure their systems of finance and delivery so that health care demands of the people are not subject to the year-to-year struggle with government budgetary allocations for health care.

CAPITATION SCHEMES: HEALTH MAINTENANCE ORGANIZATIONS (HMOs)

A group insurance market would be helpful in most developing countries, but as the previous section has described, governments can directly stimulate the growth of these markets. Capitation schemes have great promise in the developing countries. And as we have noted, the schemes can originate out of pure private sector initiative or they can be government-stimulated with spillover effects to the private sector. Capitation schemes contain the major incentives economic theory says should prevail for efficiency gains. First, a population group is insured on some actuarial basis such that all benefits (defined by government or private markets) are received for a fixed period of time (usually a year but renewable). Second, providers (government, private or both) are paid per enrolled person to administer the benefits to this population; the payment is fixed for the benefits, no more, no less. The providers are, therefore, at risk and, in theory, their incentive should be to provide all the care needs within the capitated amount. If the providers are for-profit groups, then they retain the difference between the capitated amount and the cost of all services for that population. On the theory that incentives and risk/reward yield efficient outcomes, then capitation schemes are to be recommended as a way for governments to stimulate both public sector growth and to reform their own public service systems. It may be useful, therefore, to look further into the potential of capitation schemes. One capitation scheme in particular, the HMO, has begun to reshape US health care markets. HMOs do have some potential in the developing countries but it is possible that not all countries will be able to utilize this concept. Nevertheless, the concept of prepaid, or capitated, health finance has considerable potential in the developing countries. The previous section of the paper argues that these developments can occur exclusively in the private sector, exclusively in the public sector, or what is more likely, in some combination of the two.

A priori, there does not seem to be any reason why the HMO concept could not succeed in the developing countries. HMOs have worked in the United States. But even in the United States, it is not often clear why one HMO succeeds and another fails. And there is great variety among HMO types in the United States (Anderson 1985, Luft 1983).

The important point is that what might be transferred is the HMO concept, rather than any specific design. Simply put, what you might want to establish is an arrangement appropriate to the local environment that offers effective incentives to a provider organization (insurance company, clinic group, etc.)—delivering comprehensive ambulatory and inpatient services—to deliver these services in a cost-effective manner. Those who describe the US experience with HMOs frequently point out that any particular HMO design that works well in one area may not be appropriate for another area.[62] It might be argued that in developing countries there are better opportunities to forge successful HMO arrangements, since: (1) with government control of a large proportion of the health services delivery apparatus, HMO experiments can be developed more readily; and (2) with younger modern health delivery systems and weaker, less entrenched private medical sectors, the government may confront fewer obstacles to establishing a legal and regulatory framework that can offer incentives for cost-effective delivery of services. It is possible that HMOs have not—despite their efficiency-favorable incentives—produced more dramatic cost-containment effects in many US areas up to now because, as long as they constitute a small fraction of the US health services delivery system, their latitude for combatting

---

[62]In addition to the managers, who bring it all together, there are obviously three key groups whose satisfaction and cooperation are critical: consumers, physicians and hospitals. For each of these entities there must be some net benefits to being in an HMO relative to the existing system. For consumers, the satisfaction criteria would include financial cost of services, comprehensiveness of services, geographic accessibility of services, quality of services, and waiting time for receipt of services. For physicians, satisfaction criteria include the amount of earnings obtainable, number of hours worked, ability to practice high quality medicine without concern about ability of patients to pay, and ability to minimize adverse selection bias. For hospitals, achievement of high bed occupancy rates and assured reimbursement for services utilization would be sufficient incentives. Conditions that are conducive to HMO development might include dissatisfaction among key players, including government, with the existing finance and delivery system in a country. Although the ability of potential HMO arrangements, in less developed countries (LDCs), to deliver what is desired is obviously a complex issue, depending (at least) on managerial expertise and the regulatory environment, there seems no a priori reason why the HMO concept could not succeed in LDCs.

some of the broad inefficiencies of the current US system is limited. Earlier introduction of HMOs into a medical market could, conceivably, produce greater benefits.[63]

Our experiences in Jamaica (Helminiak 1986) and Indonesia (Helminiak and Andreano 1987) suggest that there is widespread interest and some experimentation with HMOs. In Indonesia we encountered two HMO initiators. One, an individual entrepreneur, had directly contracted with private health providers and was marketing his capitation plan to the employees and families of four private companies (14,000 persons). A second, hospital-sponsored arrangement appeared to be largely the result of the director of a private nonprofit hospital in Jakarta, which also operates six community health centers. Although the membership of the latter HMO had only been extended to employees of the hospital, plus families (5,000 persons), the director was eager to expand the arrangement; he had held exploratory talks with a private firm that was interested in joining and had discussed with a commercial insurance company the possibility of the latter marketing the plan. There is also a capitation-basis outpatient clinic in Jakarta that had about 5,700 members, mostly enrolled by their employers. We have been told there were a number of similar outpatient prepayment schemes in Jakarta.

Indonesia, in 1985, announced that health services benefits directly provided by companies to employees outside of formal insurance arrangements—were to become taxable. By appreciably raising the costs of company self-insured health plans, a strong price incentive was established for shifting to formal insurance arrangements. A recent proposal by the Tugu Mandiri Insurance Company and Pertamina, the state oil company, suggests that providing health services to employees directly through company operated services, may now, with the new insurance and tax law, make it strongly to the company's financial advantage to convert into a separate HMO entity. The new tax law effect was estimated to raise the cost of Pertamina's direct provision by 60 percent (Axene et al. 1987). Obviously, the results of the Indonesian experiment will be of great interest.

In Jamaica, an insurance company, Life of Jamaica, established an HMO in Kingston and Montego Bay. Traditional third-party health insurance is already well established in Jamaica, it covers about 20 per cent of the population. Also in Jamaica, the United States Agency for International Development (USAID) supported an analysis of a Ministry of Health (MOH) proposal to establish an HMO in the Jamaican parish (province) of Trelawny, a poor rural area with a population of 70,000. Trelawny was apparently selected because of its grass roots

---

[63]HMOs and all prepaid health plans in the United States do economize on the most expensive part of health care, hospital services. The number of hospital days per 1,000 members in a typical HMO is about 400. The number in a conventional fee-for-service insurance plan is about 800 hospital days. See Luehrs and Hanson (1984).

concern over deteriorating health services and its willingness to be involved in the proposed sort of pilot scheme.

The Trelawny plan was for a private nongovernmental organization to take over the existing network of 21 MOH health centers plus one hospital in Trelawny and to privately contract with ten physicians and one dentist. Members would be voluntarily enrolled, paying a monthly premium. The MOH would pay for the portion of the Trelawny population considered unable to contribute. MOH payments were expected to be made for about 28,000 to 30,000 persons (those now eligible under a food stamp program), out of the total parish population of 70,000. (The analysis suggested that MOH payments might actually be necessary for as many as 50,000.) It was estimated that 10,000 persons in the parish had the resources to enable them to make monthly premium payments. Those not joining the plan would be able to use the plan services on a fee-for-service basis. The proposal was to negotiate a lump sum payment to the physician group, on a periodic basis, which was to ensure their not earning less than pre-plan (Zukin and Weinberg 1986).

Consistent with the points already made, the document analyzing the Trelawny plan notes that in regard to HMO feasibility "there must be the awareness of an unsatisfactory situation or a problem with the status quo that requires solution". There must be a sufficient degree of approval by organized medicine to permit the program to function, possibly constrained, however, by various restrictions and limitations. The posture of government is also a critical factor (Zukin and Weinberg 1986, pp. 7.1-7.2).

The analysis noted that as of March 1987, no organizations or individuals capable of developing and implementing the proposed plan had yet been identified; the Jamaican health insurance firms were considered to have the best chance of success, though they had not directly operated facilities. The positive factors were the supportive position of the government and its willingness to contribute significant resources as well as community interest and support for means to improve their health care. Negative factors were the failure to identify an adequate source of revenues to support the plan and the uncertainty as to whether a competent management team could be assembled to develop and operate the plan.

No doubt there are other attempts at HMO development in the developing countries. Certainly, HMOs and other capitation or prepaid health schemes have great potential for application in these countries. HMOs in particular seem to have the properties necessary to achieve the net efficiencies described earlier and on balance are amenable to government subsidy intervention to achieve net equity goals as well. There are questions, however: Can capitation schemes such as HMOs develop spontaneously in the private sector in the developing countries? Can governments really foster their growth? Can governments apply the concept to public services and blend them with the private sector? Over the long run, will capitation schemes have applications in rural as well as urban areas? If government policy is to remove constraints on private sector growth, is using government leverage to foster private capitation scheme growth a wise use of government's limited policy resources? Are the benefits of capitation schemes greater than the costs? Can governments insure competitive market conditions so that capitation schemes can autonomously achieve the desired net efficiency? How large a share of the total health care market can capitation schemes capture in the developing countries? Will their market share be sufficient to influence, at the margin, net efficiency in other private and public financing and service delivery systems? Can HMOs and capitation schemes extend government resources and move a developing country closer to an optimum production level with respect to efficiency and equity objectives?

These are all weighty and important questions. But, if theory is any practical guide to policy and if private sector growth has the potential to expand health output without sacrificing efficiency and equity objectives, the evidence to date suggests that capitation schemes are well worth an experiment or two in the developing countries. The research evidence to date is limited and heavily dominated by experience with such schemes in the industrialized countries. The natural experiments underway need to be studied. But new experiments need to be framed in country circumstances that will permit analysis of the country-wide impacts of such virtues and their cross-country replicability. This is certainly an opportunity for the international lending agencies to leverage their limited resources in ways that could benefit health care systems in the developing countries.[64]

DRUG COSTS AND THE PRIVATE SECTOR

Another area worth examination is the high proportion of drug costs in both private and public systems. It is well known that a preponderant amount of drug expenditures in the public as well as the private health sector are associated with drugs that provide no therapeutic value. This is probably due to both the minimal

---

[64]If HMO developments in a country proved significant, the distinction between pure public goods and the merit principle might be blurred. HMOs do deliver preventive services—they have an incentive to do so—and this suggests that a fine line exists, in theory. between public goods and merit goods. Theory is helpful here but not decisive. Evidence from the United States shows HMOs deliver two types of services one would think are public goods. preventive care and health education. Experience with the health cards in Thailand also suggests that the private sector can deliver some traditional public goods. The point is that capitation schemes do have ample properties to embody many of the so-called pure public goods and can assist in the reallocation of resources in the public sector.

pharmacological knowledge of consumers, especially when self-prescribing is substantial, and to the grossly inadequate pharmacological knowledge of most individual physicians. Physicians may also feel frustration at their inability to effectively deal with many health problems and suffer a desire to offer the patient something tangible, regardless of whether it has real therapeutic value. The hopeful rationale of physicians may be that the drugs offer a placebo effect on the patients' ills. Placebo effects may also "rationally" explain a large portion of the self-prescribed drugs purchased in the developing countries. It seems highly likely, however, that the placebo benefits are not worth the costs incurred. In any case, some of the inappropriate drugs are actually harmful and a more rational drug policy could perhaps offer cheaper as well as safer placebos.

Policies being discussed in this paper are meant to suggest alternative financing and delivery options in the developing countries. But drug costs, perhaps accounting for as much as 40 to 50 percent of all health expenditures in the developing countries, offer a large potential for improvement in allocative efficiency. The question posed here is, can an alternative financial system capture drug costs as part of the process? The partial answer to this question, at least based on Western experience, is yes. Using the price system, that is, establishing significant drug fees, can foster the right incentives to limit inappropriate expenditures on drugs. But the best apparent arrangement for promoting costeffective dispensation of drugs in the developing countries would be to include drugs in capitation schemes such as an HMO benefit plan, where those dispensing the drugs were at financial risk/reward for appropriate utilization. It would seem logical for the HMO to seek to reduce the major amount of therapeutically worthless expenditure on drugs that presently exists in LDCs by improving the pharmacologic knowledge of its physicians, who might also be financially motivated to dispense drugs more carefully. Similarly, the HMO would be motivated to learn and offer the most cost-effective versions of those chemical combinations that do have therapeutic (or placebo) value.[65]

---

[65]In addition to including drugs as part of capitation schemes, there are some other remedial measures. These might include direct interventions at the process level (the usual, more obvious approach). Process interventions include educational procedures to enhance pharmacological understanding of dispensers, establishment of national drug formularies (limited to therapeutically valuable. cost-effective drugs and which emphasize generics), efforts to lower importation costs through centralized bulk procurement and competitive tenders (or, where feasible, local manufacture), and seeking to limit self-prescription of those drugs likely to lead to inappropriate utilization.

Other Supply Side Policies

We do not have much new information on other supply side policies. The World Bank and others have called for full cost pricing, especially for medical education. The main point is this: If governments are to permit private sector growth and continue supply side manpower subsidies, they are transferring resources from the public to the private sector. Is this what is wanted? There is some optimum level of subsidization of manpower production for national (or equity reasons) and public net benefits derived from this policy. Political difficulties will often frustrate policy changes of such significance. Yet a key, if not the key, input in any health system is the adequacy of supply of medical personnel, especially physicians. Country situations will vary, of course, but as a general rule there is some advantage to governments that are pursuing a policy of private sector expansion to see that physician supplies grow appreciably; some subsidy may be necessary to achieve this. However, the expansion of physician supply (using almost any level of government subsidy to do so) would be counter-productive unless supply expansion is linked to explicit policy objectives. In any case, to continue subsidization of physician supply without a complementary policy on the demand side (health insurance) is not likely to be optimal.

To get as close as possible to achieving net efficiency in health sector, governments must insure that competition exists both among service providers and in the insurance market. Competition on the personnel supply side, that is, in the production of medical manpower, is not necessarily urgent, though in many countries such conditions already exist. There are three major areas of concern for government in maintaining an environment in which competitive conditions prevail: (1) consumer information; (2) maintaining free entry into the sector; and (3) preventing monopoly control of any market or sub-market. Consumer information is necessary if informed price and quality choices are to be made. Deficient information has two aspects to it: (1) as a source of market failure and thus a departure from Pareto optimality; and (2) in leading persons to demand fewer services than government deems should be consumed (the merit good principle). In the developing countries the merit good principle may be a more powerful reason for government provision of consumer information than it is for correcting a potential source of market failure.[66] Still, the potential for

---

[66]The importance of imperfect information in health care market failure is conjectural. Mark Pauly indicates that it may be of lesser importance, except for those services, which are produced and consumed relatively infrequently (Pauly 1982). Pauly's focus is on advanced countries. but the point may be applicable to developing countries as well.

government's increased provision of consumer information for both reasons is a valid option in the developing countries.

Maintaining free entry will require governments to keep licensing, trade and professional barriers to the minimum that is sufficient to insure acceptable quality. Free entry will also require governments to have an explicit supply side policy regarding medical manpower, that is, whether or not to charge full costs for education. An ample supply of physicians, especially where capitation schemes dominate the private sector, will be required. Government manpower policies, therefore, have to be comprehensively thought out and not formulated on an ad hoc basis.

Preventing monopoly control means that governments will have to be sure that some effective antitrust legislation is available in order to keep mergers, consolidations and predatory pricing—all potential effects in a growing private sector—from distorting competition in all health care markets.

EQUITY AND COST CONTAINMENT ASPECTS

We have noted, and our simple theory predicts, that policies to pursue expansion of the private health care sector will involve some trade-offs between what we have called net efficiency and net equity. In Appendix 1 we have elaborated further on distribution between public and private markets. The previous section of the paper is based on the assumption that private financing and delivery systems yield the greatest net efficiency. However, where there are market imperfections or a failure in equity one can only say that public intervention might improve the situation. If the public intervention is to improve service distribution or financial equity, there may well be trade-offs with respect to some of the efficiency elements. In such cases, the kind of public intervention may be very important. For example, direct public provision of services should be compared with some more innocuous (less disruptive of competition and price incentives) forms of intervention; for example, contracting out services to the private sector, public regulation, direct budgetary support, or partial price subsidies on either the demand or supply side. As a rule of thumb, theory suggests that the least intrusive form of intervention sufficient to meet public concern should be preferred.

Private sector growth will generate at least two potential areas of concern for government and both are equity related: (1) controlling costs in the private services; and (2) maintaining standards of quality in the delivery system. Cost containment is a major issue in the developed countries; policies followed in those countries have not been entirely successful. However, cost containment policies in the developed countries have stemmed more from efficiency concerns than from equity: cost containment policies in the developed countries have aimed to squeeze out inefficiencies on the production and utilization side. For the most part these policies have not succeeded in cost containment (expenditures continue to rise) and have only partially succeeded in improving net efficiency (Andreano 1984). In the developing countries, the cost containment problems encountered will be quite similar to those of the developed countries, except that equity more than squeezing out inefficiency will usually dominate. A well developed and growing private sector, given the usual assumptions we have about income-demand and supply-price elasticities, is likely to produce some escalation in costs. If competitive market conditions do not fully prevail, or if the financial system produces reduced access to services, governments will be obligated to intervene to contain cost escalation in the private sector. We will expand on both points by drawing on some simple analytical arguments.

Cost containment may mean either: (1) reduction of inefficiencies in the production of health, so that either (a) the same amount of gain in health status can be achieved through use of fewer resources, or (b) continuing advances in health status enhancement can be achieved with fewer additional resources than are otherwise necessary; or (2) reductions in the amount of resources devoted to the health sector regardless of whether offsetting efficiency gains are possible. This second version of cost containment will tend to be confronted in the developing countries; especially where the economy has suffered a sharp recession that has necessitated reductions in the resource allocations to all sectors. A less common circumstance for the second version is the presumption that the health sector is overfunded vis-à-vis other sectors. The second version of cost containment (regardless of the circumstances bringing it about) will still require an exercise in allocative efficiency—selecting the areas within the health sector that are to receive fewer resources and determining the resource reduction incidence for these areas so as to minimize the reduction in health status.

The first version of cost containment involves efforts to improve both health service production efficiency (reducing the unit cost for the production of given health services) and also all of the various forms of allocative efficiency— efficient resource distribution between different modes of health status production and efficient intensity of utilization of mode and delivery systems to alternative health status concerns.

Most discussions of cost containment probably involve the first version. Here again, efforts can be directed at either the level of individual processes or at altering the institutions or systems that generate these processes.

Individual process level efforts include programs (such as those now being conducted in Malaysia) for improving the competence of managers working in specific modes. Research and education can also be directed at seeking to improve our knowledge regarding possible enhancements in allocative efficiency. On the other hand, one can seek to alter the financing system, delivery system, and the "real system" so as to produce an environment more conducive to efficient health status production.

If one looks at cost containment policies used in the developed countries, four interpretations seem possible as ways to categorize such interventions:

1. The total resource allocation to the health sector is too large (i.e., resources should be shifted from health to other sectors). In other words, there is intersectoral allocative inefficiency: marginal social benefits are less than marginal social costs. For the developing countries the problem is usually suggested as the reverse, that is, relatively more resources should be allocated to the health sector.
2. Of the resources being allocated to health, fewer ought to be supported from general (tax) revenue funds, with the difference being made up by alternative funding channels such as user charges. This could be either a political issue (less government involvement, more liberty) or an efficiency hypothesis (tax/ general revenue funding contributes to inefficiency).
3. Health sector resources are being used inefficiently in the production of health status enhancement.
4. Health care services are financed or distributed inequitably.

In our view the fundamental problem in the health sector is, in fact, the efficiency problem: To the extent that the efficiency problem is resolved, concerns about category (1) above would disappear and concerns about category (2) would either disappear or become less important. Equity is probably subsidiary to efficiency, and, to the extent that equity is perceived as a significant problem, it needs to be carefully considered. Also, to the limits of feasibility, pro-equity efforts should attempt to proceed in areas where efficiency trade-offs are minimized. As yet, it is not possible to assert conclusively that the "indirect" approaches to improving efficiency in the health care sector are themselves less efficient measures than those that seek to restore market price and competitive incentives to the sector, though a good guess is that such is the case.[67]

---

[67] In one Asian country we were recently told that most medical providers believe "cost-effective medicine" means "low-quality medicine". This view is widespread. However one should emphasize that the relevant output of medical services is not simply "outpatient visits", "inpatient admissions", or "inpatient days", but rather improved health status; that cost-effective medicine thus means improving health status by any given amount, at the lowest resource cost. So the correct standard is not "high" or "low" quality of medicine, but the appropriate quality of medicine that will maximize the health status or quality of the population. Confusion occurs, of course, when we often use intermediate output measures (outpatient visits, inpatient days, etc.) to measure efficiency. But this is due to a lack of workable output measures expressed in

259

To move from the analytical back to the real world, the developing countries that opt for policies to strengthen or expand their private sector will ultimately face this dilemma of cost containment. At the least, governments should be prepared with alternative payment systems, such as diagnosis related groups (DRGs), where government market leverage opportunities exist. And at the most, governments may have to consider use of tax policy, regulation of fees, rates and capital, and other interventions that keep the incentives of providers and consumers biased toward efficiency objectives. For equity, governments may also need to evaluate the use of subsidies for groups without access (financial or service) or for maintaining access. Where government and private health care systems compete, the outcome one wants to avoid is having a dual system of care—one for those who can afford it and one for those who cannot.

A risk in sacrificing equity in terms of quality of care is also likely to be faced where private sector growth is largely unconstrained and where competitive market conditions do not automatically insure that acceptable quality of care levels will be maintained. This is an extremely vast subject and all one can do is suggest some general lines of approach. If capitation schemes and market competition on the provider side prevail, some interfirm rivalry and peer group pressure may be sufficient to maintain quality. Government intervention may, nonetheless, be required and there are many forms such intervention may take, including price/quality control through such programs as DRGs, peer review organizations, monitoring and inspection of facilities, and certification and decertification of providers and institutions.

SUMMING UP

This paper has explored a number of ways to inject the private health care sector into the health care environment of developing countries. We started with some simple theory, outlining choices and trade-offs, and ended with some cautions regarding public side interventions. It should be made clear that this paper is not intended as one of advocacy: one has to know what the problem is before one can advocate a solution. Theory showed us many problems and many possible ways of dealing with problems. The policies outlined here should work, but the circumstances will vary from country to country. And to make policy work requires a great amount of front-end research. If the problem is inefficiency

---

terms of health status improvement. Thus when we use these intermediate output measures we must remain sensitive to the possibility of the proxy relationship proving inadequate, for example, where the effective quality of an outpatient visit was obviously reduced relative to a more costly alternative, a cost-effectiveness comparison would obviously be compromised.

in public services, then private sector interactions of the type described here could help. But that is not the only policy road one could travel. If the problem is that governments will not allocate any more resources to public systems, then private sector growth offers some resource substitution opportunities. If the problem is underfunding of the health sector (in terms of intersectoral allocative efficiency), allowing growth in private source financing may again provide an answer. If the problem is equity (in all the dimensions we have defined it), then private sector growth may not help at all.

The point is that private sectors are already large in many developing countries: Should government policy be to make them larger? If the answer is yes, then what do governments perceive as the problem this policy will solve? If private sectors are small relative to the public sector, do governments wish to increase the private/public proportion? Again if the answer is yes, what problem is this going to solve? The beauty (and also the deficiency of economic analysis) is that it can offer, as many policies as there are problems. Clear statement of "problems" are lacking in the rhetoric of Health for All and in policies advocating major structural and financial reform in the health systems of the developing countries. Are there too few public resources for health? Are there too few resources relative to education? Are there inefficiencies and inequities on the public side? If so, are the relevant options and the necessary trade-offs relative to these options being realistically examined?

The existence of a large private sector, or stimulating the growth of one or more variations of the policies proposed here, will solve some of these problems but not all. And private sector growth will involve trade-offs that governments may find difficult to make. We should be cautious in pushing or advocating policies in the developing countries. International agencies such as ADB, USAID, WHO, World Bank, and others are suggesting similar policies. But the gap between what looks good on paper and what any given country can or should do is still as great as ever.

What we have tried to suggest in this paper is that if one wants to use the private sector there are ways to do so. But we need more evidence than currently exists to push this policy in every country and every situation.

The international agencies can do something very concrete to narrow the gap between theory and practice. In the area of the private sector we have noted a number of natural experiments underway in the developing countries. These should be studied thoroughly and we should find out about other natural experiments that are not so well known. Second, the international agencies can assist governments in formulating real experiments, such as the work USAID is doing with HMOs in Indonesia. Third, the international agencies must do a better job of collecting data on the health system in the developing countries so that other scholars can have access to these data. For individual researchers like us it is impossible to collect, categorize and analyze world data. Most useable data are in unpublished country reports and the international agencies must do a better job of putting such data in forms that the research community can use.

Finally, although throughout the paper some sense of neutrality has been attempted, our own experience is that for most of the problems countries are likely to center on, utilizing private markets and the principles of market behavior will generally result in net benefits to the country. If we did not believe that, we would not be economists. But that does not mean that caution should be thrown to the wind!

APPENDIX 1

PUBLIC OR PRIVATE PROVISION OF HEALTH SERVICES?

The typical rationale for public intervention in private markets is market failure; private markets are not optimizing social goals. The sources of market failure in health care markets include the following:

(1) Public good status for some services: here, consumption of the good is not rival (i.e., the marginal cost for incremental consumers is zero) and it is not possible to collect payment or exclude nonpayors.
(2) Positive externalities associated with the consumption of certain services: here, a private calculus of marginal costs and benefits leads to a less than socially optimal amount of consumption.
(3) Natural monopoly in the production of services: here, increasing returns to scale precludes the benefits of market competition.
(4) Failure of market emergence, as exemplified by the case of the failure of private insurance markets in the United States to serve all health care risk areas.
(5) Asymmetric and imperfect information by consumers.

In addition to these potential sources of market failure, public intervention may also occur to improve upon the current distribution of services (geographic as well as by income class) and to compel the consumption of certain services (i.e., certain health services are "merit goods").

Public good and externality arguments suggest a public role for basic sanitation services, mass campaigns, individual immunization programs, health education efforts, and perhaps even health research (basic and applied). Natural monopoly factors might be relevant for smaller hospitals serving rural markets. Asymmetric and deficient information can be viewed both as competitive market failure (i.e., departure from Pareto optimality) and as leading consumers to demand fewer services than government believes is in their best interest (i.e., the merit good principle).

Public sector activity in health, however, seems to be based less on market failure arguments than on equity concerns of governments. The equity factor involves two separable aspects: (1) equity of distribution of health services, and (2) equity in the financing of health services. That is, government might wish to assure that all who require certain health services—regardless of geographic locale or income status—have equal opportunity to receive them; and government may additionally wish to assure that, in the population as a whole, including both the sick and the healthy, the need for health services by some does not impose a disproportionate financial burden on any. If demands for health care services were highly priced and income-inelastic, private market health service delivery might result in reasonable equity of health services distribution, but produce poor financial equity.

There are two points of view on the merits of social redistribution in the form of health care services. The standard view in economic theory is that redistribution in the form of any given good or service is socially inefficient, since the transfer of equivalent general purchasing power would allow the recipients to decide how their satisfaction can be maximized, whether by purchasing health services or by other goods or services. An alternative view is that societies (which dictate the form of transfer) have a preference for affecting specific forms of consumption behavior; they experience less of an external diseconomy (dissatisfaction from inequity) due to general poverty than due to specific attributes of poverty, such as ill health in segments of society.

The primary argument in favor of private sector provision of health care involves the presumption of greater efficiency. Three areas of efficiency that appear relevant are: (1) production efficiency, *(2)* utilization efficiency, and (3) financial or funding efficiency.

It is widely believed that the private sector can produce health care services more efficiently, that is, at lower unit cost to the consumer than the public sector. This greater production efficiency is assumed to result from the profit incentive.[68] Theory suggests that private producers of health services will be lured by profit and forced by competition to produce quality services at lowest cost. Where, on the other hand, health care services are predominantly offered by the public sector, incentives to offer high quality services at minimum cost will be diminished by the absence of a profit-reward structure. Low production efficiency in the public sector does not guarantee displacement of the less efficient producers by more efficient producers. (These are aspects of the "real system" discussed in Appendix 3.)

The counterargument is that, as indicated earlier, elements of market failure make the private market solution less than desirable for some services (mass campaigns, basic sanitation, individual immunizations et al.); and for most other services (including most curative services) imperfect information may substantially diminish the efficiency effects of the private sector.

Unfortunately, empirical evidence on comparative production efficiency of private and public sector health service delivery is essentially anecdotal. Serious empirical investigation in this area would be valuable; however, significant measurement problems need to be resolved. The definition of "efficient" needs to be carefully considered in any comparison between public and private delivery formats. Quality of output naturally affects the unit costs of output. Depending on

---

[68]Where nonprofit activity is also predominant, a utility-maximizing model yields nearly the same predictions about behavior, as does a profit-maximizing model.

whether the delivery institution is private or public, quality may systematically differ along a number of dimensions.[69] Efforts to statistically control for such difference are not readily dealt with.

When there is public sector financing of health services, the utilization efficiency of health services may well be influenced. To the extent that such financing results in an increased divergence between marginal social benefits and marginal social costs for health care services at the delivery margin, there will be resource efficiency losses. In more casual terms this is sometimes discussed as the extent to which health care services utilization is necessary or frivolous.[70]

Another efficiency criterion for comparing different institutional structures for health care services delivery is that of financial or funding efficiency. The collection and transfer of the financial resources to employ productive factors in health services production—through tax collection/budget mechanisms, user fees, or coverage charges—will yield varying fractions of the collection amount to the actual employment of production factors. Here again there is a great deal of anecdotal evidence, which has not been well sorted. In the case of public sector provision, much undoubtedly depends on the degree of decentralization. And, where user charges are—at least in principle—employed, it is widely observed that the collection process tends to work best where revenues are retained in the delivery agency (or, at least, at the local government level), rather than being remitted to a central treasury.

The last, and somewhat questionable, criterion for choosing between public and private sector provision is that of aggregate funding availability to the health sector. What balance of public versus private sector provision is likely to yield the greatest aggregate funding of health services may be argued to be an inappropriate objective. According to this view, the emphasis ought to be on obtaining the optimal provision structure in terms of the various health sector

---

[69]The concept of systematic differences in output quality between public and private sector providers generally has been discussed be Weisbrod (1988), who hypothesizes that when public and private producers of some good or service coexist, they will systematically tend to produce qualitatively different output and to serve different groups of the population.

[70]There arc three aspects of utilization efficiency (or allocation efficiency within the sector). One aspect concerns whether the most efficient modes of resource conversion to meeting health needs are employed. This is separate from the production efficiency issue described earlier, which considers whether for a given service mode (e.g., hospital outpatient services), service units are delivering this particular service at lowest unit cost. Another aspect concerns whether given modes of health services delivery are being utilized by individual members of the population at optimal levels. A third aspect concerns whether modes of services and particular delivery systems are directed to disease groups or population groups where they can best diminish the constraining effect of disease on the economic development of the country.

efficiency and equity criteria. In an "economically ideal" world, the amount of aggregate health sector funding would be determined on the basis of allocative efficiency between sectors. As noted earlier, a public sector role in health services provision is argued because externalities and information imperfections may lead the private sector to under-produce at least some services. But it is not clear whether government fiscal realities result in funding of certain, or any, health services to the point where marginal health sector benefits are equal to opportunity costs.

APPENDIX 2

AN OVERVIEW OF THE ANALYTICAL COMPONENTS IN EVALUATING HEALTH CARE FINANCING AND DELIVERY SYSTEMS

The accompanying diagram (Figure 6) seeks to distinguish alternative analytical areas with respect to the evaluation of national health care financing and delivery systems. In Box A, we locate the various public, private and public-private mixes of financing and delivery systems. Individual formats (e.g., MOH services, compulsory insurance, voluntary insurance, and fee-for-service) are not listed. Much of the work of WHO has involved the designation of taxonomies for the range of financing and delivery options and to identifying the status of the present system (generally in terms of expenditure allocation) of some countries.

In Box B (Figure 6), we have the evaluation criteria for judging the desirability of the alternative financing/delivery approaches of Box A. Six principal objectives are noted and each interact differentially depending on the particular financing and delivery approaches a country may take: (1) health service production efficiency, (2) health service utilization efficiency (three forms), (3) funding efficiency, (4) financial (funding) equity, (5) health services distributional equity, and (6) aggregate sectoral funding (intersectoral allocation efficiency).[71] The alternative approaches will offer various trade-offs between the individual criteria.

---

[71]For any health care system, the *financial or funding efficiency* is a function of the level of administrative costs in the collection and transfer of resources to the particular system relative to the fraction of collected resources available for the production of health services. For example, in some health insurance arrangements in developing countries, collection costs in rural areas might approach (or even exceed) revenues collected. Administrative procedures influencing collection incentives for example, whether user charges are retained or remitted to a central treasury, are important, as are opportunities for graft and corruption in collection procedures.

Efficiency of health services production (or operation efficiency) is measured in terms of the unit cost of production of individual health services. Factors will include management competence and incentives, the size and complexities of bureaucracies, the adequacy of accounting systems, and incentives for diligent work by delivery personnel. (These are all aspects of the real system.) Where financial planning and budgeting are deficient, health facilities may be constructed but left largely unused owing to inadequate provision for recurrent budget funds; this is one of the most typical inefficiencies found in developing countries.

Utilization efficiency (or allocative efficiency within the health sector) has three relevant aspects: (1) are the most efficient modes of resource conversion to meeting health needs employed (e.g., hospital outpatient departments vs. PHC units)? (2) Are

Efforts of the World Bank have focused on the clarification of evaluation criteria, as well as on the economic theory (Box AB1), which seeks to link the alternative approaches of Box A to the objectives of Box B. The theory linking system approaches and objectives, though roughly suggesting in what directions—relative to individual efficiency and equity objectives—different system approaches are expected to take us, still leaves us with considerable uncertainty about precisely what might be achieved or lost in real world shifts between alternative financing and delivery approaches. Thus, for example, theory may indicate that certain approaches offer better opportunities for some elements of efficiency and poorer opportunities, perhaps, for equity elements and possibly for other efficiency elements as well. But what are the actual amounts of the individual trade-offs and what are the net benefits, if any" (And how acceptable are the efficiency vs. equity trade-offs W the society?)

To understand very much about the real relationships of alternative financing/delivery approaches to the efficiency and equity objectives, we require murk expanded empirical investigations (Figure 6, Box AB2), especially in the area of comparative studies between countries.

National decision makers who are challenged to implement new financing anti delivery system approaches in order to achieve one or more of the objectives listed in Figure 6, Box B may frequently feel constrained owing to some of the factors listed in Box C. Generally, such constraint: include political pressures opposing the shift (even though it might ultimately be beneficial to the nation), the limited competence and expertise of sector administrators to design and implement the shift, and the lack of good information related to the desirability

---

given delivery modes being utilized by individual members of the population at optimal levels (necessary vs. frivolous use)? (3) Are modes of services directed to disease groups or population groups where they can best diminish the constraining effect of disease on economic development of the country? (This aspect may be controversial.)

Financial equity (or funding incidence) involves how the funding of the particular system impacts the financial status of country residents, relative to national financial equity objectives.

Equity of health services distribution involves the level of equality of access to health care services among the population. (The fact that many countries offer in-kind redistribution of health care services is evidence of a much tighter standard for health services distribution equity than financial equity.)

Aggregate to funding level of the health sector is a frequent evaluative criterion of systems from the point of view of health sector administrators, who generally consider a system favorable insofar as it increases aggregate sector funding. The appropriate criterion is, however, that of *intersectoral allocative efficiency*, which will not necessarily argue in favor of the system that offers the highest aggregate funding of the health sector, unless one is convinced (as most health sector administrators perhaps are) that the sector is underfunded in terms of allocative efficiency.

and requirements of the shift. (Appendixes 3 and 4 expand on these points.) More research regarding relevant constraints and practical measures for ameliorating them would be extremely useful.

Figure 6: An Overview of Analytical Components in Evaluating Finance and Delivery Systems

A	AB1	B
Macro Financing and Delivery System Approaches	T H E O R Y	NATIONAL OBJECTIVES (CRITERIA FOR EVALUATION
Public vs. Private Financing		1. Health service production efficiency 2. Health service utilization efficiency 3. Financial (funding) efficiency 4. Financial (funding) equity 5. Health service distribution equity Aggregate sectoral funding (intersectoral allocative efficiency)
	AB2	
Public vs. Private Delivery (and combinations of both)	E M P I R I C S	

E
THE REAL SYSTEM

C	D
Constraints (or Preconditioning Factors)	Tools and Strategies for Implementing Approaches

1. Political constraints
  a. Shaped by historical inertia
  b. Organization of pressure groups
  c. Social-cultural factors and traditions re health and health services
  d. Political dogma
2. Competence/expertise of sector administrators
3. Information constraints
	(Some Examples)
	1. Health insurance
	2. Capitation scheme
	3. Health cards
	4. User charges
	5. Decentralization of services
	6. Non governmental or private sector opportunities, etc.

An area of important pragmatic research, blending theory and empirics, is the design of efficient tools and strategies for the actual operation of individual financing/delivery approaches. The design and evaluation of such tools and strategies (Figure 6, Box D) may be one of the more fruitful areas of current study.

Finally, attention also needs to be given to the "real system" (Box E) (see Appendix 3). The real system for each country will identify the unique system of attitudes, relationships and incentive responses of the key actors in the national health sector (administrators and managers, physicians and other service provision personnel, plus health care consumers), plus the underlying processes that need to be dealt with, or adapted, in any proposed reconfiguration of financing/delivery systems. (The innovative design of tools and strategies of Box D should reflect an appreciation of the real system.)

271

APPENDIX 3

NOTES ON THE "REAL" SYSTEM OF HEALTH CARE

When economic analysts examine a health care system because of some breakdown, fault, or unexpected problem we tend to rely on certain basic economic theorems to figure out what is wrong and devise a policy solution to fix the problem. In certain instances this approach has been exceedingly fruitful: indeed, much of what passes for health policy in America today can be said to be derived from this approach.

From our own experience, the conventional approach of economics does carry one quite far whether the unit of observation is the US health care system, the health system of some other industrialized country, or even one in the Third World. It is even useful where the type of health care system varies from the national health service (or fully public) to the centrally planned, or open and private health care systems and their hybrids that can be found all over the world. But there is a level of analysis that goes a few steps farther. This "real" system, as we call it, incorporates some pure economic concepts but unites these with an institutional process that always seems to be at work in any health care system.

It is our belief that the "real" system is basically very simple in concept but powerful in its application. In country after country health care systems have some endemic or systemic problems that make decision makers and policy analysts focus attention on "what's wrong and how can it be fixed?" In our judgment stripping away a system to basic elements that govern behavior and influence the performance of the system and the resources the system requires will be helpful in devising better public policies.

At the core of the real system are the way incentives and disincentives for behavior are shaped. Assume that a given health care system has workers (providers), consumers (patients), institutional providers (hospitals), and governments and their agencies. The forces and processes within these groups that shape incentives and disincentives for behavior are what one means by the real system. Conventional economic concepts such as benefits and costs can help us explain responses to incentives and allow us to draw certain conclusions about behavior. In one sense, the real system may be just another way of elaborating benefits and costs. That is true, but there is more. We see incentives in these groups shaped by a complex and interactive set of forces, including:

(1) management and leadership styles;
(2) career paths, civil service rules, work rules;
(3) the flow, cost and control of information;
(4) educational backgrounds and styles of education;
(5) risk-taking behavior, risk aversion tastes;

(6)   myopia with respect to the social rate of discount; attitudes toward time;

(7)   zero sum games;

(8)   resistance or acceptance of change;

(9)   perceptions of health issues vertically, horizontally, or intersectorally; and

(10) the level of current technology available, or capital/labor ratios.

The forces and conditions that shape incentives of workers, consumers, institutions and governments produce the outcomes of that system. When to the real system one adds the system of finance used to allocate resources, the two together—the interaction of the real and the financial system—produce the current health care system.

Let us just give one illustration of the ten elements we have listed. A manager of an enterprise at any level has much to do with shaping the incentives and performance of others—workers and other managers, and consumers. In Third World contexts managers, even if well trained and capable (which is seldom the case), face the typical manager's dilemma: how to achieve the task with insufficient resources? Resources are never sufficient, so managers devise their own games and their own rules. A manager dedicated to the task will make internal priorities of resources to accomplish enough of the task to be judged as performing "successfully". If the manager is neutral with respect to the task and its accomplishment, the games and rules will be devised to give the appearance of "success" with sufficient explanations at hand to rationalize the actual or real lack of success. Since managers of health care in Third World contexts are seldom performance-evaluated, the games and rules devised by the manager rub off on all those (individuals, institutions, etc.) the manager is responsible for and who are essential to the achievement of a task or goal. The incentives and disincentives for real, as contrasted with apparent or nominal, performance by managers and the managees are shaped by the current environment in which the manager operates. What happens if the manager does not succeed? If nothing happens, that constitutes a strong element in the behavioral incentives of the manager. If something does happen (discipline, removal, lowering of service grade, etc.) that too sends a message.

If one looks, therefore, at a health care system that may be "failing" or is beset with "problems", instead of looking only at the total amount of resources available and the allocation of those resources, look again at what is motivating the managers of the system. Their incentives and styles are transmitted to the employees and institutions. All managers devise their internal performance rules and priorities; some will do this in ways that make them perform successfully in reality as well as appearance; others will do so only in appearance. Some managers succeed despite severe resource limitations. What conditions seem to explain that? Are they just better than the others? Were their rules and games more successful in extracting resources from other weaker, less success-oriented managers? The insight of the real system of health care is that one looks behind the surface of managerial performance. In virtually every health care system we have seen, even where all is in shambles, there is still one person, one institution, one manager who is succeeding. If one were to total all the costs and benefits of the actions of the most successful entity or person, it might be helpful in translating these to others. But, it is our judgment that the successful manager in a world where few else are succeeding has an explanation for behavior that transcends conventional appearance. What internal allocation rules did that person devise to get around resource and personnel deficiencies? What systems of rewards and punishments did that person devise to get others behind the successful attainment of the task or objective? How did the system imposed on managers make some do well and others fail? In short, what we are asserting, not as theory but as observation based on long, practical experience, is that a careful and detailed analysis of a system's managers and their style will go a long way in helping one understand what is happening (for good or bad) within a health care system.

For all other elements of the real system, a system of rewards, incentives and disincentives for behavior become embedded because of some institutional process. Often it is the perception of an institutional process as much as the actual process that conditions behavior and contaminates outcomes. To accomplish change in any system, but especially a health care system, one must strip away the surface appearances of performance (or absence of performance) to focus on the variables that condition behavior of the key actors in the system. Rational behavior does not always follow when benefits exceed costs. Institutional and cultural restraints shape the process environment by which the key actors perceive the benefits and costs. If countries are going to ride the horse of private sector growth to higher levels of social welfare in health care, they must be advised of some of the limitations imposed by the real system.

APPENDIX 4

A PRIMER ON "CHANGE" IN HEALTH CARE SYSTEMS: ON GETTING THINGS DONE

In speculating on the main themes presented in our paper it seems clear that any expansion, co-optation, or suppression of private sector growth in the developing countries has the potential to produce very dramatic and potentially threatening changes. Theory tells us what seems rational and optimal; the real system often negates rationality and optimality. We thought it might be useful, especially to those both in the private and public sector, to set down some elementary thoughts on the concepts and consequences of "change". What follows we call a primer—the first principles—of policy analysis. The primary target audience for this primer is those decision makers in the developing countries that now have to cope with changes of a momentous kind. Real resources for Health for All in most countries will be stagnant. There will be policy prescriptions—change—recommended on all sides: by international lending agencies, by WHO, and by erstwhile advisors and the like. There is some guidance from economics that decision makers can ponder to help sort out change. Here is a modest attempt at some guidance.

LARGE PROBLEM/SMALL PROBLEM/OBJECTIVES AND INTENT

It is often just as easy (or difficult) to tackle large problems as small ones. Sometimes it is not possible to distinguish between the two! The main point is to be clear about the problem or the process one is intent on affecting. You will not be able to initiate a process of change if you are unclear or imprecise about what you wish to change, why it must (should, could) be changed, and what would happen if it were not changed.

Offensive vs. Defensive

It is usually easier to stop something from happening, or keep it from changing, than to begin something new or change something old into something new. Innovation has rewards but is difficult to achieve; the status quo is safe and everyone can assess the benefits and costs of a proposed change against what it may mean for them in terms of the present status quo. Thus, it is harder to accomplish what we call offensive or new—changes than to keep those changes (that we call defensive)—from occurring.

Why is that so? First, the status quo is easier to defend than some new, as yet uncharted new state of affairs. Consequently, to start something anew runs directly against already established coalitions. The reason the status quo persists is usually because some equilibrium has been reached among contenders. Everyone has sorted out benefits and costs and a stable, even if sub-optimal, solution persists. Thus, a power grouping already exists, that is one definition of a status quo. Along comes an offensive, that is, a new portended change. If it threatens the existing power groups (i.e., if the net costs of the change exceed the net benefits), such groups will already know, without their having to be mobilized, that they best fight the new change. Defense will usually win. And there are several lines of approach for such winning strategies:

1. Find the "weakest" link in the new, proposed offensive change. That could be a person (the one pushing the change), a projected result from the change (not only will it not work, but even if it does it will not produce the result those pushing the change say it will produce), cost of the change and expected benefits against the relevant comparable parameters in the status quo, employment effects (some people will be put out of work by the change), income redistribution effects (some persons, groups will gain more at the expense of others), and so forth.

2. Attack the "weakest link" (any or all of the above) with countervailing power, that is, mobilize the coalition that preserves the status quo, or at least those parts that would be "hurt" the most. This can be done formally or informally. Formally, a defensive strategy goes public, tries to make counterpoint arguments, holds rallies, talks to politicians where they (the status quo) have complementarity of interests, and so on. Informally, the attack takes place out of public view—back home we call this "the hallway gossip". That is, exaggerated rumors start to appear, unattributed to anyone: effects of the change become exaggerated and editorials or political speeches are made perpetuating the exaggeration. In either case, control of information and some actual "numbers", whether real or not, can go a long way towards convincing decision makers that the change will not be desirable.

3. Another avenue of approach for a defensive strategy is to find a compromise solution or prepare a counter change. Here, you take the view that the proposed change is likely to be adopted and what you seek is to minimize "damage" to you. In western parlance this is known as "cutting your losses" reaching a compromise solution that modifies the change. Compromise solutions only work if the defensive group has some power leverage, that is, something with which to compromise. Counter proposals have a similar interest; this shows you are not against

the change but want the change to take place in the correct (i.e., your) way.

Zero Sum Worlds

Any change involves a benefit to someone (person, country, or institution) and a cost to someone else. For any policy change, there are always winners and losers. Resources are fixed, needs for resources infinite. To expand the private sector means the incremental amount of resources will not be available for use elsewhere. What is available for one activity is thus not available for another; some win, some lose. Those on the loss side can become a barrier or hurdle to those on the win side who want to maintain and implement their gains. Generally, opposition to new policy changes will coalesce around those who lose the most. In the case of certain elements in the health sector, major policy changes can be prevented from being successfully effected if the "loser" has substantial political savvy and clout.

THE ACTORS/THE PLAYERS

In any policy formulation activity, any change to be achieved from the status quo involves a process of identifying the leading players in that activity. A policy to push expansion of the private sector will affect many individuals and their careers, private and public institutions, other government ministries, politicians and bureaucrats. It is a good idea to construct a matrix of the actors or players in a change activity. In developing a national health policy change, one might construct a matrix like the one shown in Figure 7. This matrix is only meant to be illustrative. Its key points are that at the initiation of a change, whether a process or a specific project, it will help implementation of the change if one first identifies all the relevant parties (institutions), and determines their direct or indirect involvement with the change, and determines whether or not they stand to gain or lose from the change.

Assessment of Interests

A step in the process behind (beyond) the matrix is to formally assess the interest involved by going into greater detail as to where the actors line up with regard to the change proposed. This could also be put in matrix form, but we shall resist because we are not proposing an easily formalized process. Rather, the point is that some of the actors will be for the change, some will be against. What one must now do is detail why this is so. What are those opposed going to lose? Is it important enough to make them (it) actively oppose the change? Is there some small rearrangement that could be incorporated to turn their opposition (active) into support (passive or active)? And on the other side, of those actors likely to gain from the change, are these the right ones? Will their active support be helpful or harmful to effecting the change? That is, do we want them to be passive or active supporters? Among the actors (active and passive) who support the change is there likely to be inter-institutional conflict, personality clashes, or repressed anger from previous battles won and lost when the sides the actors were on were different? Also, part of this assessment of interests is to examine all the key actors to look for some opportunities to form coalitions of actors to accelerate the change.

Coalitions

After assessing interest, counter-interests, and opportunities of the key actors it is then useful to think of forming coalitions. Coalitions are grouped interests, whether of individuals, agencies, or other institutions. Coalitions can be formed to push for the proposed change, but one must remember that coalitions can be formed against the change. It is generally true, though, that no policy formulation—no change in an activity—can succeed without a coalition of support. Strong individuals can overcome weakly organized coalitions; but a strong coalition can defeat a strong individual virtually any time and in any type of situation. Both individuals and coalitions require reinforcing support whereas strong individuals cannot. The point to be stressed here, however, is that coalitions will be (and need to be) formed and especially so if one is promoting a new policy change or if one is trying to defeat it. These coalitions can be active or passive, they can be overt or covert, they can be temporary or permanent, and they can be destructive or constructive. What are some hints to be kept in mind in forming coalitions? First, a coalition must be representative of the particular society, that is, to have only those who actively benefit from the change in the coalition is not likely to succeed unless most, if not all, of the following are present:

- Access, or representation, of those who control financial resources generally, and best of all, specifically (i.e., fiscal and budgetary).
- Political power to enforce decisions and to neutralize the potential and actual opposing coalitions (and/or individuals).
- Ability to mobilize public support for the change activity and to represent the coalition in public forums to mobilize support.
- The coalition should have the means to enforce its actions beyond having the political power to do so. Generally, for the coalition to succeed it must control sources and access to information about the activity or intended change.

- The coalition must speak with one voice (preferably one person) rather than multiple persons, though in certain circumstances that may not be possible.

There are other things one can mention; the coalition formed should be flexible enough to maximize entry. There is no point in excluding entrants, even disruptive ones; that is often a successful way to co-opt potential opponents. In the end, the formation of coalitions will be based on an alignment of interests, sometimes counter interests, of groups seeking the expected change. Individuals are important because they activate the coalitions. Every successful coalition has at least one individual who pushes the coalition to exert its interest.

STRATEGY

To enact a policy change, no matter how small, still requires a strategy for implementation. All of the actors can be identified and their interests assessed. Coalitions can be formed, but it still remains to use this knowledge and the accumulative experience represented to select a strategy of how to get the desired change enacted.

There are two dimensions here: (1) what organizational form can be most effective in implementing the desired change, and (2) what elements of form and power group analysis are necessary and sufficient to succeed in effecting a change.

There are very few simple rules: one often does not know in advance what will work. And often a strategy thought to be excellent will fall flat for reasons no one foresaw. There is very little guidance one can give, but a few points can be noted. The classical strategy is to form committees and let the committees formulate a plan of action. Often one has a Steering Committee where all the principal players and actors are represented. This can be the basic coalition but it is more often not the coalition used for action. In the classical pattern, committee structure and responsibilities are formulated from top to bottom in a rough hierarchical pattern. The main deficiency of the classical pattern is that it diffuses responsibility. It also increases the span of control. In addition, subgroups are clever and strong they can push well in advance of other, perhaps more important, parts of the plan of action. That can be sometimes desirable but usually is not what one wants. The point is that the classical committee structure strategy tends to give independent life to some, if not all, of the committees of groups formed. That is usually not desired, but it is inevitable and it can wind up costing more in time and money to achieve the desired change. A variation of the classical approach where responsible individuals are designated to report to some steering group often works better than committee or subgroup structures. But this approach, too, has some of the same problems of span of control, independence of action, and inflexibility. It also puts a heavy burden on selecting the right persons.

Formulation of a strategy depends on how one assesses what the opposition will be. (This point must be kept separate from how difficult or easy the intended change may be for that particular country, region, or community.) If the perceived opposition is active, vocal and organized with the political and bureaucratic power to support its opposition, then the group(s) pushing for the policy (change) must assess their strength against the opponent's strengths. Here, tactics rather than strategy become relevant; if we do A, what will they do? If they do B, what will we do? How can we do A and prevent or neutralize them from doing B? If the opposition is potentially strong but not yet organized, the strategy must not contain elements that force the opposition to coalesce. Nor must tactics pursued permit still potentially stronger opposing coalitions to be formed. The principle one wants in a strategy (and its underlying tactics) is to minimize actual and potential conflict with the opposition and maximize either their support or their neutrality. Indeed, in formulation of the policy (or change) one may (if possible) shape the intended change in such a way as to let the expected opposition obtain some benefits from the change and not just bear all costs from it.

Other possible elements of a strategy, whatever the individual tactics employed, could be:

- media use if available
- national and local meetings
- parliamentary or legislative body endorsements where appropriate
- statements by political leaders
- commercial advertising in the manner or means appropriate to the country
- business leaders' endorsements
- various forms of public forums

It is important that the strategy for initiating or implementing a change decide whether the profile is to be "high/visible" or "low/quiet". The point to emphasize, however, is that merely lining up the key actors ("political will") behind the policy will not insure that it is achieved. A mechanism or structure for its achievement will be required. And this discussion of strategy suggests that a somewhat calculating assessment of who benefits and who does not is required. Then the elements and organizational structure best suited to the country, its culture, and its politics, should be formed. What we have set down here hardly exhausts the possibilities.

KEEPING ON TRACK

One could do all of the above well and still not achieve the intended change. There is still a loop-back that requires constant monitoring of achievement and failures of the policy, and reaction and response to the policy; in short, keeping on track. There are various ways that this has been done, historically. Oversight groups, sometimes drawn from the key actors, sometimes not, are most frequently used. In broad terms, such groups test which way the wind is blowing and keep the principal players on track and tuned into how the intended change is proceeding. The oversight group could be, and often is, contained in the Steering Committee, where the classical approach to policy formulation and change is in use. Keeping on track could also be the task of a single individual, though a good rule to follow is that more than one opinion should be sought about how well (or how badly) activities are faring. The key danger points in keeping on track are usually breakdowns in logistics, information and in the chain of command and responsibility. In every policy there is a "flashpoint" and keeping on track can keep the "flashpoint" under control. The key point of keeping on track is knowing in advance what might go wrong and trying to plan for it; prevention is cheaper than correction after the fact. But it is most often true that things go wrong when you least expect them. This is when opposition to a policy change has the best chance to coalesce. Specific problems encountered in a policy change offer opposition actors and coalitions an opportunity to say: "See, I told you so!" "Now, why not do it my way, as I told you in the first place!" Problems in implementing a policy change are what the opposition seek to find, and unless the initiation of the policy change can correct, neutralize or eliminate major problems, such change will fail on two fronts: (1) on their own, because the activity does not succeed, and *(2)* because the opposition will accelerate the failure by seizing and mobilizing their opposition around the failures. In the latter, sometimes the problems need not even be as significant for the eventual success of the change. But if they hit the right power group, trouble will occur.

SUMMARY

What has been discussed is general and it is impossible to anticipate in advance every variation on what has been outlined. Circumstances vary widely based on culture, economics and politics. But something close to the elements discussed here happens in all societies whenever the policy formulation is at stake or when change is contemplated. There is no single way of achieving change. What we have suggested are things to take into account; everything has to be adapted to local circumstances.

It may seem out of place in a paper of this sort to include an appendix dealing with how to manage and cope with change. But the pending policy menu in alternative financing schemes for health care in the developing countries have potential for change of afar-reaching nature. We have said in the main body of the paper that the gap between theory and practice is large; these notes are intended to partially fill this gap.

REFERENCES

Anderson, Odin W., Terry E. Herold, Bruce W. Butler, Clair H. Kohrman and Ellen M. Morrison, *HMO Development: Patterns and Prospects, A Comparative Analysis of HMOs*, Pluribus Press, Chicago, 1985.

Andreano, Ralph, "Una vision general de la economia de los servicios sanitarios: una perspectiva internacional en los paises industrializados" (An Overview of Health Services: An International Perspective in the Industrialized Countries), in *La Reforma Sanitaria en Espana, a Debate*, Madrid, 1984, pp. 111-123.

Axene, David, Allan Fairbank, Harold Hunter, Jeremiah Norris, Susan C. O'Byrne, Robert Rosenberg, Elizabeth Wainstock and Michael Wood, "A Business Plan for Tugu Mandiri of Jakarta, Indonesia to Establish a Health Insurance and Health Maintenance Organization", *The Resources for Child Health Project*, John Snow, Inc., Arlington (Draft).

Bicknell, William J. and Ann G. Lebowitz, "The Public's Health and Private Health Care: The Private Sector in Developing Countries", Boston University, 1981 (Typescript).

Culyer, A.J. and Bengt Jonsson (eds.), *Public and Private Health Services*, Basil Blackwell, Oxford, 1986.

de Ferranti, David, "Strategies for Paying for Health Services in Developing Countries", *World Health Statistics Quarterly*, Vol. 37, No. 4, 1984, pp. 428-442.

Health Affairs. Special Issue: HMOs, *Health Affairs*, Vol. 5, No. 1, Spring 1986.

Health Economics Research Unit, "Editorial: The Health Divide—The Policy Gap", *Health Economics Bulletin*, University of Aberdeen, June 1987, p. 1.

Helminiak, Thomas, "Economic Efficiency of Health Care Delivery and Finance in Jamaica", Report prepared for USAID, Jamaica, September 1986.

Helminiak, Thomas and Ralph Andreano, "Financing Health Services: Some Speculations and an Example from Indonesia", Paper prepared for the World Bank, Population and Human Resources Department (PHN Technical Note 87-22), December 1987.

Luehrs, John and Dale Hanson, "HMO Competition for Wisconsin's State Employees", *Business and Health*, Vol. 1, No. 9, September 1984, pp. 36-39.

Luft, Harold S., "Health Maintenance Organizations," *Handbook of Health, Health Care and the Health Professions*, David Mechanic, (ed.), Free Press, New York, 1983, pp. 318-351.

Pauly, Mark V., "Is Medical Care Different?" *Issues in Health Economics*, Roice D. Luke and Jeffrey C. Bauer (eds.), Aspen Systems, Rockville, 1982, pp. 3-24.

Shepard, Donald S., Guy Carrin and Prosper Nyandagazi, "Self-Financing of Health Care at Government Health Centers in Rwanda", Prepared for Resources for Child Health Project, Arlington, Virginia (AID Contract No.: DPE-5927-C-00-5068-00), January 1987, (Revised Draft).

United Nations, *National Accounts Statistics: Main Aggregates and Detailed Tables*, United Nations, 1986.

Wasow, Bernard, "Insurance in Korea", *The Insurance Industry in Economic Development*, New York University Press, New York, 1986.

Weisbrod, Burton A., *The Nonprofit Economy*, Harvard University Press, Cambridge, 1988, (Forthcoming).

Wodarczyk, W. Cezary, "Health Insurance an Antidote to Bureaucracy", in *Health Care—Who Pays*, World Health Organization, Geneva, 1987, pp. 80-82.

World Bank, *Financing Health Services in Developing Countries: An Agenda for Reform*, World Bank, Washington, D.C., 1987.

————, *World Development Report, 1983*, World Bank, Washington, D.C., 1983.

World Health Organization, *Economic Support for National Health for All Strategies, Background Document* (A40/Technical Discussions), World Health Organization, Geneva, 1986.

————, "Financing Health Development, Options, Experiences and Experiments," (Document WHO/HSC/87.1), World Health Organization, Geneva, 1987.

Zukin, Paul, and Theodore J. Weinberg, "Proposed Trelawny Health Plan: Preliminary Assessment of a Managed Prepaid Health Service Organization for Trelawny Parish." Prepared for Ministry of Health, Jamaica and supported by USAID, Health Management Group, Ltd., Piedmont, March 1986.

www.ingramcontent.com/pod-product-compliance
Lightning Source LLC
Chambersburg PA
CBHW020731180526
45163CB00001B/196